A MENACE TO OUR HEALTH:

A history of epidemic diseases in South Africa

Julie Dyer

Copyright © 2014 Julie Dyer

All rights reserved.

ISBN: 1503096580
ISBN-13: 978-1503096585

CONTENTS

Abbreviations		
Acknowledgements		i
Preface		iii
Introduction		1
Chapter 1	A Blot on the Colony: Leprosy and Robben Island	3
Chapter 2	'A Menace to Our Health': Syphilis	27
Chapter 3	Quarantine and Vaccination: Success against Smallpox	62
Chapter 4	Plague: The Origins of Apartheid Segregation	82
Chapter 5	Typhoid: A Problem Relocated.	103
Chapter 6	Typhus: 'Devermination' and DDT	128
Chapter 7	Migrant Labour and the Pandemic of Influenza.	143
Chapter 8	Cholera and the Rural Poor	166
Chapter 9	The Curse of the Bushveld: Malaria	179
Chapter 10	Measles: A Harrowing Toll	208
Chapter 11	A Century of Poliomyelitis	223
Chapter 12	Diphtheria: Indifference and Immunisation	242
Chapter 13	A Menace to Whose Health? Conclusions	255
Bibliography		265
Index		278
About the Author		286

ABBREVIATIONS

DDT	The insecticide Dichloro-Diphenyl-Trichloroethane
EPI	Expanded Programme on Immunisation
EZ	Edmonston Zagreb (measles vaccine)
HIV	Human Immunodeficiency Virus
INAH	Isoniazid (the antibiotic)
LSDI	Lubombo Spatial Development Initiative
MMR	Measles, Mumps, Rubella (vaccine)
MOH	Medical Officer of Health
NGO	Non-Governmental Organization
PAS	The antibiotic Para-Amino Salicylic acid
SADC	Southern African Development Community
SAMJ	South African Medical Journal
STD	Sexually Transmitted Disease
STI	Sexually Transmitted Infection
TB	Tuberculosis
UNISA	University of South Africa
VD	Venereal Disease
VDRL	Venereal Disease Research Laboratory
WHO	World Health Organisation

ACKNOWLEDGMENTS

I would like to express my gratitude to all those who assisted me in this endeavour, in particular Kammy Naidoo, Pranisha Parag and the late John Morrison of the Bessie Head Library in Pietermaritzburg. The assistance of the staff in the various libraries and institutions used for my research, in particular the Bessie Head library, the University of KwaZulu-Natal libraries and archives in Durban and Pietermaritzburg are also acknowledged. I also wish to acknowledge the continuing moral support of my children, Jack and Carmen, and my parents, Brian and Greta, for everything.

Map following page:: South Africa in 1914, http:/insertmedia.office.microsoft.com
Photo of author back cover: Jack Dyer.

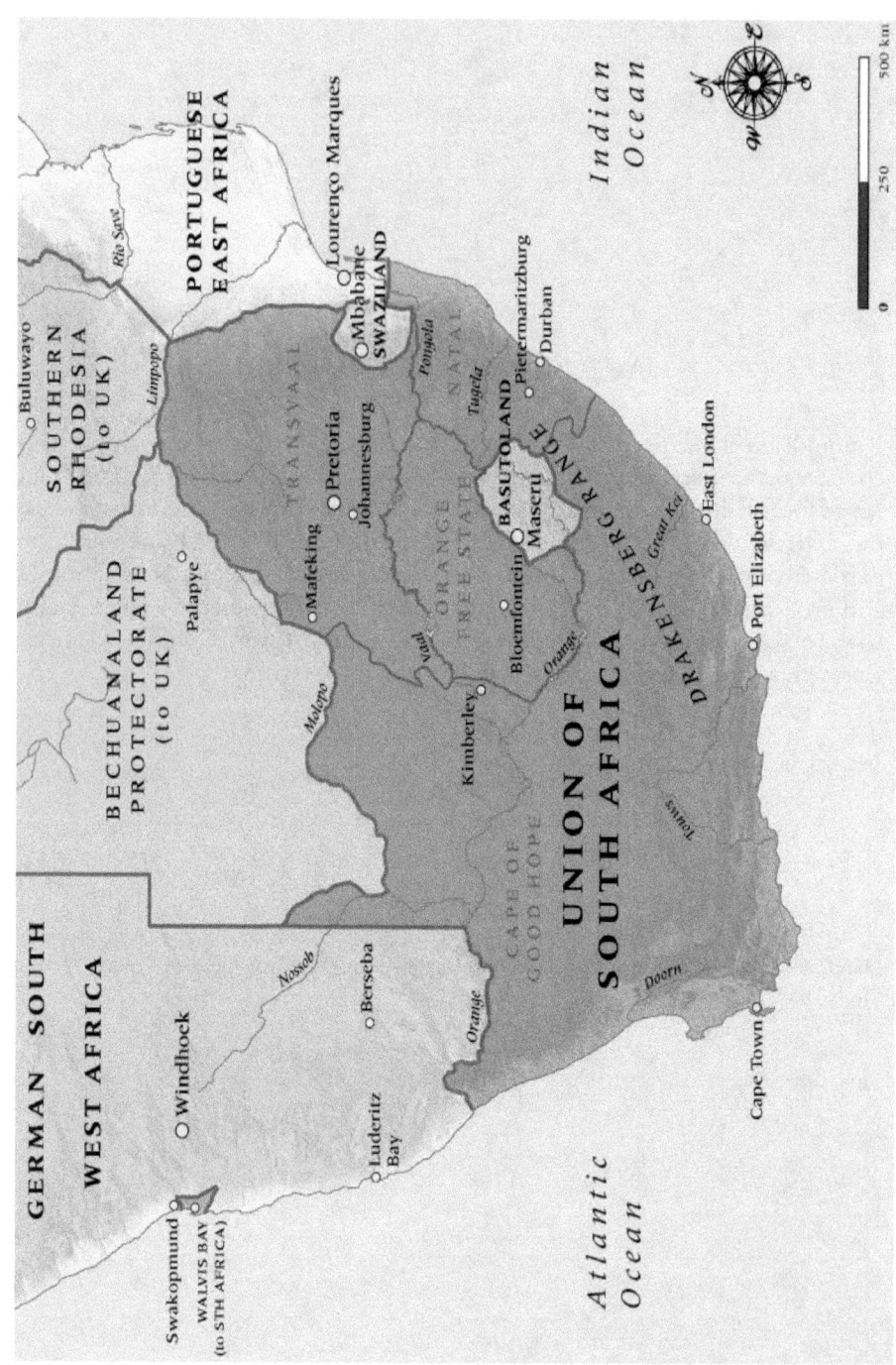

PREFACE

This is a history of some of the major epidemic diseases which occurred in and impacted upon South Africa throughout its complex and controversial history – from the earliest written records in the 17th century, through to the end of the 20th century. It is written by a medical specialist in public health, who also has an interest in social history and the ways in which disease influenced, and was influenced by, society. This interplay between disease and society is of particular relevance in South Africa, where nothing in its development or history is simple: where, due to its multi-cultural nature and certain peculiarities of its past, what may appear straight forward on the surface has multiple layers, ripples, contradictions or turbulence lying not far beneath.

It is impossible to capture all this in a single attempt, and behind many a paragraph are untold depths of stories which could present and analyze an issue from several different perspectives. No one person can hope to see all the different sides. I hope, however, to bring forward some of the facts, fiction and forgotten history of many of the epidemic diseases which raged through this country at various stages in its past, and which gave shape to the country it was to become.

One of the dominant threads running through South Africa's history is the division of society into named 'racial groups'. These names and classifications changed through the centuries, but this classification remains a feature even now, in the decades past the political and social changes in 1994. These descriptive terms are unfortunately necessary when writing about the country and its past as the classification system was integral to its development. The European settlers were historically called either European or White, the latter term being prevalent today. People originating from the east were generally termed Indian or Asian, fairly interchangeably, along with the now offensive term 'coolie'. Original, indigenous inhabitants were given various descriptive names over the years, most of which are now considered offensive – 'Hottentot', 'Kaffir', 'Native', 'Bantu', - along with the terms Black and African which are still in use today. Nowadays the term Black can be interpreted to include those of Indian or mixed ancestry, but this use is not applied in this book. People of mixed 'race' are termed Coloured, a word originally also applied to Africans. This is a term long in use and still in use today although somewhat controversial, and not always acceptable to those to whom it is applied. As this book quotes extensively from original historical documents these racially offensive terms will be found. These have been retained within the quotations where necessary to give an accurate depiction of the attitudes of the time. It is to be hoped that no offense is taken as certainly none is intended. In similar vein the historical spelling and grammar of that era have been left in the original form within the quotations.

INTRODUCTION

We live in an age in which antibiotics, vaccines and progress in public health have almost completely defeated the fatal infections of the past. The plague, smallpox, typhus, poliomyelitis and diphtheria have almost faded from memory. Typhoid and cholera are removed from our cities and leprosy is a distant legend; but these diseases, along with diseases still present such as syphilis and tuberculosis, were integral to the history of South Africa. Landscape, settlement, occupation, industry and the politics of segregation were shaped repeatedly and in varying ways by the dread diseases and society's reactions to them. These same factors also contributed to the epidemic diseases – both their intensity and distribution – and hence are deeply interwoven into the fabric of South Africa's developmental processes. This book is written to remind us of the past dread diseases and the fear and devastation they caused; to explain how their incidence was shaped by the peculiar colonial, racial and industrial background of the country; to relate how they were controlled and in many cases defeated; and to discuss how they affected South Africa's development into the country it became - particularly in the period up to the year 1994 which signified the transition to democratic governance.

The great epidemic diseases seem to have been largely absent from South Africa before the arrival of European settlers. Early descriptions of the country, whether by those who came by sea to the Cape or by those travelling overland to the interior, are generally consistent in finding that the indigenous populations were particularly healthy, with the only major pre-existing disease being malaria in the north east of the country. Conversely, tales by the earliest arrivals from Europe by sea also agree that most of the ships came with large numbers of sick aboard – and were in fact desperate to land in order to off-load the ill, feed them and return them to health before setting sail again. Ships arrived from both Europe and the East and thus infectious diseases were effectively spread between three continents. Johan Nieuhof said in 1654: 'The Draek [a ship] now first came in to the Bay and had 50 sick lying in their bunks and 26 dead, the rest being so weak with scurvy and other sicknesses'. Wouter Schouten said of the ship the Amersfoort in 1665: 'We understand ... that the plague raged not a little in that ship, about 60 men lying sick in their berths, and that the thirty-eighth man had been buried that day on the Robben Island'. George Phenney aboard the ship Sceptre in 1695 gave another typical report: 'this day sent 25 of our sick men ashore.

Yesterday came in a Dutch ship at anchor off Penguin Island from Holland who in his passage lost 96 men and all the rest sick but 4 or 5'. Skipper Leendert van Deiji of the Peperboom in 1699 reported '6 deaths during the journey and 150 sick, mostly with scurvy...now there were only 64 sick to send ashore'.[1] Little wonder that epidemics of infectious disease were launched onto the shores of South Africa by the adventurers and colonizers. From then on the history of the spread and control of these diseases was intertwined with the peculiar social and political history of South Africa, with the approach to epidemics differing according to who was directly or indirectly affected – whether indigenous African populations, immigrant labour or the European communities.

This book chronicles the history of 12 of the widespread epidemic and/or infectious diseases which affected the country over a 350 year period and attempts to detail where they came from, how they impacted upon South Africa and how they were all, in succession, largely overcome – at least for now. Most of these diseases were regarded with great terror as many of them caused devastation through illness, death, disability or disfigurement up until the period when vaccines, antibiotics or other technological innovations gradually brought them under control. This history relates how both the medical profession and society-at-large reacted, with some comparisons made to other, more established countries. Many of the measures taken were drastic, draconian and experimental, influenced partly by a lack of understanding of the cause and means of spread of disease, up until the middle decades of the 20th century. There was often scant regard for human rights of the afflicted and, while this needs to be considered in the light of the times, with its imperfect knowledge and lack of vaccines or antibiotic treatment, the approach was often highly discriminatory in terms of race or gender. The modern epidemic of the present, which continues to engage South Africa and it still evolving, is of course HIV/AIDS, which has been an epidemic of an entirely different nature and has been responded to in a very different way to the dread diseases of the past. This disease is not included here – firstly due to the fact that it is a modern epidemic, which has been most devastating in its impact post-1994, and which is still developing and changing year on year. While it has been a disease of great political, social and health impact in South Africa it has also been covered in numerous other works.

1. Raven-Hart R. *Cape of Good Hope 1652-1702: the first 50 years of Dutch colonisation as seen by callers,* Vol 2; A.A. Balkema Cape Town; 1971.

1   A BLOT ON THE COLONY: LEPROSY AND ROBBEN ISLAND

While leprosy does not occur in epidemics, being rather a slow-onset condition which does not easily spread from one person to another, the disease is included in this book for the fear and dread that it evoked before reliable treatments were discovered and the drastic and often controversial measures taken to control it. Its chronic nature, with the possibility of eventual gross disfigurement and loss of limbs, was sufficient in earlier times to cause ostracism and abandonment of its sufferers forcing them to be outcasts from society, living only with each other and eking out a miserable existence as best they could. The first mention of leprosy in South Africa comes from 1756 when a Jean Marnay and Jacques Maree of Franschoek were found to be suffering from it, with their daughter Maria Maree developing it in 1757: 'Her nose was swollen and covered with blue or purple blotches, and on her feet were raised red spots similar to smallpox'.[1] Four doctors were sent to confirm the diagnosis. It appeared that the disease had come from arrivals of the 17th century, Huguenot refugees. The sufferers were quarantined on their farms with their families. They were instructed to isolate themselves completely and notices were put up to warn the public. After their deaths the disease seemed to disappear for a while and leprosy was unheard of amongst the indigenous inhabitants.

    The cause of leprosy at that time was unknown. Dr William Falconer in England 1791 was confident that it was due to the 'sudden application of cold to the body when in a heated state', hence those considered particularly susceptible were those working near fires, such as blacksmiths, or engaged in 'violent exercise or labour …. such as huntsmen, porters and such like'. Women similarly susceptible included cooks, laundresses etc, particularly if they pursued their labour for some time after drinking cold drinks – including water, milk, and beer. However, despite trying many chemical and bathing remedies, Dr Falconer was unable to pronounce confidently on any cures[2].

    There is mention of lepers being housed at a Moravian Mission at Sunday's River near the eastern city of Port Elizabeth from as early as 1786. No further cases in South Africa are mentioned until 1804 when

Catharina Smit, on behalf of her husband, asked for exemption from paying rental on her farm Hemel-en-Aarde on the grounds that her husband had been suffering from the 'disease of Lazarus' for the past six years. In 1808 a Dr Liesching discovered a small group of impoverished people living in unhygienic conditions in the Overberg mountain range who had contracted the disease. By 1813 leprosy was made a notifiable disease, having spread across the Cape area. In that year lepers were put into quarantine in huts near Caledon's hot springs and the Moravian station of Genadendal. By February 1817 the disease had spread to such an extent that a leper colony had been established at the farm Hemel-en-Aarde, a remote spot in the mountains near Hermanus in the Cape, and they were moved from their homes to the colony. Lord Charles Somerset proclaimed that 'the distressed sufferers are frequently left in a state of abandonment which it is shocking to humanity to reflect upon'.[3] Lepers from all over the country were sent to the colony, and over 400 lepers were kept there during its 28 years of existence.

However an inspection of the colony by Dr James Barry, Colonial Medical Inspector, in 1822 found the lepers in a pitiful state, with inadequate food and an absence of medical treatment. At that time there were 150 people at Hemel-en-Aarde. Their clothing was dirty and they were emaciated, and Dr Barry immediately took steps to increase their rations. He visited again in 1823, when the management had been given over to the Moravian brother Leitner and his wife, and found it much improved. The Leitners' intention was to keep the minds of the lepers occupied with religion and industry to lessen their misery. Barry also set aside two or three wards at the Somerset Hospital for their care and treatment. For the Institute he prepared strict rules for the treatment and care of lepers, including bathing, changes of linen, contents of the diet, dressing of sores and the giving of 'a sufficient quantity of wine to the sick'. However Barry's reforms were resisted by the missionary couple running the institution, the Leitners, to such an extent that he later wrote 'the number of insuperable objections to the present local situation of the leper hospital renders it impossible in my opinion ever to carry into effect any plan for the benefit of the patients there – during the space of six years little has been done either to ameliorate the personal situations of the lepers, or to prevent the spread of this horrible malady in the Colony'.[4] This Dr Barry was a very interesting character who was found, after death, to actually have been a women who passed through her entire medical and military career disguised as a man. Perhaps her true gender accounts to some extent for her extreme sensitivity to the plight of the lepers, unusual in that era. In 1825 a Leprosy Commission sat at

Swellendam to enquire into the disease which was believed to be contagious, although segregation was not rigidly practised except through ostracism and abandonment. At that time there was also another institution at Uitenhage in the east of the Colony. Up until then the disease had been the responsibility of local authorities, but in 1827 it was accepted as a debit against Government Treasury.

The 1838 Voortrekkers and their servants, who left the Cape to escape British rule and the abolition of slavery, migrated across the country into the interior of the continent, spreading infection with leprosy to the native tribes of the Transvaal and Orange Free State where it was previously unknown. In Natal the disease appears to date from 1843 when two Zulu servants returned from Grahamstown, but it may have also been introduced by Arab traders along the east coast of Africa. Leprosy was said to have spread to the then Basutholand (Lesotho) in 1862-63 when Griquas trekked in from the Free State, although one case was reported from 1842.

In 1845 the lepers of Hemel-en-Aarde were transferred to Robben Island which was used as the leper settlement of the Cape. The island had been recommended by the colonial secretary, Mr Montague, who on a visit to the island had noticed it's 'healthy position and its fitness as a hospital for those whose complaints rendered it necessary for them to be removed from the less afflicted of their race.' He commented in his report 'as the salubrity of Robben Island has long been acknowledged, and there is abundance of stone, lime and labour on the spot to erect the necessary buildings, I would strongly recommend for your Excellency's serious attention the expediency of removing the leper and pauper settlements of Hemel-au-Aarde and Port Elizabeth to Robben Island, also the pauper establishment of Cape Town and the lunatics at present confined in the Somerset hospital at Cape Town.'[5] This suggestion also coincided with Montague's proposal to return the Island's convict population to the mainland for use as free labour by sending them to convict road stations in the interior. The prisoners' labour became more useful for colonial expansionism than the lepers, the lunatics and the chronic sick.

However not considered at the time was the difficulty of finding a suitable medical person to manage the facility and it was later found impossible to get a married physician to reside there, only an unmarried one, a Dr Birtwhistle. In 1852 and 1853 there were Commissions of Enquiry into the conditions at Robben Island. While serious allegations were made, in particular regarding the Superintendant Dr Birtwhistle, improvements were slow in coming, with the Superintendent, 'a man under whom such treatment and cruelties have taken place,' due to be left in situ until the facility could be moved to the mainland. Sir A. Stockenstrom raised the matter in Parliament declaring himself astonished that the government was allowing it to continue. He stated that there were 'no less than three hundred of the most unfortunate wretches on the face of the globe, afflicted under the dispensation of an inscrutable Providence, by some of the most fearful visitations of which human nature is susceptible, and that these unhappy beings, maniacs, lepers and chronic diseased …are left under the despotic direction and treatment of a man under whose management, as was proved among other matters two years since, one of the patients had been kept in chains until he was dead, and buried in chains,' an act justly described as an act of barbarity. In 1852 eleven charges of a serious nature were brought against the Superintendent and a Commission of Enquiry was called, which found him guilty of three serious offences, yet he was left in place. A second Commission of Enquiry urged that he be dismissed yet still no action was taken. The Report was considered in Parliament in September 1854, where one member commented that allowance should be made for his having been single and 'surrounded by madmen and lepers,' whereas others agreed with the Report's recommendation that the facility be moved to the mainland where it could better be inspected and controlled.[6] A motion was passed supporting its removal to the mainland, but it was to remain on the island for almost eighty more years.

At that time there were around 20 buildings on the island housing 66 lepers, along with 106 'lunatics' and 129 chronic sick. However many were neglected and forsaken, looking after each other as best they could. The 'lunatics' did much of the labour. Dr Matthews, visiting the following year in 1855, described the situation of the lepers thus: 'I saw human beings kennelled worse than dogs. In a long, low thatched shed some 40 poor creatures were stowed away. Both varieties of the disease, the tubercular and anaesthetic, could here be studied. Some I saw with their faces shiny, discoloured and swollen, others with both hands and feet dropping off joint by joint; one man especially attracting my attention, whose nose, eyes, tongue and cheeks had all rotted away.' He continued 'these woe-begone creatures were allowed to go to the mainland if they wished once every three months, according to the criminally absurd enactments then in force. Of this opportunity many availed themselves, never returning, but sowing the seeds of a disease hereditary and possibly contagious as some believe it to be, broadcast through the land with impunity'. The tragic circumstances were further described: 'I found the bathroom and the kitchen to be identical, one place only being provided for them in which to live, eat, drink and sleep...the miserable sufferers themselves could be seen rolling about in squalid filth, their clothes soaked and besmeared with the discharges from their festering sores. No one seemed to have power or inclination to manage them; neglected and forsaken they were left to the charge of fellow lepers as helpless as themselves'.[7] Yet this report was only a year after two Commissions of Enquiry had been held into the conditions there. At that time nearly three fifths of the lepers on the island were Khoi indigenous people. In 1859 there were only three white lepers there with Khoi and Black lepers making up the balance of 47.[8]

Small settlements were also established near Port Elizabeth and other large towns across the country. During 1874 a Medical Board reported that lepers were to be found all over the country and encouraged the retention of lepers nearer their home towns, suggesting they reside in cottages under the direct supervision of the Magistrate and District Surgeon, but towards the end of the century the disease had continued to spread. In 1879 another Commission was appointed to inquire into the 'Lunatic Asylum' at Robben Island with a view to relocating the facility to the mainland. In giving evidence to the Commission the Island Chaplain warned that, in leaving the lepers behind alone 'they would sink into a chronic state of neglect and abuse.' At that time the mode of spread was still uncertain, with opinion divided as to whether or not the disease was contagious or hereditary. The Chaplain expressed uncertainty in this regard, citing many conflicting medical reports and recommended that they be forbidden to marry, as he leant towards the contagious view. He reported his view to the Commission that the Island was not a suitable place for them as 'none but the utterly helpless and destitute would remain on it' if the asylum was removed. He felt the island were not suitable for any permanent residents and recommended the entire facility be removed.[9] Dr Ross, the Superintendent of the Robben Island Infirmary, stated in 1885 'I am now more than ever convinced that it is not desirable to locate any more lepers on Robben Island.' He continued 'the buildings hitherto allotted to their gradual diminution and extinction have long been a disgrace to the country and are literally fit only to be burned down.' They were replaced by a set of wooden huts which were considered only a slight, improvement on the previous thatched barns. Dr Ross noted that their placement on the island deprived the lepers of gardens, education, and industrial pursuits. He described them as gambling and loafing about on the beach, and being a 'turbulent, quarrelsome and insubordinate lot...gregarious, barbarous and insolent'. He recommended the use of Langubulele's farm on the mainland, and maintaining a modest establishment for the segregation, employment, treatment and industrial training of the lepers.[10] Nonetheless it was to remain the leper settlement for the Cape until 1931, with on average 15 to 25 patients admitted annually.

During 1883 a Committee sat to consider the spread of leprosy which was increasingly affecting European and coloured people and it was recommended that an Act be drawn up which would give powers to compulsorily segregate and isolate all lepers. In 1884 the Act for the segregation of lepers was passed by the Cape Legislative Assembly (Act No 8 of 1884) entitled the Leprosy Repression Act, empowering the Governor, on the certificate of a district surgeon or any other medical practitioner to the effect that a man or woman was a leper and the disease communicable, to authorise his or her removal to Robben Island and to force them to remain there for life. Despite having concerns about the conditions on the Island Dr Ross said of the Repression Act that:

> Unless it includes a denial of all civil rights, the bastardy of all children born to lepers and confiscation of their property for their public and special support and treatment in Lazarettos and Lodges, [it] will never succeed in stamping out the sexual propagation of this horrible disease.[11]

The strict segregation of the sexes was also recommended in order to prevent children being born who would contract the disease from their parents and perpetuate it. The Act was finally promulgated in 1891 and enforced in May 1892.

In 1886 leprosy was reported to be very prevalent in the Division of Herschel, an African reserve near Aliwal North in the interior. Dr Matthews reported it as being found over the whole Cape colony at this time, including the areas of Fort Beaufort, Malmesbury, Saldanha Bay, Caledon, Calvinia, Clanwilliam, Hopetown, in Fingoland and Namaqualand, and through into Natal. Other reports were of lepers in Cape Town and other areas who were fishermen or small traders and of a group in Rondebosch who refused to go to Robben Island. Even after the new Act some cases were concealed by doctors and relatives, or evaded detection by moving frequently. Some escaped from the Colony and the Orange Free State and hid in the then Basutholand (now the country of Lesotho). Other richer folk fled to England. While the causative organism, Microbacterium leprae, had been identified in leprosy sufferers by Hansen in 1873, attempts to cultivate it in the laboratory were met with difficulty and debate still raged as to the communicability of the disease. Some, including a Dr Keith Guild, District Surgeon of

East Griqualand, considered it a form of tertiary syphilis. It was reported as being prevalent in the Transkei scattered through the district and it was thought it would be 'a great advantage if these unfortunate people could be isolated and prevented so far as is possible from marrying into healthy families'.[12] The Leprosy Act was amended in 1894 to increase the control with the Robben Island lepers no longer being allowed to leave the island to vote, to kiss or otherwise touch their visitors.

In Natal a Commission on Leprosy was established on 27th January 1885 by the Governor, Sir Henry Bulwer, to institute an inquiry as to the extent of the disease in Natal, to consider the best means of dealing with those affected by it and to consider measures to check its progress. Its Report was published in the Natal Government Gazette of 28th September 1886 in which it was noted that leprosy was widespread across the Colony but slowly increasing. Its spread was thought by the Africans to be by hereditary transmission, which the Commission agreed with in many cases. There were two stories regarding its commencement in Natal, which was affected later than other provinces. One theory was that it had been brought back by two men of the Amapapeta tribe who had returned from living for two years with women in Grahamstown in the Cape, who became lepers after they returned and from whom it then spread. Sir Theophilus Shepstone, who had been Secretary for Native Affairs in Natal for many years, also gave evidence to the Commission, and concurred that it had commenced in the Amapepeta tribe from around 1843, with the first death being that of the chief's eldest son, Bafakee, in 1846 and had spread to other tribes from around 1870. He reported that the disease had originally been attributed to the action of witchcraft instigated by revenge for the refusal of the Amapepeta Chief to permit his son to marry a particular girl belonging to another tribe.[13]

The Commission considered it implausible that it spread through some methods suggested 'such as bad sanitation, diet of salt meat, salt fish and vegetables in an unwholesome state, none of these causes being applicable to natives in this Colony' as their homes were considered healthy and they did not eat putrid meat or fish.[13] The Commission cited the work of Dr Carter in India and Dr Hanson who favoured the contagious theory of spread. It also cited a report from Dr Wynne, Medical Officer at the Robben Island Leper Asylum at the time, who thought its transmission through animals was possible, describing 'two pigeons suffering from leprosy, the bowed legs and incurvated claws, with nodular or hypertrophied articulations'. He also stated that leper mice had been caught in the wards, along with pheasants and turkeys. Leprosy was also known among the indentured Indian labourers, presumed to have been brought from India. However it was thought not to have spread from them to the indigenous population 'as there is no sexual intercourse between the races, nor can they have done so by contagion or infection, the Native having an intense objection to touching an Indian or his clothes'.[14]

Increasing social contact between Europeans and Africans started to raise fears that it would spread to Europeans, in particular from African nursemaids. Discussions with various Chiefs and Headmen were held and detailed accounts given of cases of leprosy and their symptoms, followed by the spread of the disease. Reports were of copper-coloured spots appearing on the skin, swelling and ulceration of fingers and toes, followed by the affected digits falling off and then the hands and feet, ending with death after a period of several years. Cases were reported from several areas of Natal, including Alexandra County and Zwartkop outside Pietermaritzburg. It was said that the disease was spread after marriage to an affected person and was incurable and that segregation of lepers was held to be the only means of arresting the spread of the disease, commencing with the Amapapeta location. Segregation of families should then be effected, with no inter-marriage between those inside the leprosy location and those outside. It was suggested that they should be exempted from taxation, as they would not be in a position to earn money, and be under medical supervision. The Commission made no recommendations in respect of Indian lepers as it was understood that the Indian Immigration Board returned such lepers to India. The report of the Natal Commission, which was published in the Natal Government Gazette of September 23rd 1886, was followed by the drafting of the Contagious Diseases Bill, which was debated in the Legislative Council in December 1886 although not passed.[15]

In September 1889 an anonymous, detailed and descriptive letter was submitted to Blackwood's Edinburgh Magazine raising attention to the conditions of Robben Island, described as an 'island of desolation'. The author travelled there on 'a dirty little tug' and found no jetty, so passengers were transferred to the island on the backs of the convicts who waded thigh-deep in the water. At that time there were approximately 130 lepers, 230 lunatics, 30 convicts and 160 police and ward-masters on the island, the appalling conditions of which are put down to 'the parsimony of the Colonial Officials'. First some of the patients are described:

> His arms are pulpy and inflated, and the skin resembles the rough rind of a boiled orange. His earlobes are dangling down in grotesque lumps; huge

knobs are disposed about his cheeks; his nostrils are swollen monstrously; the nape of his neck is scarcely to be distinguished; and shocking, shocking beyond my powers of description, is a gigantic excrescence on the side of his head, which has disfigured him almost beyond recognition as a human being ... would indeed that he were wholly dead! [16]

Of another it was said:

> Legs, or rather what remains of them, drawn up, and their extremities resembling round rulers, arms in a far worse condition – they are now scarcely longer than from an ordinary shoulder to elbow-distance; in fact they are perfectly useless, shapeless stumps, with rudimentary fingers but perfect finger-nails projecting from a small knob at the base of the stump, which once represented a hand. Truly here is absorption of a man's corporeal being; his very collar-bones and shoulder-blades seem to be in process of diminution; he is undergoing a living death, and that 'the beautiful living death' might be quickly sent to him is the most merciful prayer which can be breathed.[17]

He then proceeded to inspect the leper wards unaccompanied by the attendant doctor and is appalled at his discoveries. [Although anonymous it is assumed that the author was male due to the shooting of animals he describes on a walk around the Island and his killing of a large snake.] While some of the wards are not too bad in construction and cleanliness, although basic and without comfort, others he finds appalling:

> I find human ingenuity could surely scarcely contrive anything more vile and discreditable. Decrepit outside, ruinous within, deficient in the commonest furniture and fittings, fourteen beds are crowded into a totally insufficient space, the miserable rickety bedsteads mere masses of foul rags, and fouler mattresses, on which are stretched patients in the most advanced, helpless stages of the disease unprovided, so far as I could discover, with ordinary hospital appliances ... the very ground is destitute of boards and consists of bare earth trampled into hollows, over which ... numbers of large loathsome snakes crawl at night in search of mice. Is this disgraceful cabin a Cape Government Hospital, or is it a lazar-house which even the pariahs of the East would scorn to inhabit?[18]

The blame was clearly laid with the Cape Government who were not assigning funding to the Leper Establishment. The author talked of the lepers' virtual incarceration on that terrible island, and asked 'is it too much to ask that the bitterness of their lot should be alleviated, so far as is practicable, by at least a moderate expenditure of money and labour? At all events let the foul wards I have described be instantly demolished'. He also asked where were the clothes, washhouses, kitchen, library and reading room; where were the clean airy wards and gardens; where were the resources for employment and amusement, and 'where above all, that solicitude, tenderness, and consolation which would render it less hard for them to die?' One of the lepers approached him and asked for help in drawing attention to their plight and for help 'explaining how miserable we are. We have nobody to speak for us. I am scarcely at all ill, yet I am compelled to remain here. My wife and children are on the mainland. I have not seen them for years. Indeed I am unhappy – ah, so unhappy!'[19]

The article prompted a flood of correspondence and newspaper articles: 'such a general outburst of sympathy with the sufferers and of indignation at their treatment as has rarely been elicited by any magazine article'.[20] Articles were written in the British Medical Journal, the Morning Advertiser, the Glasgow Herald, and the New York Herald expressing the deepest concern and also relating similar tales of their own experiences of the Island. The comments of J.W. Matthews, a former member of the Cape Parliament, were repeated, as in the comments cited above, in the Evening News and Post. The Morning Advertiser stated that they could not have believed that so inhuman and disgraceful a state of things could have been permitted to exist in any British colony. The Glasgow Herald added 'the Leper Establishment at the Cape remains a blot not only upon the colony, but upon the fair fame of British Philanthropy'. The anonymous article was reproduced in the New York Times with the Editor commenting:

> The descriptions of the prevailing oppressive silence in the horrible wards of an hospital unfit for the lair of wolves; the references to the monotonous talk that on thresholds of death sometimes broke that silence... and the unanswerable indictment of foul neglect and inhuman management by Cape Town authorities, clearly demand instant attention from philanthropists in Parliament or in that wider House of Commons, the great British Commonwealth of souls.[21]

In November 1889 Blackwoods published an update of the affair based on further submissions by the original author from the Cape. Many of the allegations had been refuted by the Cape authorities, even denying that the inmates were being detained against their will. The ex-Colonial Secretary, Mr Tudhope, wrote 'The government had no power to detain the lepers compulsorily on Robben Island'; also adding that they 'have permission to wander about the island, to fish and to amuse themselves in any reasonable way'. He also stated that 'the lepers themselves were of the very lowest class of the people – black people ... the condition of the lepers is infinitely superior on Robben Island to that in which they would exist in their own homes'. The anonymous author vehemently contradicted these assertions, commenting 'I do not think it will be considered that black people have a less claim on our compassion than white people, but I declare the statement to be painfully inaccurate. I declare that I myself saw sufferers there of all shades from half-breeds to whites. Of pure blacks there were comparatively few'; and 'can anyone in his senses argue that these lepers would voluntarily remain to undergo the horrible miseries confessedly entailed on them by their residence in this Inferno, if they had the power to leave it!'[22] Following this, public agitation in Cape Town had resulted in a deputation of citizens appointed to visit the Island on October 1st, after which it was reported that the Colonial Secretary was taking steps for the removal of some of the inmates from the Island and for increasing the accommodation, although by November no evidence of this had yet been seen.

Notwithstanding all the controversy and promises Robben Island still had 553 lepers in 1900 who, during that year, also suffered an outbreak of smallpox causing 21 cases with eight deaths. The Asylum was under some strain to cope as one of the doctors had been taken away to deal with the plague camp at Uitvlugt outside Cape Town and others had gone on active service in the Anglo-Boer War. An outbreak of dysentery also caused six deaths. Treatment of leprosy was mainly with chaulmoogra oil and creosote although other drugs were tried. Chaulmoogra oil had been around for many years, and was derived from a tree (Taraktogenos kurzii) growing in parts of Burma and Assam, India. Other related oils used included hydnocarpus oil. In addition tracheotomy was often resorted to in cases where the larynx was being destroyed by leprotic growth. The doctor commented that he often observed general improvement afterwards with nodules on the face and limbs sometimes even disappearing, which he put down to the effect of increased oxygenation of the blood causing the absorption of leprous tissues and bacteria.

While conditions were still poor on the island improvements to the buildings were continually put off on the grounds that it would be shortly relocating to the mainland. The male wards were described as overcrowded and poorly ventilated with limited bathroom accommodation and no isolation facilities. The poor ventilation and overcrowding were thought to contribute to the high death rate from tuberculosis with one third of the deaths in that year, 34 out of 92 in total, being due to it. Sanitation was also poor with refuse being collected in a cart and tipped into the sea at a spot about half a mile from the female wards. The rubbish, including used bandages and dressings, was then thrown back up on to the rocks by the sea, to which crowds of sea birds came flocking. The male lepers worked and were paid as ward assistants, in the kitchen, the laundry, and as tailors, shoemakers etc. The female wards were in better condition than the male, and they also worked as attendants as well as in the laundry, kitchen and sewing room. They made all their own clothes, sheets and pillows etc along with clothes for the men. Seven children were born that year to female patients, fathered by male lepers, ascribed to them being able to climb over the fence between them. Along with a further eight children who didn't yet have leprosy it was recommended that they be removed without delay to either a home or people on the mainland: 'that they shall indefinitely remain here is too painful to contemplate'.[23]

Around this time discharges started to occur of arrested cases which were thought to be no longer infectious, with five discharged in 1899 and 12 in 1900. This was a new event in the history of Robben Island and gave the patients new hope, encouraging them to persevere with the treatment offered. The concept of total segregation was still discussed however, with Dr Gregory, the Medical Officer of the Colony commenting in 1909 that modified segregation as practiced in some other countries would be futile as in South Africa 'you have a very different population to deal with. A people largely composed of native and coloured, unreliable, indifferent to the dangers of the disease, ignorant and devoid of the simplest knowledge of hygiene'.[24] The Orange River Colony Leprosy Act was passed in 1909, following closely on from the Transvaal Acts of 1904, 1907 and 1908. The divisions between White and other patients increased from around the late 1890's and by 1904 there were around ten cottages for use by lepers who paid, along with special new wards for non-paying European lepers. The paying system was abolished in that year with all White patients being treated equally and treatment became along the lines of race rather than financial status.

Leprosy remained prevalent across the Cape with the District Surgeon of Herschel reporting 87 on his Leper Register in 1902, up from 57 the previous year. The District Surgeon warned of the need to remove them to the Emjanyana Leper Institution in order the clear the district of the disease. As the disease was often unreported in its early stages he wanted to make a search for lepers in order to certify, register and remove each case. The Emjanyana Leper Institution had been started in the Engcobo district of the Transkei in 1892 with sufficient accommodation for 1,080 African patients. By 1900 it had 315 lepers of whom 171 were males. The mortality rate was high with 60 dying during the course of the year. Practically all the work at the Asylum was done by the lepers themselves - cooking, nursing, washing etc - who were paid small salaries for their labours. The Asylum kept their own cattle to supply milk to the residents and some for sale along with other farm produce such as corn, potatoes and lemons. The patients added their own traditional treatment to that supplied by the Medical Officer, but the Medical Officer reported that neither their treatment nor his appeared to make any difference to the course of the disease.[25]

The Bochem Leper Institution was started in 1914 on a site 55 miles northwest of Pietersburg, in the Transvaal, for the purposes of a station for the treatment of sick Africans, on the same site as the Venereal Diseases Hospital. The Mkambati Leper Institution was opened in 1920 in the Lusikisiki district of Pondoland. At that time there was still debate as to the cause of the illness, with suspicion still placed upon the eating of putrid fish or meat. It was suggested that as the Bushmen didn't eat fish they must have been infected another way. As their traditional hunting grounds had been destroyed by commercial farmers the Bushmen were said to have changed to mutton. Meijer, commenting on the period of the late 1800's, postulated that this then 'caused the farmers to hunt the Bushmen who were then obliged to turn to other things, such as squirrels, mice etc. This source of supply being small, they had to economize with their food, carrying it about with them for a considerable time, during which it got putrid. This diseased meat may have been the cause of the leprosy'. He thought that the farmers were at little risk as they always ate fresh meat.[26] Others' argued strongly that leprosy was being spread by smallpox vaccination and that only its cessation would stop the onslaught of the disease. Whatever the cause, there was little available in the way of treatment in the 1920s. Chaulmoogra oil was recommended by some, which gave good results in some cases and no results in others, particularly those with nerve damage.

On 14th February 1918 a Parliamentary Select Committee was appointed to enquire into and report upon the measures to be taken to improve the conditions governing the treatment of lepers in the Union. It looked into the five institutions of Robben Island, Bochem, Pretoria, Emjanyana and Amatikulu existing at that time, which contained a total of 2,332 patients. At Pretoria there had been an investigation into maladministration just the year before which had lead to the removal of the lay Superintendent and the transfer of the Medical Officer, at whose hands some patients alleged they had got worse instead of better, to Robben Island. The lay Superintendent had been replaced with a Medical Superintendent under whom the cleanliness, sanitation and treatment had improved. Alongside these five institutions there were at the time nine known lepers isolated at their own homes and it was suggested that there were probably well over a thousand African lepers in communities in the Cape Province and Transkei alone. The Committee visited the Island and heard numerous grievances from the patients, most of which included that they wished to be removed back to the mainland. They complained that it was harming their health through the brackish water, the winter fogs giving lung trouble and the glare of the sun on the white sand harming their eyes. It was said by the European patients that 50% had tuberculosis and 20% were blind as a result of the conditions. They also complained that their relatives were loath to visit as they had a dread of the place which was added to by the large number of lunatics and criminals also placed on the Island. They said the Island was a dumping ground for murderers and criminals of the worst type and that murders and rapes had taken place. The European patients objected to having to endure some of restrictions that were placed because of the African patients and the Coloured and African inmates wanted the privileges that the Europeans had. One European stated that in England he had been allowed to stay in good hotels and be treated in general hospital wards with a certificate stating that he was no danger to the public. He then came out to South African and was sent to Robben Island where 'living is an animal existence – eating, drinking and sleeping. It is most demoralising and our lives become very embittered'. The women complained about the dangers of the criminals on the island and about ill treatment by the nurses. One reported:

> When I want to put my clothes on I have to pay another patient to do it. I have to pay 2 or 3 shillings a month to other people to assist me in dressing. I have to work for the money and when I have not got any money I have to remain as I am. Although I have no hands I make up the beds and I sweep and scrub and clean the windows'.[27]

The matter of moving the settlement to the mainland had been considered in two earlier Commissions of 1904 and 1909 but the Committee still did not support it, although it did consider that the White patients could be removed to Pretoria where their facilities were better with each patient having their own bedroom and kitchen. The idea of a settlement on the mainland had always been resisted by local people on various grounds – one was that it would allegedly interfere with the purity of the water supply. A suggestion that Pretoria lepers be allowed to visit the spa resort of Warm Baths was similarly opposed. The nine lepers isolated at home had to observe strict conditions of segregation with separate utensils, clothing and bedding and no contact with any other person, including spouses and children, beyond talking. However the disease was generally accepted to be not highly contagious and it was reported that in the recorded history of the institutions there had only been two cases of supervisory officials contracting leprosy – one doctor who was known to have eaten and drunk with the lepers and later died of the disease, and one overseer from the Pretoria Institution who was later admitted as a patient on Robben Island. Methods of spread proposed included through close contact, sharing utensils, sharing food on a plate and by insects. The leprosy bacterium had been found in house-flies and bugs through feeding on sores or biting lepers and this was suggested as one of the routes by which leprosy was spreading in African kraals, where bugs were said to be numerous. Others thought this unlikely given that employees in the institutions were not getting the disease. The hereditary route was thought less likely as babies separated from leper mothers at birth did not develop it. By this time the idea that it was spread by fish was said to be 'as dead as dead can be'.[28]

Each Province of the country at that time had separate Acts dealing with Leprosy and providing for separation of sufferers, but all of them did allow relatives to visit occasionally and provided accommodation for them at the Institutions. The spread of leprosy in the Transkei and 'Native Territories' caused much worry as it could spread not only among Africans, but also to the European population and through them to the rest of the Cape. Sexual relations between patients also worried the Committee members with Dr John Dunstan, a medical inspector commenting 'my experience as a medical man is that when a man has got phthisis or some fatal disease, or a woman is similarly afflicted, the sexual instinct is very strong. It is the same with the feeble minded. The feeling of unfitness to compete and to continue the species is a great incentive to propagation'. He proposed that this be explained to them in lectures to encourage them to withstand these subconscious urges and understand their duties to the State and that sterilisation could also be a possibility.[29]

In 1919 when the National Department of Public Health was established the administration of leper institutions was not taken over by them, but remained under the control of the Department of the Interior.

The first Secretary for Public Health had given evidence before the Select Committee of the House of Assembly on the Treatment of Lepers in 1918 and again to the Cabinet Finance Committee in October 1922. He made several points in his submissions, including that the high expenditure on this disease was out of all proportion to its public health importance in comparison with disease such as tuberculosis and syphilis. He felt that there were a large number of cases in leper institutions which were no longer infectious and should be re-examined as to their need for continued segregation. The methods of dealing with it needed to be modernised, a technical Leprosy Advisory Committee was required and a new Leprosy Act and the institutions should be transferred to the Public Health Department. These proposals were subsequently approved by the Government, and transfer to the Health Department agreed with effect from the 1st April 1924.[30] Leprosy was declared a notifiable disease in 1921, and 108 cases were notified in that year. A subsequent medical board undertaken before the transfer to the Public Health Department found that of 2,501 cases examined in Institutions 693, or 28%, no longer required isolation on the grounds of infectivity or danger to public health. The new Act repealed some of the harsher provisions of the earlier Leprosy Repression Act by providing for the discharge of the arrested cases.

The first meeting of the Leprosy Advisory Committee appointed under Government Notice No 1898 of November 1924 was held in 1925. In a report given in 1925 by Sheldon of the Union Health Department he recommended the closure of the Robben Island institution and the transfer of the patients to the West Fort facility at Pretoria. At this time there were 2,163 lepers detained in the country. More cases were being discharged back into the communities as they were deemed no longer infectious, although it was hard for them to make a living outside. Between 400 and 500 a year were still being admitted. It was estimated that there were 2,264 lepers still 'at large' in the community and 905 discharged cases, giving a total number of 5,332, or a rate of 0.74 per 1,000 population. There was, however, a tendency of lepers 'to wander to escape detection', so exact numbers were unknown. The highest incidence in proportion to the population was in the rural area of Impendle in Natal, adjacent to Basotholand (Lesotho). The only proposed reason for this was that it was rather remote and could be being used as a refuge by those in Lesotho, as generally the rates tended to be lower in the higher, dry areas of the country. The contagious theory of spread was favoured, with it being thought to be primarily due to direct inoculation of the organism into the skin or nasal mucous membrane.

There was also evidence that it could also be spread by arm-to-arm smallpox vaccination. The bacteria could reach the skin through fingers, clothes or insects and then be introduced by scratching any itchy lesion. However it also required the person to have lowered resistance due to ill health, poor diet, syphilis, unfavourable climate or poor hygienic or economic conditions. The climatic conditions at Robben Island were one reason why it was thought it should be closed, being humid, windy, and with the strong sun glare and sand which were unfavourable to the disease.[31]

In 1927 there were 107 patients at Bochem and 153 at Robben Island, of whom 22 were European. The Government had turned down the proposal to relocate them to the Pretoria Institution. There were 594 patients in Emjanyana, 231 in Mkambati and 416 in the Amatikulu Leper Institution. All of these institutions were on farms with the aim of producing meat, milk and vegetables to reduce the running costs. Efforts were made to reduce the time between diagnosis and admission, with depots being constructed in African areas for temporary detention being removed to an institution by motor ambulance. It was estimated there were between 1,500 and 2,000 unreported and undiscovered cases in the African districts.

In 1930 the Secretary of the British Empire Leprosy Relief Association, Robert Cochrane, submitted a report on Leprosy in South African to the Department of Public Health. He visited the West Fort institution at Pretoria, and found it to be efficient and well organised with up to date treatment protocols and good results. Over 50% of patients improved to the extent that they could be employed in some useful occupation. He also heard that altogether eight staff had contracted the disease from patients over the years since it opened. 90 of the patients were European and he commented that leprosy occurred most frequently among poorer Europeans, who tended to develop it rapidly and who passed quickly into a contagious stage, which supported the notion that they should be segregated in a leprosarium rather than isolated at home. He stated that the conditions under which Europeans lived at West Fort were excellent with every comfort and that their relatives received an allowance. Leprosy among Europeans and Coloureds was by then decreasing, and only found in those living under conditions of poverty and poor hygiene. He then visited Emjanyana in the Transkei which he stated had good accommodation with an excellent diet ration – in fact the meat ration was considered 'rather high'. He commended the treatment given and their experimentation with 'shock-producing drugs', Hydnocarpus oil and 'massive doses of Alepol'. Dr Cochrane then moved on to Mkambati and the detention camp at Salisbury Island in Durban bay, where patients were sent before transfer to Amatikulu. Amatikulu had twelve square miles of land where the lepers were accommodated in 'native houses' or traditional dome-shaped, wattle-and-daub huts. He noted that at all institutions babies were separated from their mothers at birth, then kept in a crèche until two years old after which they were sent to relatives. He recommended that, if there were no adequate crèches, they should rather stay with their mothers until two, as without good crèche facilities 'the chances of survival are very meagre'. Overall he commented that the African leprosy problem, although more serious than for Europeans, was of minor significance compared with syphilis, tuberculosis and malaria. Leprosy was favoured by the presence of other diseases in the community such as syphilis, intestinal disease and other chronic infection. Because of the sparseness of the population and the lack of a health service Cochrane supported institutional treatment but also recommended education and an organised 'native health service', and the extension of the 'native typhus visitors' to include all infectious diseases, with first-aid trained Africans in all villages.[32]

At the International Leonard Wood Memorial Conference on Leprosy in Manila in 1931 Leprosy was reclassified into two main groups: *Neural*, which showed signs of nerve involvement, loss of sensation and paralysis with their consequences – contractures and ulcerations - and *Cutaneous*, which had lesions in the skin. These might also have a lesser degree of neural involvement. By the 1930s the idea that leprosy was transmitted by eating rotten fish had fallen out of favour and it was seen as a contagious disease. Of 372 cases at West Fort in Pretoria all except five gave some history of contact with a leper, 64% had contact with someone within a house-hold and most of the remaining 36% had some other form of contact. The actual manner of transmission was still unknown however, although prolonged contact with an infected person was recognised as necessary. Many experiments were conducted internationally to try and solve the problem - an injection of leprous material into a condemned criminal in Hawaii had resulted in disease, but such experiments were not always successful. Danielson injected himself and nine other volunteers without success, and other experiments were conducted by injecting lepers with material. Mostert, appointed at West Fort as a Leprosy Research Officer for the Union, noted that the state of health of the recipient was important as 'the disease occurs chiefly among people low down the scale of civilisation with poor resistance', the result in particular of a deficient diet, along with squalor, overcrowding and lack of personal hygiene. Those aged less than 20 years were also more susceptible. Weather was also a factor, with it being commoner in hot, high rainfall countries. The preferred treatment in Pretoria was still hydnocarpus oil which was less likely to give reactions than Chaulmoogra oil, was cheaper and easier to obtain. It was given subcutaneously and was of varying effectiveness. Also under trial were synthetic dyes such as trypan blue, brilliant green, methylene blue and mercurochrome. The latter was successful in the treatment of nerve pains and clearing up septic conditions when given by injection. The other dyes were of variable effectiveness, the most effective of which, trypan blue, was too toxic for regular use.[33]

The closure of Robben Island as a Leper Institute was recommended again by the Leprosy Advisory Committee in 1930 and finally agreed in that year, with the date set for 31st March 1931. That left five leper institutions in the country where all lepers were compulsorily segregated – at West Fort in Pretoria (which in 1933 had 107 Europeans and 860 non-Europeans), at Bochem (with around 90 Africans), two Institutions in the Transkei at Emjanyana (632 Africans) and Mkambati (252 Africans), and at Amatikulu in Zululand with 269 Africans. Approximately 600 to 800 people a year were admitted, who had the chance of release if their condition became arrested, following the introduction of a policy of 'probational discharge' of non-infective lepers in 1922. Following release they were followed up under surveillance unless the condition completely disappeared. Around 20% to 30% of all inmates were discharged each year. Annual visits were made by medical boards to decide who would be allowed to return home without danger to the public. The District Surgeon was informed and sent a chart of the patient so that he could do periodic examinations and send the patient back if the condition worsened. Drewe at Mkambati felt that the segregation of lepers in institutions improved their mental wellbeing as they no longer had to hide their disfigurements and became more self-assured. They also provided the opportunity for good nutrition, cleanliness and general hygiene, which is in marked contradiction to the state of the leprosy institutions in the 19th century. Chaulmoogra oil was still in use, applied topically as a lotion, as well as orally and by injection. Those resistant to the use of the oils were tried with a 'protein shock' treatment, which involved injections of sterilized milk, up to 10cc given intramuscularly.[34] Other treatments continued to be tested, but gave disappointing results. The Department of Health considered that 'Chaulmoogra oil and its derivatives still hold the place of honour among drugs in our armamentarium against leprosy'.[35]

The Pretoria Leper Institution as West Fort was used for the practical training of medical students in the recognition and treatment of the disease, which was credited with increasing the early recognition of leprosy and enabling earlier admissions into institutions, with the time between onset and admission estimated to be around six years in 1935. The Department of Health plotted the relative incidence of cases between 1901 and 1930 on a map of the country, which gave some interesting findings. The highest incidence was found in the area around Klerksdorp which was ascribed to the establishment of a refugee camp there during the Anglo-Boer war. Other areas of high incidence were the west coast region of the Cape and the area running from Heidelberg across Standerton towards Swaziland. Also with a high incidence were the Waterberg, Middleberg, inland areas of the Transkei and southern Natal (Polela and Himeville) and Port Elizabeth and East London. Certain areas were notable by their lack of the disease, in particular the coastal areas of Natal and the central Cape/Karoo. There appeared to be no geographical association between leprosy and other endemic diseases such as malaria.[36] Over the years the number of inmates declined as did the type of patient. There was a considerable reduction in European and mixed race patients such that the problem by the late 1930's was largely confined to Africans, who comprised 92% of institutional residents.

Treatment regimens were described as making considerable progress by the early 1940's, but still depended on chaulmoogra oil by injection and by mouth, to which were added injections of iodised ethyl-esters into the lesions which caused disappearance of many of the lesions and a significant cosmetic improvement. In 1941 the Minister of Public Health re-appointed a Leprosy Advisory Committee to sit for the next five years. By 1945 the mode of entry of the leprosy organism, known as the bacillus of Hansen, into the body was still unknown, with entry through the oro-pharynx or through cuts and abrasions considered possible routes. It was also acknowledged that the disease was associated with poverty, malnutrition and overcrowding and that the incidence was more than eight times as high in Africans as in Europeans who comprised only 3% of the 2,214 inmates. Different types of leprosy - lepromatous (where the patient had a poor immune response), tuberculoid (where the patient had a strong immune response) and indeterminate - were recognised. While it was considered that the lepromatous patients should be given rest, good food and fresh air in order to build their resistance, Drewe reported that they were unable to do this due to 'lack of room and the poor mentality of the patient'. Various attempts at other treatments were tried, including injections of dyes such as lithium carmine, and acriflavine, with little success.[37] However, by 1947 it was found that there was new hope with the sulphonamide drugs, with the National Leprosarium at Carville in America finding good responses to treatment with three sulphonamide drugs, although between 18 months and five years of treatment was required. Another positive development was that people were getting diagnosed with the disease at a much earlier stage - less than two years into the illness compared with an average of six to eight years in earlier times.

Segregation was still the norm for the initial period of treatment in the early 1950s, at which point the incidence in South Africa was estimated at 0.77 per 1,000 people. There were approximately 6,000 patients in total of whom 2,000 were living in the five institutions and of whom 56 were European. The majority of patients were able to be discharged within 12 months of their diagnosis. By this time the institutions had somewhat improved, with schools provided, land made available for farming, sports and pastimes provided. Sulphonamide drugs had improved the prognosis considerably over chaulmoogra oil with the death rate at West Fort cut by 50% since their introduction.[38] Internationally trials of Isoniazid (INAH) were also taking place with mixed results. Streptomycin and Para-Amino Salicylic acid (PAS) were also tried with some beneficial effects. Discharge rates were steadily improving and the numbers of patients absconding were falling with only 25 absconding from West Fort in a five year period. Fear of admission was no longer causing concealment of the disease with only 17 of 500 patients surveyed giving this as a reason for delay in coming forward. The majority of late presentations were due to delay in diagnosis by the doctor (17%), delay by a traditional healer (14%) or failure to recognise the seriousness of the disease and seek any help (49%). The Minister of Health, Mr de Wit Nel, stated in Parliament in 1958 that the government's efforts to combat leprosy had met with great success, particularly since the commencement of treatment with sulphone dating from 1947. As a result it was no longer considered a serious national health problem with an incidence of 0.14 per thousand. One of the five leper institutions had been able to close due to lack of patients, and two others had been converted for the accommodation of tuberculosis patients.[39]

The number of new cases of leprosy fell steadily from the time antibiotic treatment was introduced until by the 1970's there were only around 100-200 per year, mostly coming from Natal, the Orange Free State and the Southern Transvaal. By the 1980s West Fort Hospital was the referral hospital nationally for leprosy patients where diagnosis was confirmed and treatment commenced, but few were being admitted for more than six to eight weeks – the time taken to render them non-infective. The introduction of multidrug therapy had greatly improved the leprosy situation, with registered total cases in the whole of the African continent having fallen from 987,607 in 1885 to 352,222 in 1992.

In South Africa by 1988 there were only 962 registered cases in the country, a prevalence of 2.7 per 100,000 people, one of the lowest in Africa. Annual notifications of new cases had fallen to 120, with a male to female ratio of 1.5:1. 68% of the caseload for that decade was from the Transvaal (now Mpumulanga) and KwaZulu-Natal Provinces - the 'leprosy belt'. 98% of the cases were Black South Africans with the disease presenting most often in adulthood, between the ages of 20 and 55. By this time cases in the west and south of the country, including the Cape and the former Transkei, had dropped to a negligible level with only a handful of cases a year. In 1990 only nine cases were notified and the disease – once considered one of the most fearsome and dreaded diseases due to its appalling disfigurements - had virtually disappeared from the South African landscape, its defeat being mostly due to the prompt and effective treatment regime using antibiotics which cured the disease long before the complications set in.

ENDNOTES

1   Laidler P.W. and Gelfand M. *South Africa, its medical history, 1652-1898: A medical and social study*; C Struik, Cape Town, 1971: 58

2   Smuts F.; *Stellenbosch three centuries*; The Town Council of Stellenbosch; 1979: 243

3   Laidler P.W. and Gelfand M.; *South Africa, its medical history, 1652-1898: A medical and social study*; C Struik Cape Town, 1971:174

4   Searle C. *The history of the development of nursing in South Africa 1652-1960*; The South African Nursing Association; 1980: 70

5   Matthews J.W. *Incwadi Yami or Twenty Years Personal Experience in South Africa; 1887*; Africana Book Society, Johannesburg 1976: 345

6   Stockenstrom A. Parliamentary Debates, Cape of Good Hope, 1854 published by The State Library, Pretoria, Reprint 33, Volume 1 1968, debates dated 11th September, 14th September, 22nd September and 16th August 1854, pages 299,301,317,418.

7   Matthews J.W. *Incwadi Yami or Twenty Years Personal Experience in South Africa; 1887*; Africana Book Society, Johannesburg 1976: 355

8   *Report on the General Infirmary Robben Island for 1859*, Published, 1860, G 11-1860:3
9   Baker J. *Submission to the Commission Appointed to enquire into, and report upon, the best means of moving the Asylum at Robben Island to the Mainland;* Saul Solomon and Co 1880:13
10 Ross W.M.H. *Robben Island Infirmary Annual Report for 1885*, Cape Of Good Hope, WA Richards and Sons, Cape Town, 1886 G2/1886: 9-10
11 Ibid, 9-10
12 Nankivell J.H. 'Report of the District Surgeon, Transkei' *Blue Book of Native Affairs 1882,* Cape of Good Hope, Volume 1 part 1,WA Richards and sons, Cape Town: 20
13 'Report of the Commission on Leprosy'; Government Notice No 434 of 1886; *The Natal Government Gazette* September 28 1886: 900
14 Ibid, 894
15 Haydon F.S. Acting Colonial Secretary; *Debates of the Legislative Council Colony of Natal; First session Twelfth Council*, Volume IX; WM Watson Pietermaritzburg; 1887: 494.
16 Anonymous 'Lepers at the Cape: wanted, a Father Damien' *Blackwood's Edinburgh Magazine*, Sept 1889, no DCCCLXXXVII Vol CXLVI: 295
17 Ibid, 296
18 Ibid, 298
19 Ibid, 293-299
20 'Lepers at the Cape: wanted, a Father Damien'; Correspondence and Editorial Comments, *Blackwood's Edinburgh Magazine*, October 1889, noDCCCLXXXVIII Vol CXLVI: 576
21 Ibid, 576-580
22 Anonymous; 'More about the Lepers at the Cape, Memorandum for the information of the readers of 'Blackwood's Magazine''' *Blackwood's Edinburgh Magazine*, November 1889, No DCCCLXXXIX Vol CXLVI:743-746
23 Colonial Secretary's Ministerial Division, *Reports on the Government and State-Aided Hospitals and Asylums*, WA Richards, Cape Town, 1900, G41-'1901
24 Gregory Dr. in *Report of the Select Committee on Robben Island Lepers*, 1909, Cape Town, A12-1909: 22
25 Emjanyana Leper Asylum in: *Reports on the Government and Aided Hospitals and Asylums*, 1900, WA Richards, Cape Town, 1901, G41-'1901: 154-156
26 Meijer H.B.W 'Reminiscences of Leprosy and Plague', *South African Medical Record,* 21(20) 1923:475-476
27 Watt T. *First and Second Reports of the Select Committee on Treatment of Lepers*, Cape Times Ltd Government Printers 1918, S.C.10-'18: 63
28 Ibid, 40
29 Ibid, 33
30 *Annual Report of the Department of Public Health*, Union of South Africa, 1939, Government Printing and Stationery Office Pretoria, UG 57-'39: 36
31 Sheldon H.F. 'Leprosy', *South African Medical Record*, 23(20) 1925:447-453
32 Cochrane Robert G. 'Report on Leprosy in the Union of South Africa', in: *Annual Report of the Department of Public Health*, Union of South Africa, 1930, The Government Printer Pretoria, UG 40-'30: 59-65
33 Mostert H.v.R. 'Leprosy: some aspects of modern research', *South African Medical Journal*, 9(13) 1935:459-463

34 Drewe Frank, 'The Treatment of Leprosy', *South African Medical Journal*, 10(19) 1936: 655-658
35 *Annual Report of the Department of Public Health*, 1937, Government Printer Pretoria, UG No 52-'37:38
36 *Annual Report of the Department of Public Health,* Union of South Africa, 1935, The Government Printer Pretoria, UG 43-'35, 29 and annexed map.
37 Drewe Frank, 'Some of the Problems of Leprosy' *South African Medical Journal*, 19(21) 1945:408-310
38 Davison A.R. 'Leprosy in South Africa *South African Medical Journal*, 27(32) 1953:659-661
39 De Wet Nel M.D.C. 'State of the Union's Health: Minister's Review', *South African Medical Journal*, 32(35) 30 August 1958: 876

2   'A MENACE TO OUR HEALTH': SYPHILIS

Syphilis is not often thought of as a devastating epidemic disease, but in South Africa it was to become regarded as a terrifying threat to society and health and one of many contagious or infectious diseases that played a significant role in shaping the country's history. Venereal or sexually transmitted diseases were mentioned from the earliest settlement at the Cape of Good Hope, probably introduced by passing sailors. It is thought that there was no syphilis among the indigenous population before Europeans came, amongst whom it had spread in epidemic form from 1493, and that it spread concurrently with European penetration into the country. Others however, suggest that it had also come down from the east coast of Africa due to trading contact with Arabia, Asia and Egypt, which had been occurring for many centuries. The Contagious Diseases Commission of 1906-1907 found that there were several African names for syphilis, but that they referred to a new disease brought in from elsewhere.[1] In IsiZulu it was known as 'isifo sabelungu' (disease of the white man) whereas in Malawi it was known as 'the disease of the Arabs'.

As soon as the first sailors arrived at the Cape the venereal diseases they brought with them started to spread to the indigenous population through sexual contact. An attempt was made in 1681 to prohibit 'immorality' between Europeans and other races, whether slave or free, and to minimise contact with the first reference made to a brothel in that year. But the attempt was soon forgotten. Slaves started arriving from 1657 and the East India Company had maintained a 'slave lodge', which also received sailors and soldiers as lodgers. Through this means venereal diseases spread to an extent where they became almost ineradicable. Very little direct reference is made to it in the early records of that era, although a Report of the Commissioners of the Hospital in 1710 refers to an inspection of the Hospital, commenting 'all the sick, excepting the syphilis patients, were mixed up together, especially those suffering from dysentery and other bowel complaints. It is interesting to note that the syphilis patients were separated, as unlike many other diseases of the time this was not directly infectious without close personal contact.[2]

Gonorrhoea was said to very often affect sailors, soldiers and slaves 'who are in all cases infected by the dissolute female slaves'. There were suspicions that 'these harlots, without being infected themselves, have a trick of infecting those who have not paid them well enough, or those with whom they cohabit but from whom they do not receive enough pleasure'.[3] What was possibly gonorrhoea was thought by Mentzel to be common amongst female slaves, but that it should be common amongst White women 'seems to me mysterious and doubtful'. Information on this was judged difficult to come by, as it seemed unlikely that the women would confide these intimate secrets to the 'inexperienced young bachelors' who were the surgeons in the hospital.[4] Certainly venereal disease in slaves could be punished harshly – a case in 1792 relates how a slave Stijn was thrashed with a sjambok (whip) for having venereal disease, after which she took to bed and shortly thereafter died.[5]

A determined effort was made to diminish venereal diseases in the early 19th century through the control of prostitutes, based on the complaint that the vagrant 'Hottentots' (Khoikhoi), the slaves and also free women were responsible for much of the disease amongst the troops, yet it is notable that early travellers into the interior in the early 19th century stated that the disease was largely unknown. A proclamation was published in the Kaapsche Courant in December 1803 that any affected soldier would in future be asked from what woman he had caught the disease. If she were Khoikhoi she would be put in the Slave Lodge until cured and then restricted to the country beyond the Salt River. If she were a slave she would be cured at her own expense and then given corporal punishment, and if she were a European she would be cured at her own expense and then kept on bread and water for ten days. A second offence would lead to imprisonment. Wandering Khoikhoi women who were unemployed could be taken in for examination. There is no mention of any penalties for the men.[6] The blaming of women, in particular sex workers, for the spread of sexually transmitted diseases, and the ignoring of the role of men who drove the industry and took diseases back to their wives, is a common theme throughout the history of these diseases in South Africa.

The next attempt to deal with the issue was the Contagious Diseases Act of 1868 (Act 25) which was enforced at Cape Town, King Williamstown, Grahamstown, Simonstown and Port Elizabeth and aimed at the control of brothels. There was strong opposition to the Act as it was claimed that the police stigmatized respectable women and that it exposed poor women to insult. Even early writers on the disease continued to stigmatize prostitutes while Sax, although sympathetic to the Africans who had experienced the spread of this hitherto unknown disease from foreigners, commenting of the high levels of infection in the late 1800's said 'the enormous incidence of syphilis among troops was in no small measure due to coloured prostitutes'.[7] The Act was based on similar legislation in Britain and had the effect of institutionalizing prostitution. It provided for the registration and periodic examination of prostitutes and their 'voluntary treatment' in Lock Hospitals if found to be diseased. Similar legislation had been passed in other colonies including Malta, India and Australia. Pressure for an Act at the Cape came partly from the War Office which claimed that British troops at the Cape were being decimated by venereal disease and threatened to withdraw them from Cape Town. Within a year of passing the Act an abolition campaign was started lead by a politician, Saul Solomon, calling itself the Association for the Repeal of the Contagious Diseases Act. The Act was withdrawn in 1872.[8]

During the 1800's the arm-to-arm vaccination for smallpox was being introduced which was thought to be possibly a way in which syphilis was spread without sexual activity. Up until the discovery of the organism that causes syphilis in 1905 there was still limited understanding of the mechanisms of spread of syphilis and gonorrhoea. While it was understood to be transmitted sexually and congenitally it was also widely believed that it could spread through non-sexual contact, such as the kissing, breast feeding or hugging of children, or the sharing of glasses, pipes, clothing etc.[9] Early treatment was with mercury which was used for almost 400 years, given by mouth, by inhalation, or by injection, although the narrow margin between treatment and toxicity meant mercury poisoning became common and for many the cure was worse than the disease. Potassium iodide was introduced in Europe as a treatment in 1834.

The development of the diamond and gold fields in Kimberley and the Witwatersrand in the centre of the country lead to large numbers of both European and African migrants being attracted to those areas. From then on syphilis became an ever increasing problem across the length and breadth of the country. Between 1871 and 1895 approximately 100,000 men came to the mines, leaving their families behind and living in overcrowded male compounds for up to 18 months at a time. The conditions were ideal for the spread of sexually transmitted diseases with use of prostitutes and heavy drinking common. They then returned to their homes in the rural areas and villages to spread disease to their wives. With the growing mining industry followed the expansion of the ports and secondary industries, all of which grew using African labour, drawn from the rural areas to rapidly expanding urban and peri-urban areas where the bringing of families was not permitted. Harrhy, writing from Barkley West, talked of the early studies of the Frontier Medical Association showing that by the mid 1880's syphilis was widespread among the black population. Harrhy started a free dispensary and reported treating hundreds of cases, although many of these cases may have been yaws which at that time was not able to be bacteriologically distinguished from syphilis.[10] District Surgeons and Native Commissioners were similarly giving reports of the increasing incidence among the black population.

In 1888 the Cape Colony's 1885 Act for the Better Prevention of Contagious Diseases was promulgated, following scares about the increasing incidence of syphilis which was reaching epidemic proportions. This required prostitutes to be registered and periodically medically examined with those found diseased to be detained in hospital until cured. Minor panic about syphilis spread through the Cape and the Act proceeded without the same agitation as previously, although there is evidence that the disease was to some extent being confused with yaws. By December 1891 there were 196 prostitutes registered under the Act. Many of them moved to the mining towns in the interior. The Cape Government established 'Lock hospitals', appointed special medical officers and instituted a system of free treatment of Africans by district surgeons throughout the Cape.[11] Similarly in 1886 a Contagious Diseases Bill was introduced into the Natal Legislative Assembly. While the capital city of Pietermaritzburg had supported it as a way to prevent infectious disease coming into the city, there were also those who saw the city as a centre of disease to which it was dangerous to send their farm workers, for fear of them becoming contaminated. The presence of large numbers of African prostitutes, estimated at 200, were presumed to be giving rise to the spread of syphilis and gonorrhoea which were thought to be spread by 'inoculation' to European children and thence women, presenting a danger to the health of that population. For this reason certain Members of the Legislative Assembly were strongly in support of the Bill.

The debates of the all White-male Natal Assembly give an interesting example of the perspectives of the time. Member F.W.B. Louch stated:

> the evidence of medical men for the last hundred years proves...that after the second or third generation from the impregnation of syphilis, insanity and

consumption are the natural results of this terrible disease. I am assured also that the Native servants being diseased it is really most difficult now to protect little children, and I believe unfortunately that there are many children of the white inhabitants of this City who are affected with this disease. Not only that, but... some ladies are suffering actually from disease. They have probably got it from the child.[12].

The concern was that male nursemaids could spread the disease to children through oral contact, with medical men claiming that African male nurses infected white children when they kissed them. Not all Council members were in favour of draconian control measures however. Mr J. Robinson stated 'so far as I can make out this Bill is one to protect and propagate a social evil rather than a Bill to prevent the spread of disease ... it has social and moral consequences which cannot be contemplated at this moment'. Mr J.L. Hulett described it as an attempt to bring about a 'system of espionage and a system fraught with a very large amount of evil and injury to the whole country'. He noted that the disease was virulent, but had been present in the Colony for at least a quarter of a century. One of his objections was that 'under this Law any woman may be subjected to the greatest amount of indignity and lifelong misery through circumstances possibly beyond her control. Power is given to certain individuals upon certain information to bring up a woman...and on suspicion she may be compelled to be examined by a medical man. It is known that a very large amount of injustice and wrong has been done to many women in England under the provisions of a law similar to this'. However his objections were not totally out of sympathy to women, but also out of a concern that prostitutes, if uninfected, would be given free licence to offer themselves to the young men of the town which would 'bring publicly to the notice of the community this social evil which men endeavour to keep out of sight'. H.E. Stainbank commented 'the only really good argument that has been used in favour of the Bill is that we have brought this disease amongst the Blacks, and therefore it is necessary to cure them, and especially in reference to innocent children'. He continued 'this bill applies entirely to one class of the community. A man may spread the disease broadcast and there is no penalty to be enforced upon him. He can do it with impunity. ... If there is to be a bill at all it ought to apply, so far as it goes, to both classes [male and female]'.[13].

The debates continued into the following year. The Bill was subsequently amended to refer to any person suffering from any venereal disease and re-introduced as a Bill for the Better Prevention of Certain

Contagious Diseases. It was almost identical although covered both males and females. The idea that gentlemen could also be reported and subject to medical examination concerned some members. The Bill was passed by the legislature and submitted to Lord Knutsford, the Secretary of State for the Colonies. However Knutsford refused to assent to it, noting that in England the compulsory medical examination of women had been condemned and given up.[14]

By 1891 agitation had started again against the Cape Act but attempts to have it repealed failed and then were distracted by the outbreak of war. Repeal failed due to the innate caution of many Members of the House who felt that the Act was better than nothing in dealing with the evils of prostitution and venereal disease and in fact new regulations were introduced in 1898 by Cape Town Municipality prohibiting the keeping of brothels in the city, although this left the women without a fixed place to reside and made them more reluctant to appear for examinations. Along with the social disruption caused by the war it also had contributed to a growing phenomenon of prostitution between White prostitutes and African men which scandalized the House of Assembly:

> There were certain houses in Cape Town which any Kaffir could frequent, and as long as he was able to pay the sum demanded he could have illicit intercourse with these white European women. This was a matter of the gravest importance, for once the barriers were broken down between the European and native races in the country there was no limit to the terrible dangers to which women would be submitted.[15]

The causal organism of syphilis, the spirochaete Treponema pallidum (originally called Spirochaeta pallida), was discovered in 1905 by Schaudin and Hoffman from a genital sore on a prostitute, and a year later the Wasserman test was devised as a way to diagnose the disease in the laboratory. Meanwhile syphilis continued to spread, emanating from the Witwatersrand in response to the vast number of men moving about the entire southern African region to and from the mines. The Commissioner for Native Affairs in the Transvaal reported in 1904 that the disease was very prevalent and the Resident Magistrate in the Eastern Division of the Transvaal reported that it was worse every year. In 1906 the Acting Lieutenant-Governor of the Transvaal appointed a Commission to consider to what extent contagious diseases were prevalent amongst the native population of the Transvaal (The Contagious Diseases Amongst Natives Commission), and to submit a definite scheme for the treatment of such diseases 'suitable to the conditions of life of the said population'. The term Contagious Diseases was defined as syphilis, gonorrhoea and soft chancre – 'a contagious venereal ulcer...arising from contact with the discharge from a similar ulcer'. It was noted that there were also African names for these conditions and that they seemed to have been coined for a newly introduced disease, as they were not found in the original languages. While all three conditions were prevalent it was syphilis which gave the most concern due to its systemic and long term side effects. The disease was noted to be of recent origin in the Transvaal having spread out from the mines to the kraals by Africans from the mines, in particular from Kimberley, where it was said to be 'exceedingly prevalent and is spread by the class of coloured and native women engaged in the pursuit of prostitution'.[16]

Evidence was given to the Commission that it was unknown to Xhosas and Fingoes (tribes) twenty years earlier and unknown prior to 1876 in Basutoland (Lesotho) where it was given the name 'makaola', which apparently translated as 'to cut off the end of the penis'. Chief Molaba of Mpahlela's Location in the Zoutpansberg said specifically that it was first seen in 1884, being brought by a man who came from Kimberley. When people saw it spread they thought that it would be cured by vaccination and they vaccinated themselves with matter from those that suffered from syphilis. Following this it was said that there was hardly a woman with a baby who was not suffering from it. Dr Veale reported from the Waterberg that the tribes who had the most to do with Whites were badly infected. The worst was Zebediela's tribe and of those few were free of infection. Again the locals reported that it came from Kimberley. Dr Mehliss, in charge of the Rietfontein Lazaretto to which syphilitics from all over the Transvaal were sent, concurred that it seemed highly prevalent on the Waterberg as well as Pretoria. In the mines around Johannesburg however the disease was not reported to be highly prevalent. Dr Turner, who examined thousands of Africans for the Witwatersrand Native Labour Association, thought the infection rate was as low as 5 per 1,000, and other doctors working on the mines agreed that the rate was very low. Still the reports from the rural areas gave very high rates with doctors in the Pietersburg, Potgietersrust and Klerksdorp areas estimating rates as high as between 70 and 90%. In the Zoutpansberg it was said to be causing lameness, blindness and disfigurement and overall the majority of cases seen were in the late secondary or tertiary stages.

The Commission summarized that the disease was certainly very prevalent and greatest in the western and north-western parts of the Transvaal. Reports were given of infection of white children through kissing by syphilitic African nurses and it was stated to be clear that the prevalence of syphilis amongst natives was a serious menace to the health of the population of the Transvaal. The Commission concluded that the disease had spread from Kimberley in about 1881 and had since become widely prevalent except for the Shangaan and BaVenda peoples. Spread by infected knives during circumcisions and use of shared utensils or other indirect means may have played a minor role. The recommendations included the adoption of a special Contagious Diseases Act similar to that in the Cape to cover the labour centres (curiously the Cape Act did not apply to the Cape labour centres including Kimberley); that all Africans should be examined at the Pass Offices for syphilis and that nurses [child minders] should be similarly examined before employment; that specified health facilities be established and that district surgeons be provided with potassium iodide for free treatment.[17] By 1910 Africans found to be suffering from syphilis in the Transvaal were either returned to their homes for treatment or sent to the Rietfontein Lazaretto. State-Aided institutions were provided in the Northern Transvaal at Elim and Bochem hospitals. In the Orange Free State syphilis was also considered to be in need of urgent attention with the Magistrate in Senekal estimating in 1910 that 75% of the population were affected. Resident Magistrates and Health Officers from all over the country at that time reported it as being one of the major health problems of the period with fears that it was weakening the population as a whole and the Magistrates in the Orange Free State were recommending the establishment of segregation camps.

In Britain a Royal Commission on Venereal Disease sat from 1913 to 1916, the results of which made it compulsory for all County Councils to provide free diagnosis and treatment of venereal disease. It was estimated at that time that at least 8% to 12% of the male population of London had acquired syphilis. In South Africa only Johannesburg had implemented a similar policy. In the opinion of the medical profession in the Eastern Cape these principles were in 'refreshing contrast to those which would seem to have animated the framers of the Contagious Disease Act of 1885' which was still in force in the Cape Province, which aimed at the control of prostitutes and instructed the Cape District Surgeons to cure them and their contacts within two months. The doctors condemned the Act as superficial and ineffective, with inadequate resources allocated to the task. The Wasserman test had to be paid for at great cost by the patient, and the District Surgeon services were inaccessible. They remarked:

> In contrast... the Royal Commission treats of venereal disease not so much as a by-product of irregular sexual connection, but as a grave menace to public health. The whole population is endangered, and that for more than the present generation. It is only necessary to refer to the state of the native population who provide us with nurse-maids and domestic servants, who wash our clothing and handle our bedding and food in a dozen ways.[18]

Syphilis was considered by some to be 'the most efficient cause of the degeneration of a race' and Brock gave an estimate of 80% of mineworkers having had syphilis. He felt it was possibly a chief cause for the great prevalence and high mortality from tuberculosis in Africans engaged in mine work on the Rand, giving rise to a fibrotic condition of the lung which contributed to tuberculosis. However it was more likely that the particular lifestyle of workers on the compounds at the mines greatly predisposed them to both conditions. It was also thought by Brock to be a predisposing factor in leprosy and probably cancer.[19] The Tuberculosis Commission of 1914, in examining the cases presented by Dr Brock, were not completely convinced of his allegations, but agreed that syphilis could be a contributing factor.

The Contagious Diseases Act of 1885 continued to be a source of much controversy. During the Anglo-Boer (South African) War the presence of large bodies of troops in the country was seen to attract numbers of 'loose European women, mostly of Continental origin', to the seaports and the larger inland towns, to which they resorted for the purpose of prostitution. 'The brazen manner in which they paraded the streets and accosted men, extending their attentions also to natives and other persons of colour' became a public scandal and in 1902 and 1903 brought about legislation for the 'suppression of immorality'. This made sexual intercourse between a White woman and an African for gain liable to severe punishment in the Cape and Orange Free State. This was apparently to stop White women being 'brought into contempt in the estimation of Coloured or native males'.[20] Similar legislation was in place in the Transvaal where a petition was submitted to the British King, signed by members of the United Political Associations, 46 Chiefs and 25,738 Africans on various matters of concern. These included a concern that the Transvaal immorality law was discriminatory in that section 19 of Ordinance 46 of 1903 placed special penalties on Africans to prevent intercourse between the races and 'outrages on White women', but African women were not similarly protected from White men. The death penalty was applied for all cases of 'outrage or attempted outrage by natives on White women', whereas the reverse attracted brief imprisonment. The response from Britain, however, was supportive of the defensive explanations offered by the Governor of the Transvaal.[21]

After the War, during which there was a large increase in the prevalence of venereal diseases in Cape Town, the Cape legislation was strengthened to penalize the keeping of brothels. Progress in the implementation of the Contagious Diseases Prevention Act of 1885 was reported upon in the Cape by Medical Inspectors who reported that the Police were being increasingly stringent in chasing foreign women away from the town. 474 women were examined in 1902 under the Act, and the Inspector, Dr W.M. Ross, reported that 'the women themselves do not seem physically to flourish in their calling, and exhibit a great deal of bronchitis and kidney trouble, from exposure and poor dietary habits. Their death rate is far higher than normal conditions of living would justify at the Cape'.[22] The Chairman of the South African Council for Preventing Venereal Disease, established in the early 1900's, Mr Patrick Duncan stated 'what is the woman under the Contagious Diseases Act but a machine, less than a human being, less almost than an animal, for the gratification of the lusts of those unable to control them'.[23] Colonel Gray, the Deputy Commissioner of Police for the Cape, stated 'this indulgent attitude towards the male is probably due to the fact that males made this law, and I have no doubt that if women ever get the suffrage it will be quickly repealed, and I can only say the sooner the better'. The Editor of the South African Medical Record, however, dismissed this as the view of 'an advanced feminist', and felt that the Act treated a prostitute 'as she is, a potential purveyor of diseases from commercial motives' and strenuously defended it, although accepting that it needed improving as a tool for the improvement of public health.[24]

The first public meeting of the National Council for the Prevention of Venereal Diseases was held in Cape Town on the 8th June 1917, presided over by the Archbishop of Cape Town, who felt that the Contagious Diseases Act was wrong both in principle and foundation. At that time it was thought that 10% of the population of Britain was syphilitic, and that it was the third or fourth highest cause of death. In South Africa Dr Mitchell, Assistant Medical Officer of Health for the Union, who addressed the meeting reported that the estimated levels in South Africa at that time were 5% actively diseased and another 10-15% affected. There were then calculated to be 50 European and 300 coloured women living on prostitution in Cape Town, with many more occasional prostitutes. He maintained that, as there was sufficient employment opportunities for women in the city, 'drastic measures of repression, applied to both sexes, should be taken' including free treatment and education.[25] Dr McNeillie of Boksburg stated that the disease had a terrible hold on the country, and alleged that in the Waterberg 50% of Africans were affected and that the average infection rate of the whole area was 25%. The state of affairs was one which 'constituted at all times a menace to the White population of this country'.[26]

The public fear of the disease and the mode of treatment at that time is illustrated in a report by a doctor in Umzinto, Natal who was treating syphilis with salvarsan, which required pre-treatment purging and three days bed rest. He reported

> I found Europeans insisting...on the greatest secrecy, and on the other side I found hotel-keepers growing rather suspicious, on seeing a stranger arriving, getting rather suddenly ill (the day of the purge), stopping in bed for three days (the three days after the intravenous injection) and of feeding on very spare diet, although apparently in good health and with excellent appetite. Hotel-keepers are very much afraid of the disease, and very much object to giving accommodation to anyone they suspect suffering from syphilis.[27]

He instead erected his own treatment room to which he escorted patients from the station, where they could stay incognito. The treatment of Syphilis was written about extensively by Sir Henry Gluckman, who described the disease in 1920 as 'the greatest hygienic problem of humanity', greater than tuberculosis or cancer, as it 'preyed upon man during his second and third decade, and is the result of impulses accepted as uncontrollable'. He divided the preparations of arsenic then used into two groups, the '606' group, which were related to salvarsan, and the '914' group, which were related to neosalvarsan. The 606 group contained around 31% arsenic and were highly toxic when mixed with water until alkalized by sodium hydroxide. It formed a poisonous compound when exposed to air. 914 formed a neutral solution with water, but were much more liable to become toxic on exposure to air, and had to be injected as soon as it was prepared. Other variants included the addition of phosphorus, silver bromide and antimony oxide. These arsenical preparations were found to be highly effective, and an improvement on the older mercurial remedies where there was always 'cause for anxiety as to whether the disease would be stopped before the patient was poisoned by mercury'. Mercury was still used as a supplementary drug, although opinion was divided as to the best regime.

Side effects to treatment were common and severe, including pyrexia, vomiting, headache, gastro-intestinal symptoms, coma and death. The most difficult problem was in knowing when the patient was cured.[28]

The South African Public Health Act of 1919 repealed the Contagious Diseases Act which, it was noted, gave offence to a considerable section of the public as it penalised one sex more than the other. The Public Health Act had a section dealing with venereal diseases which made it compulsory for every person suffering from any venereal disease to consult a medical practitioner and remain under treatment until cured. It made it an offence for any employee suffering from venereal disease to accept or continue in employment in any factory, shop, hotel, restaurant, house or other place entailing the care of children or handling of food or food utensils and any employer who knew of such infected employees and engaged them was guilty of an offence. If a person did not persist with treatment until cured it had to be reported to a Magistrate and the person could be detained in hospital. Powers were given to examine any person in any place where there was reason to believe venereal disease was prevalent. The Act was to be carried out by the local authorities. The local authorities were required to commence with schemes for the implementation of the Act, including the provision of treatment, clinics and if necessary accommodation. The National Department made provision for free laboratory diagnostic tests for all Doctors, supplies of medication to district surgeons and financial support to hospitals for in-patient treatment. J.A. Mitchell, then Chief Health Officer for the Union, felt that the key issue however was to prevent exposure to infection, which was a question of human nature. He stated

> People are not going to be frightened into it by lurid pictures of the effects of venereal disease or of the tortures of evil-doers in this life or in the hereafter; they are not going to be preached into it, ... they must be educated into it, not only by giving them sound knowledge of the elementary medical facts, but by dissipating and exploding the old pernicious ideas about what constitutes true manhood and about the harmfulness of continence [abstinence] and by the teaching and inculcation of principles of morality and cleanliness of mind and body.[29]

He espoused the promotion of healthy recreations, the desire to bring up healthy children, and early marriage.

The City of Pretoria opened a 'Municipal Anti-Venereal clinic for Natives and Coloured persons', with separate days for men and women/children, where the overwhelming majority of patients were found to have syphilis. The only treatments available were neosalvarsan, (given intravenously) potassium iodide, mercury ointment and potassium permanganate. The potassium iodide was decanted into a bottle which the patient had to supply and which could be anything from a gin bottle to a perfume bottle. This was given to all patients with any type of problem, venereal or not. The Medical Officer there estimated that 37% of the African and Coloured population were infected with syphilis, which was thought to be impacting on population growth. A survey done in the clinic of 1,200 adult married patients found that the average number of births per marriage was four, of which two had died, of which a large percentage were presumed to be due to syphilis. In addition to the government facilities there was increasing involvement of other organisations, including the Society for Combating Venereal Disease, the South African Red Cross Society, the Johannesburg Chamber of Mines and the Witwatersrand Labour Association. Mitchell, then Secretary for Public Health of South Africa, noted the impact of the 'diseased Native prostitute' on the high prevalence of syphilis on labourers in the gold mines and in towns, and considered that the new Natives (Urban Areas) Act of 1923, which brought about the registration of all Africans within municipalities and empowered them to control, restrict and expel them to the Native reserves, would 'prove a valuable adjunct in safeguarding the natives in the towns against venereal infection'.[30]

The implications for spouses and children of syphilitic patients were serious. Debates ensued regarding when it would be safe for a single man or woman to marry, complicated by the fact that it was hard to tell when treatment had successfully cured the patient. The only test available was the Wasserman reaction which was considered unreliable for the management of treatment. Before the arrival of the arsenicals, when mercury was used, a period of up to four years after treatment was considered appropriate. With the new drugs this was reduced to some two years. If they were already married the prevention of pregnancy was of great importance, as it seemed that if a woman contracted syphilis before the fifth month of gestation the child would always be infected. Treatment was recommended throughout pregnancy if the woman was infected.

Syphilis was also a significant cause of admission to mental institutions, with it being estimated that 7.5% of European men, 14% of coloured men and 4% of all admissions to mental institutions in South Africa in 1922 were suffering from 'general paralysis of the insane', caused by syphilis. This condition was one of progressive mental deterioration with increasing irritability, lack of self-control, loss of memory, personal neglect, depression or delusions. Physical neurological signs such as irregular sluggish pupils, changes in reflexes, tremors and seizures also occurred. The onset was slow and insidious, some 10 or 15 years after the initial infection. Very little was available for treatment of this condition, with variable results reported from the use of the arsenical drugs, although spontaneous remissions did sometimes occur. Treatment by giving the person benign tertian malaria through inoculation was considered the best available at the time and was initiated as standard treatment in Vienna. About one third were improved sufficiently to be discharged after an induced malaria attack followed by salvarsan and another third showed improvement in symptoms. This malaria treatment was described as Pyrexial treatment and had been discussed as far back as 1848 after noting a favourable impact of malaria on insanity. It was first applied in South Africa by J. Marius Moll of Johannesburg, and carried out in Pretoria Mental Hospital in the 1920's with patients being sent there from all over the country. Other methods of inducing fever had been tried, such as injections of mild, tuberculin, various vaccines and relapsing fever bacteria (Borrelia). The latter had been tried by placing blood-sucking ticks onto the patients. The use of sub-tertian malaria had been tried with sometimes disastrous results as it was difficult to terminate the fever once induced. The blood from patients with benign tertian malaria was injected under the skin or into the veins. About 12 - 16 rigors were then allowed before the malaria was terminated with either quinine or salvarsan. Mortality was around 20%, but this was not considered alarmingly high or implying that the treatment was harmful, as the lifespan of the patients was deemed only 3-5 years anyway. Studies in Pretoria gave 25% good remissions, 25% some mental and physical improvement and 25% some physical improvement only.[31]

By 1925 the rates of infection were considered greatest among the coloured populations around Cape Town. It was thought to be decreasing in the western and northern Transvaal, while the Eastern Transvaal, Zululand, and Pondoland were said to be relatively free. Mitchell felt there was an 'extraordinary tendency to exaggerate the prevalence of venereal disease amongst Natives' with statements being made in the press that as many as 50% - 60% or even 90% of Africans were syphilitic. A study undertaken in gaols, where they expected to find a high rate of infection, found less than 2% with symptoms and Mitchell concluded that it could not be said that venereal diseases were a serious menace. However opinion was clearly heavily divided on the matter at this time.[32] Regardless of the prevalence figures, the fact is that the country was treating more and more syphilis cases. Over 8,000 cases were treated in hospital and 82,679 outpatient treatments were recorded in 1930 across the country. The increase in numbers was put down partly to greater recognition of the value of treatment, but also due to increasing prevalence in the 'urbanised and de-tribalized natives, and the slackening or absence of moral restrictions amongst them'. The Department of Public Health commented further 'a large percentage of such patients are almost or entirely a-moral and many are without feelings of shame or common decency. They will often freely admit to repeated exposure to infection, or even perhaps to incest'. It noted that, while a lot of large municipalities had undertaken a great deal of treatment work, there was no evidence of a decrease in cases and the question was raised as to whether the provision of free treatment was encouraging exposure to infection and whether the state was getting value for the money spent. However they were opposed to the frequently requested compulsory examination of female African servants as they felt this would arouse intense antagonism and resistance. 'Although it is admittedly repugnant and undesirable to employ infected natives as domestic servants or in handling food, the actual danger of spread of the disease in these ways is very slight'. They were however very concerned about the risk of spread to children from their nursemaids. It recommended that local authorities could, if they wished, set up special clinics with women doctors for the examination of domestic workers if sent by their employers, but that friendly persuasion was the best approach [33]

By the 1930's there were estimated to be more than 300,000 men employed in the mining industry of the Transvaal, with a male-to-female ratio in the general population in excess of 3:1 for men aged between 20 and 40 years. The ratio was 4:1 in Durban and more than 10:1 in Springs. Kark estimated that, at any one time, some 40 – 50% of men across the country were away from their homes. In the rural area of KwaZulu-Natal where he was based he found that 80% of men between 20-40 years were away for an average period of eight months during a year. This also left young women alone at home where they might indulge in extra-marital intercourse. Kark concluded that the industrial revolution in South Africa had led to the development of an urban life based on a socially pathological system of migratory labour, which had profoundly disturbed the family stability and sexual mores of several million African people. It had created a set of conditions ideal for the spread of syphilis.[34] The Department of Public Health considered that

> When housing improves, when diets are adequate, when education in the broadest sense is disseminated, when occupation and employment of

leisure time are developed, when health services are established and expanded, and when a higher civic and social sense has arisen, then will venereal disease...decrease. Venereal disease will be a gauge of communal pride and responsibility'.[35]

It called for more research into the long term effects of syphilis on the African and their children and suggested that its treatment should be integrated into ordinary clinics and hospitals. Treatment in the early 1930's was still hotly debated, with some 14 elements having been found to be useful of which most were heavy metals, including vanadium and uranium. Mercury had been the drug of choice until the discovery of salvarsan, with large doses of mercury being given almost to the point of toxicity with it being said that 'to cure is nearly to kill'. While largely replaced by the arsenicals by the 1930s it was still found useful for those who had failed to respond to arsenic and bismuth, given by ointment and intramuscular injection.[36] Compounds of bismuth, given by injection, were of greater value in late syphilis. Interruption of treatment in the first 20 weeks was found to result in a large percentage of relapses.

Studies of the time started to show alarmingly high levels of syphilis in the general population, including children. In the late 1930s Cape Town reported some 2,000 new cases a year, with a rate more than 10 times that of England – and this was considered to be only 50% of the true rate. Over 40 new cases per 1,000 people were reported from Germiston, where a 40.5% positive Wasserman reaction had been found during routine testing of native women.[37] It was also noted that the disease presented in far more different ways than in European countries, and 'no difficulty would be experienced in filling an album with photographs of eruptions and isolated lesions that would be rarities in Europe'.[38] This was also true of congenital syphilis, which was similarly extremely high in incidence. The disease was identified, along with tuberculosis, as the country's leading health problem. Studies of men working in the mines, ante-natal patients and general outpatients using the Wassermann test were giving positive test results as high as 47% and random surveys of school children were giving prevalence figures of up to 46%. The National Department of Public Health in the 1930's was inundated with demands from the White population for protection from the African population, which was believed to be riddled with disease in general, but in particular syphilis. Wild statements alleged that up to 90% of the population was affected. Public attitudes amongst the White community were reflected in statements like those of General Jan Smuts, in his speech at the National Provincial Congress of the United Party in 1937, who stated:

> The natives of this country are becoming rotten with disease and a menace to civilisation, instead of a first class nation. The position is becoming worse and worse and venereal disease is increasing at a terrible rate.[39]

Fears were such that employees were often dismissed if they were found to have had treatment for the disease, which further discouraged Africans from seeking treatment. Demands were made for compulsory medical examination of rural and urban Africans. However such demands focused on the health of the European population, and largely ignored the crippling physical effects on the African population, with the cardio-vascular and neurological side effects of disease and its inadequate treatment.

In Parliament in 1939 Mr. Bain-Marais moved that the government appoint a commission to 'enquire into the prevalence of certain diseases, particularly venereal diseases, which are undermining the health of the native races and also that of certain other communities'. He felt that the diseases were gradually sapping their vitality and that thousands of people were suffering, but that it was not being addressed because of stigma. He cited medical opinion which suggested that venereal diseases were contributing greatly to malnutrition, reduced labour output and infant mortality and made several recommendations to improve medical care. Whether or not the disease should be notifiable was also debated at length. Calls were made for it to be a crime to fail to come forward for treatment, with compulsory examination of African men at six-monthly intervals. Others however argued against such drastic legislative action, preferring the route of voluntary treatment. The appalling overcrowding and insanitary conditions in the Alexandra African Township near Johannesburg were described as being a contributing factor. Mrs M. Ballinger commented that she hoped the debate was not going to be used as a lever to engineer a movement to turn the people out of Alexandra, but rather that there was a necessity to improve living conditions, with an improvement in housing and wages. At this time the Thornton Commission into the state of peri-urban areas was sitting, appointed by the Minister of Public Health. The Reverend Miles Cadman pointed out that the disease was 'totally unknown amongst the natives until they had contact with what we call civilisation, and so I would approach it not so much from the point of view of economics, but of humanity'. He also suggested improving recreational facilities, noting that 'for 95% of the natives when they come off work in Durban there is no provision whatsoever'. Reference was made to the use of the Native Urban Areas Act, of 1923, under which people could be 'repatriated' from towns to rural areas as a method of controlling 'undesirable women'. The final motion agreed was that 'In view of the prevalence of venereal diseases with the consequent undermining of health of the people, the Government be requested to continue its efforts to control these diseases and to that end to take into consideration the advisability of (a) appointing a medical officer to devote his whole time to the matter, and (b) appointing a Venereal Disease Advisory Committee to make recommendations to the Public Health Department'.[40]

The City of Johannesburg had started new clinics in their townships and the Public Health Department had appointed a Syphilis Control Officer whose plans included extending medical and nursing services into rural and African Territories, assisting the mission hospitals by providing drugs, stimulating local authorities to provide health services and to employ Medical Officers of Health and training district surgeons on modern methods of treatment. Education campaigns focused on attacking the identified enemies of ignorance and conduct that was labelled as socially harmful and self destructive and included pamphlets and films. One such film on the dangers of syphilis was made by the Red Cross, entitled 'Two Brothers' which related the experiences of two brothers who had been infected with syphilis while working in Johannesburg. It showed the unfortunate physical effects of untreated syphilis in one who had rejected conventional medical treatment, and the cure of the other who had accepted a course of injections.[41] Fear of the dangers of infection from African domestic servants remained high, and in some opinions grossly exaggerated. The State, on the unproven assumption that syphilis was very easily spread by servants, waitresses or waiters, nurses, or the handling, preparation and serving of food, prohibited such people from carrying out their duties while they were contagious.

Attendances at municipal clinics for syphilis remained very high with there being 23,512 African attendances in Cape Town, 13,836 in Pretoria, 13,547 in Pietermaritzburg, 10,740 in Durban and 9,486 in Port Elizabeth in 1937. Nationally the increase in attendances for syphilis from around 120,000 the previous year to 160,000 in 1937 was seen as very satisfactory and indicative of the extension and improvement of the venereal disease treatment programme, although the fragmentation of health services between the Public Health Department, Native Local Councils, and Provincial Health Departments were causing co-ordination problems. Every male African had to submit to compulsory examinations at the Pass Office on entry into town, before being granted a permit to look for work, on renewal of such a permit or when registering a service contract with an employer. The process was brought about to assuage the fears of the European community, and was generally degrading and humiliating. Men lined up in single file for public examinations by doctors, a system which was all the more embarrassing if they had an obvious venereal lesion or other genital problem. Gale in Pietermaritzburg made the point that, given the incidence of venereal disease was higher in towns, it may have made more sense to examine them on leaving to return to the rural areas and he found that the majority of cases seen were already on treatment. Out of 7,144 examinations made in the city only 54 cases were discovered of active venereal disease. He found that motivating people to come forward voluntarily for treatment was 100% more productive, and felt that the best function of the Pass Office examination was as a means to convey health education. While there was strong public pressure for the compulsory inspection of females this was opposed as being an unwarranted indignity. He associated the generally high rate of venereal disease with bad housing conditions and indulgence in alcohol, and recommended the improvement of social and recreational conditions.[42] The hospitals admissions for venereal diseases in Pietermaritzburg increased from 219 in 1934 to 1,264 in 1940.

The National Department of Public Health also had reservations about the African male screening programme as indicated on a report on the Reef Pass Offices: 'the legislation requiring the examination of male natives entering the labour areas is class discriminatory ... it is open to serious doubt whether the best interests of health are being served when but one class of the community is subjected to compulsory medical examination.' The report continued 'There is a growing number of educated and civilised Non-Europeans who feel this class and race discrimination ... these dislike not alone the discriminatory legislation but also the usual herd methods of examination, when all and sundry are stripped and examined in the mass'. The author stated that this, and its association with the police and pass issues, must lead to a suspicion that medical and health measures were not for the benefit of the African but for repressive disciplinary purposes. He also concluded that such a measure was of extremely limited value in controlling infectious disease, but had some value in facilitating medical treatment for venereal and other illnesses and health education and that the discrimination was a social danger in terms of securing African cooperation in any public health programme.[43]

Standard treatment of the time still involved injections of salvarsan.

In 1935 the League of Nations had held an enquiry into syphilis treatment and recommended two full courses lasting for 12-18 months. However the Department of Public Health did not promote the administration of a full course of injections of salvarsan but only a course of 10 injections, which was sufficient, it was mistakenly thought, to render them non-infectious but not to cure. It was thought that many Africans left the treatment centres believing themselves cured, when in fact inadequately treated disease may have left them in a worse position. Whites were given a course of weekly injections lasting 12–18 months. In addition they also continued to recommend the older, less effective and more toxic treatment for Africans using mercury. Purcell commented on the differences in treatment meted out to Africans and Whites in 1940 'the great amount of under-treatment of the diseases continues. More and more individuals are infected. The health of the country is being steadily undermined'.[44] Cluver commented also: 'this is a policy which outrages the feelings of most decent-minded medical practitioners. The idea of allowing a patient to stop treatment knowing that he will certainly suffer from gross pathologic sequelae in later years is frankly revolting'.[45] In Britain at the time the standard treatment consisted of three or four courses, rather than one. The ineffective treatment of African patients left many with damage to their cardiovascular and nervous systems as the disease progressed silently. The best possible treatment regime of the early 1940's with arsenic-bismuth was expected to give 100% cure rates for sero-negative syphilis, 90-95% for secondary syphilis and 90% for sero-positive syphilis.

The onset of the Second World War elicited editorial comment from the South African Medical Journal in respect of syphilis, noting that 'we fully realise that there is still a section of the public…that adopts the outrageously obsolete principles of the middle of the last century when it discusses or in any way deals with venereal disease. That section must be fought to the bitter end, for it has in the past been responsible for much human misery and tremendous community demoralisation'. There was a concern that, unlike other countries, South African young men were not being given information on the disease, and it continued 'every young South African who goes on active service should know not only how venereal disease is caused, propagated and treated, but how he may…safeguard himself against infection'.[46]

A study in Johannesburg into European prostitutes between 1939 and 1941 estimated there were 1,000 streetwalkers in the city, of whom the great majority were estimated to be infected with one or more venereal diseases. It was said that the incidence of venereal diseases in the city depended upon the age composition of the population and that the extent of prostitution and the incidence of venereal disease correlated to the proportion of unmarried men of marriageable age. It was estimated that 64.6% of infected men had contracted their venereal infections from prostitutes and that between 1920 and 1939 approximately 30,000 men had been infected, and prostitutes were seen as the principal disseminators of venereal disease in the community. In order to deal with the problem several recommendations were made including: improvement of welfare services, slum clearance and re-housing, raising the income of unskilled female workers such as in shops, factories etc, so that the maintenance of a decent living standard was possible without resorting to prostitution, sex education in schools and universities and the amendment of the Public Health Act to make it compulsory for a health authority to cure a patient rather than just rendering them non-infectious. The replacement of penal measures against prostitutes by educational and rehabilitation measures within an institution were also recommended.[47]

Commenting on the lack of application of prophylaxis to prevent venereal disease it was noted by Purcell that there was a current belief that venereal disease was a just punishment for sin and that preventive measures encouraged immorality, with an assumption that those acquiring venereal disease from illicit sexual intercourse were specially selected for punishment. The preventive measures suggested included chastity, reduction in alcohol consumption, condoms and cervical caps. Measures such as preventive cleaning with green soap and various ointments such as calomel and mercury cyanide as practiced in France were thought ineffective, although some maintained they were more effective if applied within one hour of exposure in highly organized bodies such as the armed forces. The practice of giving a few injections of the drug neo-arsphenamine was condemned by Purcell as it may hide the early lesions and delay diagnosis.[48] Notwithstanding the lengthy treatment regimes prior to the discovery of penicillin it was still considered by some medical experts that syphilis could be eradicated. Cluver noted in 1940 that 'without doubt the cost of maintaining syphilis in the Union is much greater than the cost of a really effective campaign to combat it would be. Think of the expense at the present moment of maintaining hundreds of persons chronically disabled as the result of syphilis in our general chronic-sick and mental hospitals'. However he also noted that the social stigma regarding sexually transmitted diseases was pervasive and responsible for a large amount of the spread of infection and that 'in no other plague have we to deal with the taints of secrecy and sin which are associated with this disease'.[49] Europeans were thought to be filled with dread at the prospect of moral and social stigmatisation and were deterred from seeking medical help by their anxiety to keep their condition secret. With Africans it was more the fear of loss of employment or of eviction from tenancy on farms. A plea was made by the Department of Public Health for a change in social attitudes and for a change in attitudes by employers: 'the employer who regards any employee who has contracted venereal disease as a moral and physical untouchable fit only for instant dismissal puts a premium upon concealment and thus actually increases the very risks he so greatly fears'.[50] The dread was not aimed exclusively at Africans – the health department noted with indignation that European children who had a positive Wassermann reaction had on some occasions been excluded from school, a response it described as 'cruel' – but certainly fear of the African population as a carrier of venereal diseases was still rife. The Department described as unnecessary some of the demands made to it 'that Natives who deliver bread should all be submitted to the Wassermann test' and then banned from this type of employment and stated that 'it is foolish to dismiss a servant simply because he is discovered to be attending a venereal disease clinic. On the contrary he should be encouraged and given every facility to attend'.[51]

In the 1940's the prevalence of syphilis infection in the Transkei on the east side of the country was estimated at around 15% and effective treatment was rarely available in this remote and rural area. Severe complications were thought to be less common than in Europeans and, ever conscious of the impact of disease on White South Africa, it was noted that syphilis was not thought to play an important part in causing the loss of shifts amongst African mine recruits. However the incidence of syphilis was very high on the mines as a study in Kimberley showed, with routine Wassermann tests giving an incidence of between 30 and 43% in African labourers. Mental disease caused by syphilis was also found to be on the increase. There was only one venereal diseases clinic in the Transkei and an attempt to start another in three huts initially failed, as the huts were almost immediately burned down, possibly due to people fearing that they would be forcibly isolated there until cured. At ante-natal clinics the rate was 34% and similar figures were reported from the town of Brandfort in the Orange Free State. The Department of Public Health commented, with a somewhat less tolerant tone than previously:

It is apparent that large numbers of the population carry on a life of gross immorality unheeded and unchecked – a life which can only lead to physical, moral and spiritual degeneracy. That is the crux of the problem.[52]

Experiments with the antibiotic sulphanilamide, discovered in 1935, had commenced in the treatment of gonorrhoea with some success. However the treatment of syphilis remained 'at best ... a long-drawn-out series of weekly or bi-weekly injections, during which time the patient is well-nigh exhausted and his doctor is hard put to it to restrain him from abandoning treatment altogether'. Experiments with arsenicals aimed at giving early, huge doses in order to shorten treatment times, such as 'massive dosage by constant intravenous drip', of which O'Malley (Venereal Diseases Officer in Cape Town) said: 'hitherto undreamt-of doses can be given in a short period without actually killing the patient ... this is quite a notable achievement'! It raised the possibility of treatment regimes of less than a week.[53]

While the treatment of gonorrhoea with the new sulphonamide drugs had been promising, by the 1940's there were already resistant cases. By 1944 it was estimated by Behr, a military doctor, that some 10-15% of cases were sulphonamide-resistant. This was thought to be due to a combination of 'under-dosage by quacks, chemists and timid doctors', the rising dominance of resistant strains of bacteria and the practice of giving sulphathiazole as a prophylactic to prevent gonorrhoea rather than reserving it for treatment. Experiments had been tried by following a dose of the drug with 'electronically-induced hyperpyrexia' where eight hours of high fever were induced in the patient, which Behr found gave a 75% cure rate and one fatality in 100 cases. He then describes the experimental use of penicillin for gonorrhoea, which he described as a drug of 'the most amazing potency', and as an 'almost miraculous drug' which had been found to have dramatic effects on many different bacterial infections. Behr gives a detailed description of the discovery and usage to date of this drug, which had first been used to great benefit during the Second World War. He then reports his experimental use of penicillin in the treatment of 41 patients with sulphonamide-resistant gonorrhoea where he describes the results as 'nothing short of miraculous: by the end of the first day's treatment the discharge was practically gone'.[54] At this stage the potential use of penicillin in the treatment of syphilis is not mentioned. The treatment of 40,000 cases of syphilis with arsenicals over a eight year period between 1935 and 1943 is described by Daneel, with high levels of complications including jaundice, exfoliative dermatitis, kidney failure, encephalitis and bleeding, which resulted in deaths at a rate of 2.5% of cases treated.[55]

In 1944 the first mention is made of trials of penicillin for the treatment of syphilis, with Moore and Mahoney in America reporting a trial of its use in 2,428 cases where a profound and immediate effect was noticed. It was noted to be effective in both early and late cases, using high doses by injection at frequent intervals.[56] However initial difficulties in culturing the organism causing syphilis had limited scientific studies on its sensitivity to penicillin and it was not listed as one of the susceptible bacteria in the early reports. Penicillin was first introduced as a possible treatment for the Allied forces during the Second World War, where 60 injections of 40,000 units were given over a $7^{1/2}$ day period. This incidentally led to a massive increase in hepatitis as the virus was transmitted from soldier to soldier on inadequately sterilized syringes. At that time penicillin, then described as one of the greatest discoveries in medicine in living memory, had been found particularly useful during the war when its use for the general public had been restricted. By May 1945 the War Production Board in America was making it available to civilian hospitals and its large-scale production was underway, aiming to increase its production to 200 times the previous year's output, and it was anticipated to be soon also available in South Africa. It was described as 'a substance with hitherto unheard of – almost unimagined – properties'. It combined 'enormous antiseptic power' with a remarkable freedom from toxicity.[57]

By 1945 the remarkable effects of penicillin had come to the public's attention and pressure was rising to make it freely available. The Natal Mercury newspaper, in an Editorial on 2nd June, commented on it having saved many lives during the war and celebrated the fact that it was now released to the general public, albeit in limited amounts, but lamented the fact that it was available on medical prescription only. They described it as 'a completely harmless drug, less toxic than aspirin', and as an 'inexpensive harmless commodity ... every effort should be made to encourage the widest possible use as a household remedy ... its control should be taken out of the hands of doctors'. This seemed to be in ignorance of the fact that it was mainly used as a powder to be reconstituted for injection, not in oral form, and horrified the medical profession who commented that it required constant expert supervision and handling (being very unstable and subject to quick deterioration) and that the patients who needed it were generally too sick to be treated without medical care. At that time it was thought that a superficial form may however become available to be 'incorporated in proved popular appliances such as toothpaste, lipstick and throat lozenges ... in such a form ... the public will have ample opportunity of buying their sixpennyworth over the counter'.[58] At that time no mention was made of one of the greatest reasons for controlling penicillin's use – that of preventing growing bacterial resistance to its effects by inappropriate and incorrect administration – which would lead ultimately to its deteriorating effectiveness and usefulness as an antibiotic.

The Department of Public Health meanwhile was warning of the dangers posed by the end of the War:

> This country, like all other belligerent countries, will be faced with many vexed social problems of which venereal disease, from an epidemiological viewpoint, is a most important one. During the period of demobilisation and the transition from war to peace thousands will be on the move and there will be the inevitable reaction from the tensions of war.[59]

This presumably referred to a potential unbridled promiscuity by returning soldiers. However as usual attention was focused not on the danger posed by the men, who could be bringing back diseases acquired overseas, but by 'promiscuous women' and prostitutes who would become 'active disseminators of the disease'.

Certainly the problem was increasing with syphilis attendances at clinics and treatment centres by non-Europeans rising from 72,256 in 1935 to 289,885 in 1946. Penicillin was still not in widespread use. The Department estimated that between 5,000 and 10,000 adult males each year became physically incapable of contributing to national production owing to syphilis alone. It commented that the most important single contributory factor was the system of migratory labour and recommended that this wastage of manpower be taken into consideration when assessing the economic value of the migrant labour system. Perhaps however the leaders of the economy considered such African labour expendable as the migrant labour and hostel system remained in place up to and beyond the end of apartheid. The conditions described by the Health Department regarding migratory African male labour – a movement of men from a simple hut with their family in an outdoor, rural setting to an overcrowded barracks with an unnatural celibate life relieved by prostitutes and illicit alcohol – continued unabated for decades.

By 1946 studies with streptomycin, another new antibiotic, were underway wherein it was found that large doses could be as effective as penicillin when tested in rabbits, but that higher doses were required. However it was penicillin that was arousing the most excitement as a way to combat venereal diseases. In America it had brought the treatment time down for gonorrhoea from 16 days to three and the addition of penicillin to the old treatments of arsenicals and bismuth had reduced the treatment time for syphilis from 24 days to 11. The faster turnover of patients had allowed more attention to be devoted to case finding and intensive public campaigns were being waged. In the state of Alabama compulsory blood tests were brought in for all persons aged between 15 and 50 years and over 270,000 people cooperated, coming forward to 370 sites for testing and treatment. 4,781 cases of early syphilis were detected, and nationally infection rates were falling.[60] Within a short period, however, concerns were being expressed about its falling efficacy and the thought was occurring that, because of the popularity and widespread use of penicillin, it may become ineffective as a remedy within the next five to ten years due to the development of resistance by the bacteria. Penicillin was considered remarkable in its lack of toxicity even in overdose, with no fatalities to treatment recorded or serious organ damage, only skin reactions, and it was felt that under-dosing was a bigger problem. The indiscriminate public use of it in the form of cream or lozenges posed a real risk in the induction of resistant bacteria. The use of arsenicals was being moved away from due to toxicity, although the use of induced malaria fevers for the treatment of neurosyphilis remained. In South Africa, however, new arsenicals were still being tested. Humphries reported on 133 cases treated with arsenicals and bismuth at the Van Dyk mine between 1944 and 1947.[61]

Efforts to create a synthetic penicillin were starting to succeed in 1947, albeit in small amounts, and excitement was rising with the isolation of different forms of the wonder drug, whose effectiveness in the treatment of gonorrhoea was now unquestioned and remarkable. It was known that treatment over a period of 15-18 hours cured 97% of all cases. A high percentage was cured after just a single dose. For syphilis initial regimes still gave 60 injections over a period of seven days, but this was reduced by some to between 10 and 15 injections at a higher dose. Arsenicals and bismuth were sometimes still added however.

Treatment of neurosyphilis was still by induction of fever, now possible with electrical induction instead of malaria, where patients were treated by keeping for long periods at temperatures of 40.5°C – an average course of treatment being 10 twice weekly sessions of 40.5°C for five hours. This treatment was 'strenuous, and probably gives the doctor and the sister-in-charge as much worry as it does the patient, but the results are as good as those of malaria, and the mortality rate practically nil'. [62] Penicillin was being tried for neurosyphilis, but usually in combination with fever therapy. In America new treatments for syphilis and energetic campaigns were making inroads, with the mortality from the disease declining continuously after the War, although the treatment schedules were still arduous. Marshall maintained that penicillin could only be properly evaluated in the treatment of syphilis after patients thus treated had been followed for at least five years. Between 10% and 20% of patients would suffer relapse and he recommended continuing to use arsenicals and bismuth in addition to penicillin.[63] However some of these relapses may have been re-infections as they were again susceptible immediately after finishing the course of penicillin. Courses were still employing multiple injections, with one presumably painful schedule involving 85 two-hourly injections. In order to reduce the number of injections efforts were made to find a form of penicillin which would last longer in the body, such as placing blocks of ice on the buttocks, mixing penicillin with blood and preparing it with arachis oil and beeswax. The discovery of procaine penicillin was a considerable improvement as it was found to last in the body for several days. The aim was to find a way to reduce treatment to a single dose. The new antibiotics aureomycin and chloramphenicol, related to streptomycin, were also found to be effective against syphilis. Due to the increasing availability of new antibiotics, in particular penicillin, with high levels of activity against syphilis the World Health Organisation was leading extensive research efforts and promoting large scale control programmes around the world. Programmes in such countries as Poland, Yugoslavia, Finland, India, Haiti, Indonesia, Iraq and Thailand had lead to great reductions in incidence.

A study published in 1949 of 1,000 African men arriving to work in Cape Town from all over South Africa found no significant difference in prevalence of a positive Wassermann test between those coming from urban or rural areas, or between married and single men, and an overall positivity rate of 7.4%. The authors commented that the investigation 'does not reveal an incidence of unsuspected syphilis amongst our Bantu population as high as suggested by the alarming, though unauthorised statements one hears from time to time. Most health officials, before the results of this enquiry were known, tentatively placed the rate as high as 20%'. They concluded that their study did not support the widely held view that syphilis was rife amongst the African population at that time.[64] A trial of treatment in 365 cases in the city was published in 1950 which used penicillin in a course of 80 injections over 7-8 days, together with arsenicals and bismuth over the next 8-10 weeks. Many relapses occurred however.[65] Still the impact of penicillin on the incidence of syphilis and the workload of health departments was dramatic and started to occur from around that time, when the Medical Officer of Health of Cape Town commented

> We owe this favourable state of affairs to the rapid curative action of the new antibiotic drugs, chiefly penicillin. Now although the administration of penicillin will not influence the promiscuous sex impulse it does cut short drastically and abruptly the infectious stage of the two common diseases, gonorrhoea and syphilis.[66]

He also suggested it could be used as a means of protection if given after exposure to the disease. In the five year period 1950–1955 in the city of Pietermaritzburg annual admissions to hospital dropped from 2,051 to 358, and outpatient attendances for sexually transmitted diseases fell from 19,116 to 2,331 due to the introduction of the new antibiotic treatments.[67]

Following on from the work of Kark, Sax looked more deeply into the reasons for the high incidence of venereal infection in the early 1950's. He found that promiscuity was of more importance than prostitution, but that such behaviour was not something which arose spontaneously. It was noted that the system of migratory labour was responsible for drawing as many as 50% of the male population aged between 18 and 54 years out of rural areas, and it was this separation which was responsible for marital instability, the breakdown of African family life and contributing to widespread promiscuity among both urban men and rural women. In addition there was a high mobility of the population within the towns, as people moved about changing homes and employment, which reduced the restraints imposed by a stable neighbourhood or group pressure. Similarly single girls were migrating to the city and getting employment allowing them increasing levels of freedom. Changes in African cultural traditions were also noted, such as the loss of initiation ceremonies within African tribes where parents had placed importance on the chastity of initiates before the ceremonies, and also the decline in polygamy. It was suggested this was delaying marriage for young women as they waited for young men to marry them, who could not afford to pay the lobola (or 'Bride price'). Delays in marriage, and the taking by men of 'informal' second wives rather than formal, may have contributed to increasing promiscuity outside of a marital relationship. The legislative requirements around accommodation for single African people in urban areas due to 'Influx control' similarly impacted on peoples living arrangements and relationships, as did the level of overcrowding in the municipal locations and the small, inadequate houses provided there for Africans. Underlying all this was the problem of severe poverty.⁶⁸

By the mid 1950's the development of long-acting types of penicillin, which could be still found in the body two to three weeks after a single dose, was reducing the number of injections required and the manufacture of penicillin in large quantities had considerably reduced its price. Internationally its use for syphilis prevention had also been tried, such as giving it to prostitutes at regular intervals, but this was not recommended as it could contribute to the development of resistant bacteria. The use of arsenicals in addition to penicillin was starting to decline and the Department of Health stopped supplying them from 1953, supplying only penicillin, and was undertaking trials of mass treatment campaigns. Penicillin had also been found to be effective in syphilis affecting the central nervous system and the induction of fevers such as by malaria was no longer thought necessary. The rapid treatment methods were freeing up hospital beds previously occupied by syphilis patients on long term therapy and were instead being used for the treatment of tuberculosis patients in places such as the Rietfontein Hospital near Johannesburg and the Amatole Venereal Diseases Hospital in King William's Town. The incidence of congenital syphilis in babies, acquired from their mothers, had plummeted with cases dropping in Cape Town from 502 in 1949 to only 21 in 1959 due to treatment with penicillin. In the ten years from 1949 to 1959 new cases of syphilis in the city fell from 2,779 to 693 – a highly significant drop when considering that the population increased by 40% in the same period.⁶⁹

Still in other parts of the country syphilis and other venereal diseases remained a problem. The Medical Officer of Health of Port Elizabeth, J. Saville Lewis, noted an increase in attendances ascribed as follows: 'the prevalence of casual sex life, prostitution and the difficulties of bringing VD defaulters to the clinic are the main causes for the spread of disease among the inhabitants of New Brighton and Kwazakele'.⁷⁰ His successor J.N. Sher warned in 1975 that any one was at risk: '

> as a result of migratory labour and split family life there is a criss-cross of infection going on between the urban Bantu and those of the Transkei. The history of VD's has shown that they are no respecter of race, colour or creed ... he or she is liable to contract the disease whether artisan or artist, peasant or poet, prostitute or professional man, king or concubine, the Colonel's lady or Judy O'Grady.⁷¹

He felt that 'the pill' and 'the injection' had made the female more promiscuous through removing the fear of pregnancy and also blamed ignorance promiscuity in the youth; the breakdown of old ideas of morality, the deterioration in home life, the 'blatant commercialisation of sex', and the 'hectic present day chase for pleasure and enjoyment at any cost'. As usual however, women came in for special mention, blaming the disco and nightclub culture 'frequented by the professional prostitute and her more dangerous sister, the enthusiastic amateur, who makes herself available for peanuts, presents and promises'. At that time Port Elizabeth was treating around 8,000 cases of venereal disease per year, of which approximately half were syphilis.

A study of four major South African cities, Cape Town, Durban, Port Elizabeth and Pretoria, showed the number of new cases of syphilis had declined to a minimum around 1978-80 in Pretoria, Port Elizabeth and Durban, but then starting to show a slight increase from the late 80's. Rates in Cape Town however continued to show further declines with a minimum in 1989. Collectively the four cities reported 11,157 cases in 1980, increasing to 15,322 by 1990, an incidence rate of 4 per 1000 population, with Port Elizabeth (the smaller of the four cities) accounting for 42% of them. This was still however a drop in the ocean compared with the levels of 50 years earlier, although it only included those treated at municipal clinics, not those seen by private general practitioners. The rate varied between cities, being lowest in Pretoria at around 1.2 per 1000 and highest in Port Elizabeth at around 9 per 1000. Rates for Johannesburg, the largest city with the highest mining and migrant population, were not given.[72] However, while new cases were increasing, the rates of congenital syphilis were dropping significantly with only 49 cases in 1990 compared with 339 in 1980, which probably reflects better case-detection and timeous, effective treatment. Attention on treatment for sexually transmitted diseases (STDs) was increasing hugely due to the growing HIV/AIDS epidemic as concomitant STDs were known to increase the rate of transmission of HIV. During the second national HIV survey of antenatal women in October-November 1991 samples were also tested for syphilis. The prevalence of syphilis infection was estimated at 6.6% across the country, varying from a low of 2.3% in the Transvaal (excluding the then African homelands) and a high of 13.9% in KwaNdebele, a desperately poor homeland situated in the mid-Transvaal. A significant association was found between HIV infection and positive syphilis serology, worse in the Cape and KwaZulu-Natal, although interestingly no specimens positive for both HIV and syphilis were found in the Transvaal, Venda or Transkei, the latter being so-called independent rural homelands. Similarly none of the specimens from Asian, Coloured or White women tested positive for both diseases simultaneously.[73]

By 1997 the prevalence of syphilis had increased to 11.2%, but by 2001 the prevalence was significantly lower at 2.8% overall. All provinces had rates under 6.2% and the decline was attributed to the intensive programmes in place for screening and treatment of syphilis as part of the national strategy to combat STDs due to the connection with HIV/AIDS. It also may be due to an improvement in the treatment regime following the introduction of the 'syndromic approach' to the treatment of STDs in the late-1990's, whereby standardised treatment regimes, covering all possible causes, were introduced at clinics for either ulcerative lesions or infections with urethral/vaginal discharges. This replaced the need to try and get a definitive bacteriological diagnosis for the patients' symptoms which was well nigh impossible in the absence of laboratories, and meant that comprehensive treatment, proven to be effective against all possible organisms, could be given by nursing staff at government clinics following simple algorithms or guidelines. Following this research undertaken in Hlabisa, a rural area in northern KwaZulu-Natal, showed that pre-1997 syphilis and chancroid were responsible for 80% of genital ulcer disease. The treatment regime introduced for ulcerative STDs, (now renamed Sexually Transmitted Infections) was then a seven day course of the antibiotic erythromycin and penicillin, which would treat those ulcers. Studies in the same area in 2001 found that the profile of the ulcers had changed, with only 25% due to those diseases with Herpes simplex virus and Chlamydia trachomatis accounting for 60%. While the new treatment protocol had apparently reduced the incidence of syphilis, this meant the protocol had to be changed to accommodate these other diseases.[74]

By the start of the new millennium syphilis had become largely under control, with neonatal syphilis having largely disappeared due to improved ante-natal care and treatment of pregnant women, and the chronic long-term complications of the disease in adults were no longer seen due to improved and effective treatment of cases with antibiotics. The mass panic and hysterical reactions that the disease had provoked in the White South African population in the first half of the 20th century were forgotten, along with the discriminatory and humiliating approaches taken towards its control. A similar phenomenon had been seen with the initial diagnoses and explosion of HIV/AIDS during the first 20 years of that epidemic and the massive numbers of deaths associated with that disease during the late 1990's and early 2000's had overshadowed any lingering concerns about syphilis. Syphilis remains present to this day however, being highly unlikely ever to be eradicated, and is of great significance due to its role, along with other ulcerative sexually transmitted infections, of facilitating the spread of the HIV virus. It also remains a risk due to increasing threat of growing resistance to the commonly used antibiotics. We cannot afford to let it slip off the public health agenda and consign it to history just yet.

ENDNOTES

1. Mitchell Dr, 'Address on Venereal Diseases' *South African Medical Record*, 15(12) 1917:186-188
2. Liebbrandt H.C.V. 'Report of the Commissioners of the Hospital' *Precis of the Archives of the Cape of Good Hope, Journal 1699-1732*; Cape Town 1896: 213
3. Mentzel O.F. *A Geographical and Topographical description of the Cape of Good Hope; 1787*; Translated by Marais G.V. and Hoge J. Edited by Mandelbrote H.J. The Van Riebeeck Society, Cape Town, 1944:256,
4. Ibid, 1944:257
5. Worden N. and Groenewald G. *Trials of Slavery: selected documents concerning slaves from the criminal records of the Council of Justice at the Cape of Good Hope, 1705-1794*; Van Riebeeck Society for the publication of South African historical documents; Cape Town 2005:602
6. Laidler P.W. and Gelfand M. *South Africa its medical history, 1652-1898: A medical and social study*; C. Struik, Cape Town 1971:93
7. Sax Sidney, 'The Introduction of Syphilis into the Bantu peoples of South Africa' South African Medical Journal v26, 27 December 1952: 1037-1039
8. Van Heyningen E, 'The Social Evil in the Cape Colony 1868-1902: Prostitution and the Contagious Diseases Acts', *Journal of Southern African Studies*, 10 (2) 1984:170-197
9. Martens Jeremy C. 'Almost a Public Calamity: Prostitutes, 'Nurseboys' and Attempts to Control Venereal Diseases in Colonial Natal, 1886-1890'; *South African Historical Journal* 45 (Nov 2001): 27-52.
10. Harrhy W.R., cited in Gilder S.S.B, 'South African patients and their Diseases in the 1880s' *South African Medical Journal*, 66 No 7 August 1984:250
11. Van Heyningen E. 'The Social Evil in the Cape Colony 1868-1902: Prostitution and the Contagious Diseases Acts', *Journal of Southern African Studies*, 10 (2) 1984:192
12. 'Debates of the Legislative Council of Natal, First Session Twelfth Council'; December 14 vol IX 1886:494-5
13. Ibid, 494-5
14. Martens Jeremy C. 'Almost a Public Calamity: Prostitutes, 'Nurseboys' and Attempts to Control Venereal Diseases in Colonial Natal, 1886-1890' *South African Historical Journal* 45 (Nov 2001) 27-52.
15. Graham T.L. Attorney General 1902 cited in Van Heyningen E., 'The Social Evil in the Cape Colony 1868-1902: Prostitution and the Contagious Diseases Act', *Journal of Southern African Studies*, 10(2) April 1984:192
16. Gregory A.J. 'Letter from the Office of the Medical Officer of Health for the Colony, Cape Town, 19th October 1906', in: *Report of the Contagious Diseases*

amongst Natives Commission, 1907, Government Printing and Stationery Office, 1138_25-3-07_750, 1907:30.

17. Lagden G.Y. et al, Report of the Contagious Diseases amongst Natives Commission, 1907, Government Printing and Stationery Office, 1138_25-3-07_750,
18. Lea J.A. et al; 'A Scheme for the Treatment of Venereal Disease'; *South African Medical Record* 16(19) 12 October 1918:296-298.
19. Brock B.G. 'Syphilis and the Commonweal' *South African Medical Record*, 15(1), 1917:19-25
20. De Villiers C.W. et al, *Report of the Commission on Mixed Marriages in South Africa, 1939*, UG 30-'39: 13-14.
21. Lagden G.Y. *Report by the Commissioner for Native Affairs, Transvaal, for the year ended 30th June 1906*, Pretoria, Government Printing and Stationery office, 1906 pA6-7
22. Ross W.H. 'Report of the Acting Medical Inspector 1902, Reports of the Medical Inspectors on the working of Part 1 of the "Contagious Diseases Prevention Act, 1885'; in *Reports on the Public Health ; Cape of Good Hope, 1902*, Cape Times Ltd; G66-1903 1903:275.
23. Duncan, Patrick cited in 'The Anti-Contagious Diseases Act Agitation', (Editorial) *South African Medical Record*, 15(9) 1917:130
24. Editorial: 'The Anti-Contagious Diseases Act Agitation' *South African Medical Record*, 15(9) 1917:129-132
25. Mitchell J.A. 'Address on Venereal Diseases' *South African Medical Record* 15(12) 1917:186-188
26. MacNeillie Dr, .Public Health of Union, *Cape Times* 30th January 1919 :24
27. Bonfa A. 'Syphilis and Salvarsan in Country Practice' *South African Medical Record* 15(24) 1917:372-375
28. Gluckman Henry, 'The Treatment of Syphilis' *South African Medical Record* 18(10) 1920:182-189.
29. Mitchell J.A. 'The problem of Venereal Disease; Address given at the Annual Conference of the Transvaal Branch of the National Society for Combating Venereal Disease, Johannesburg 24th February 1921' *South African Medical Record* 19(7)1921:122-124
30. Mitchell J.A. 'Venereal Diseases in South Africa', *South African Medical Record* 24(8), 1926:181
31. Pijper A. and Russell E.D. 'Malaria treatment of General Paralysis: a Report on 44 cases' *South African Medical Record* 1926, 24(13) 1926:292-303
32. Mitchell J.A. 'Venereal Diseases in South Africa' *South African Medical Record* 24(8), 1926:181
33. Mitchell J.A. *Annual Report of the Department of Public Health, Union of South Africa, 1930*, The Government Printer Pretoria, UG 40-'30:47
34. Kark Sydney, 'The Social Pathology of Syphilis in Africans' *South African Medical Journal* 23(5) 29 January 1949:77
35. *Annual Report of the Department of Public Health, Union of South Africa, 1935*, The Government Printer Pretoria, UG 43-'35:45-46
36. Purcell F.W.F. "Remarks on the treatment of Syphilis' *South African Medical Journal* 8(21) 1934:783-787
37. Purcell F.W.F. 'Syphilis in South Africa', *South African Medical Journal*, 14(23) 14 December 1940:453

38. O'Malley Kevin C. 'Syphilis in South Africa' *South African Medical Journal* 14(23) 14 December 1940: 459
39. *Sunday Times* 3rd October 1937
40. Bain-Marais C. 'Prevalence of Venereal Diseases' *Debates of the House of Assembly*, 34(28) April 1939: 3714-3754.
41. Jeeves Alan; 'The State, the Cinema and Health propaganda for Africans in Pre-Apartheid South Africa, 1932-1948' *Southern African Historical Journal*, 48 May 2003:120
42. Gale G.W. 'The Incidence and Control of Venereal Diseases among the Natives of an Urban Area', *South African Medical Journal*, 13(8) 1939:265-270.
43. Cited in: *Annual Report of the Department of Public Health, Union of South Africa, 1937*, The Government Printer Pretoria, UG 52-'37: 57-58
44. Purcell F.W.F. 'Syphilis in South Africa' *South African Medical Journal*, 14(23) 14 December 1940:456
45. Cluver E.H. 'Syphilis and the Public Health', *South African Medical Journal* 14(23) 14 December 1940:457
46. Editorial: 'Syphilis in the Union', *South African Medical Journal*, 14(23) 1940:452
47. Freed, Louis F. *The Problem of European Prostitution in Johannesburg: A Sociological Survey*, University of Pretoria 1942.
48. Purcell F.W.F. 'Anti-venereal Prophylaxis', *South African Medical Journal* 14(23) 14 December 1940:462
49. Cluver E.H. 'Syphilis and the Public Health', *South African Medical Journal* 14(23) 14 December 1940:457
50. *Annual Report of the Department of Public Health, 1940*, Government Printer Pretoria, UG No 8-'40:p51.
51. *Annual Report of the Department of Public Health, Union of South Africa, 1941*, The Government Printer Pretoria, UG 46-'41, p42
52. *Annual Report of the Department of Public Health, Union of South Africa, 1939*, The Government Printer Pretoria, UG 8-'45, p 1
53. O'Malley C.K. 'New methods in the treatment of syphilis' *South African Medical Journal* 15(17) 1941:343-347
54. Behr S. 'The Treatment of Sulfa-Resistant Gonococci with Penicillin' *South African Medical Journal* 18(21) 1944:369-372
55. Daneel Jos and Meyer J. 'Major complications of Arsenical Therapy', *South African Medical Journal* SAMJ 18(14) 1944:247-248
56. Moore J.E. and Mahoney J.F. et al, 'Penicillin treatment of early syphilis' *Journal of the American Medical Association*,126(2) 1944
57. Kloppers P.J. 'Penicillin: it present status and modern use,'*South African Medical Journal* 19(5) 1945:70-72
58. 'Penicillin by Prescription', Editorial, *South African Medical Journal* 19(14) 1945:241
59. *Annual Report of the Department of Public Health, 1945*, Government Printer Pretoria, UG No 6-'46, p30-32.
60. 'Bulletin from America: New Era Developing in Struggle against Venereal Diseases', *South African Medical Journal* 20(11) 1946:307-308
61. Humphries S.V. 'Report on the response of 102 Natives to Anti-syphilitic treatment,' *South African Medical Journal* 21(16) 1947:600-604
62. Behr S. 'Development in the Treatment of Syphilis' *South African Medical Journal* 21(17) 1947:648-653

63. Marshall James, 'The modern treatment of the Venereal Diseases: Syphilis' *South African Medical Journal* 23(7) 1949:113-115
64. O'Malley C.K. and Wilson A.J. 'Results of the Wasserman Test in an unselected Bantu group' *South African Medical Journal*, 23(5) 29 January 1949:73
65. O'Malley C.K. 'Penicillin in early syphilis: results obtained in 365 cases'. *South African Medical Journal* 24(8) 1950:127-132
66. *Annual Report of the Medical Officer of Health, City of Cape Town, 1950*, Cape Times Ltd, Parow 1959:50
67. *Annual Reports of the Medical Officer of Health*, Pietermaritzburg Corporation Yearbook, 1940-1955
68. Sax, Sidney, 'The Social Pathology of Syphilis among the Bantu people of the Union of South Africa' *South African Medical Journal* 27(7) 1953: 129-134
69. *Annual Report of the Medical Officer of Health, City of Cape Town, 1959*, p39
70. Saville Lewis J., *Annual Report of the Medical Officer of Health for Port Elizabeth for 1963*, Longs, Port Elizabeth, 1963:49
71. Sher J.N. *Annual Report of the Medical Officer of Health for Port Elizabeth for 1975*, Port Elizabeth, 1975:43
72. Harris B.N. 'Incidence rates of Syphilis and Congenital Syphilis in four local authorities, 1976-1980 and 1986-1990', *Epidemiological Comments* 19 (10), Department of Health, October 1992:173
73. Ballard R. 'Syphilis in women attending antenatal clinics October/November 1991', *Epidemiological Comments,* 19(10) October 1992:165-170
74. Sonko R. et al, 'Sexually Transmitted Infections' in *South African Health Review 2002*, Health Systems Trust, Durban 2003:258-275

QUARANTINE AND VACCINATION: SUCCESS AGAINST SMALLPOX

In the Journal of Zacharias Wagenaer for the year 1669, written in Cape Town, he relates that a female slave 'lying stiff and stinking with the small-pox in the slave house, had not hesitated to strangle her infant', for which she was sentenced to being 'tied up in a bag and thrown into the sea'.[1] Such was the terror induced by smallpox, an infection of the virus Variola major, which eventually also became the first and only dread disease to have been eradicated from the face of the earth. It had occurred with deadly consequences in epidemics throughout the centuries until as recently as 50 years ago in South Africa, leaving those who survived weakened and pock-marked by the disease. On May 8th 1980 the 33rd World Health Assembly declared that the world and all its peoples had won freedom from smallpox. However up until this time smallpox had not only been a dread epidemic disease, inflicting death, disfigurement and terror among populations, but in South Africa it had, along with many other public health problems, made a significant contribution to the profound social engineering that later became entrenched as Apartheid.

The first epidemic of smallpox in South Africa occurred in 1713, possibly starting around April 9th, with the death of an 'old slave of nearly 100 years' mentioned on 21 April. This was a disease often affecting sailors on their voyages to the Cape and the first infections were traced to clothing from an East India vessel which had been washed in the Slave Lodge where, in consequence, 200 slaves out of 570 died.[2] Just a month later on May 6th it was said that the Khoikhoi indigenous peoples (known then as Hottentots) had been almost exterminated by the smallpox outbreak. They had tried to flee but on May 19th it was reported that they were killed by another tribe among whom they had intended to take refuge. The disease spread rapidly and with such devastation through the town that by May 15th it was commented by Governor W.A. van der Stel that 'the burghers die of smallpox in large numbers'. By June there was hardly a family that had not lost one or two of its members, following which it spread across the country, so that by June 25th 'there were not 20 healthy people in Drakenstein'.[3] When all the planks in the settlement had been used up the dead were buried without coffins and the bodies covered with sand, but these were often uncovered and eaten by hyenas, jackals and dogs. A quarter of the Europeans in Cape Town and surrounding farms died. It was never known how many Khoikhoi died, but it was said that in their case to contract smallpox was to die and many of the Cape tribes completely disappeared.[4] Other tribes were greatly reduced in numbers. The susceptibility of the Khoikhoi to smallpox was probably not due to any peculiar immunological deficiency rendering them vulnerable, but rather to the cumulative effect of serial episodes of different new infectious diseases which had been brought by the European settlers, including typhoid and measles, which gradually undermined the population's ability to withstand continuing epidemics. In addition several years of drought and cattle disease following the 1713 epidemic also had an impact.[5]

However the devastation wrought by smallpox was considered by some to have resolved the problems of intermittent conflict between the expanding White settlers and the indigenous population who were being displaced, and solved 'the whole Hottentot difficulty ... from this time we find the Hottentots living peaceably with the Dutch'.[6] It appears to be the first instance in South Africa of an epidemic being linked to population movement and, while unintentional in this case, perhaps raised the possibility of the use of infectious diseases in South Africa, as a cover behind which to address social and racial problems.

Localised outbreaks of smallpox continued to occur, probably from infected ships, most of which did not go on to cause epidemics. Mead in 1748 mentioned such an outbreak when a Dutch ship called at the Cape with some sick men. He maintained that smallpox had originated in Ethiopia, being first written about by Arabs in the fifth century and from there spread around the world through wars, trade and, in particular, the crusades 'this being the only visible recompense of their religious expeditions which they brought back to their respective countries'.[7] He proposed that 'the purulent matter, which runs out of the pustules, being caught in the bed-cloaths [sic] and wearing apparel of the sick, and there drying and remaining invisible, becomes a nursery of the disease, which soon breaks forth on those who happen to come in contact with it, especially if the season of the year and state of the air be favourable to its action'. Following the arrival of the Dutch ship at the Cape of Good Hope, some of the crew of which had had smallpox, Khoikhoi were employed: 'some of those miserable wretches were employed in washing the linen and clothes of these men, who had had the distemper; whereupon they were seized with it, and it raged among them with such violence that most of them perished under it'. However the Khoikhoi soon understood the contagious nature of the disease, and 'contrived to draw lines round the infected part of their country, which were so strictly guarded that, if any person attempted to break through them, in order to fly from the infections, he was immediately shot dead'.[8]

'Air contaminated by putrefaction' was considered a major cause of spread of disease in the mid 18th century. Dr Pringle had observed that

> These destructive streams work like a ferment, and ripen all distempers into a putrid and malignant nature, but the air in hospitals, and crowded barracks, close transport ships and, in a word, every other place where air is pent up, not only loses a part of its vital principle, by frequent respiration, but is also corrupted by the perspirable matter of the body which, as it is the most volatile part of the humours, is also the most putrescent.[9]

He recommended that 'nothing short of scraping away the whole external surface of the floor, as well as of the walls, and thereby substituting an entire new layer of the whole inside of the house, is capable to extinguish the seeds of infection of certain diseases once sown'.

The second major epidemic of smallpox in South Africa, introduced from Sri Lanka (then Ceylon), started around May 1755 and also affected the Khoikhoi more than the European. Separate hospitals were established for Europeans and slaves, one being an empty house on the farm 'Vreedenhoff', but practically every adult who was infected died. Slave nursing attendants were appointed who worked under the supervision of the doctor, drawn from the ranks of those who had survived an earlier outbreak. Soon so many patients required admission that a second hospital was opened on the adjoining site. Of the 237 patients who were admitted to these temporary hospitals only 95 recovered.[10] During the month of July 489 Europeans, 33 'free blacks' and 580 slaves died.[11] By 31 October nearly 1,000 Europeans and over 1,000 slaves had died. The epidemic was said to have started among the slaves, in particular slaves owned by a Mr Jan de Waal who were working near the beachfront, and then spread to the Europeans who they worked for.[12] It was believed that 'evil vapours' were spread by the wind. The slaves' houses were cleansed and fumigated, and people were ordered to open the doors and windows to air their houses. The dead were buried within 24 hours in the clothes in which they died and those who failed to notify cases were fined. Slaves failing to report cases were flogged. Country residents were ordered to bury their dead on the farms rather than bringing them to Cape Town's churches, and the lending of black clothes to slaves who attended funerals was banned. By mid-July farmers were avoiding the town and the supply of food was decreasing, cemeteries filled up and corpses were buried above corpses. As the epidemic declined in town it spread up to Namaqualand and East along to Outeniqualand.[13] The first directive was issued to the Harbour Master to investigate the presence of sickness on ships as they arrived in Simons Bay and sailors were not allowed to visit the surrounding districts or to stay ashore overnight. Only the officers were allowed to leave the ships to go to the farms or towns.[14]

The various administrative measures against smallpox also affected social and cultural activities - the annual military parade was postponed and the economy suffered greatly as rural farmers refused to transport sufficient agricultural produce to the town. In addition as shop owners and bakers became ill the regulations stated that the entire business was to be suspended immediately. There was also a fear that the water could be contaminated, and the washing of clothing in the river water was prohibited. The disease finally disappeared during March 1756 and the Governor Tulbagh declared the 7th April 1756 to be a day of prayer, fasting and thanksgiving.[15]

The next epidemic came in 1767 from a Danish ship named *De Kroonprins van Deenemarken* and again was thought to be related to the bringing ashore of contaminated laundry. The experiences of the previous epidemic lead to immediate containment efforts, which restricted the dead to 280 Europeans and 440 slaves and Coloureds and very few cases outside Cape Town, but the disease dragged on until the last case in April 1769. The Diaconie of the Dutch Reformed Church played an important role in dealing with the outbreak and at an emergency meeting in May 1767 the Church Council decided to lease a number of houses and convert them into a temporary hospital, with six young slaves acting as stretcher bearers, assisting with nursing and attending to the burials of free slaves and Coloureds who had succumbed to the disease. Altogether 178 patients were nursed in the hospital of which 113 recovered.[16] Smallpox visited the Cape every seven to ten years after that with outbreaks of varying severity. Mentzel in 1787 wrote 'Smallpox in epidemic form breaks out only every forty or fifty years according to statements of the Hottentots and recent experience'.[17] The only treatment measures available were isoation and quarantine. Between the epidemics of 1755 and 1767 the Khoikhoi tribe was almost destroyed. Many of the survivors fled inland and by 1787 only about 56 Cape Khoi were seen to be remaining around the Cape Flats.

Smallpox was very prevalent also in Europe at that time but

inoculation, in the manner known then, was not widely practised. It had been brought back from Constantinople to London by Lady Mary Wortley Montague around 1721, although it had been known in certain parts of Wales since the previous century.[18] It was reported from Algeria in 1769 that smallpox was prevalent in 'Algiers, Tunis and Tripoli, and fully as destructive. In order to avoid the bad consequences of the natural disorder many people have recourse to inoculation'. The person wishing to be inoculated would go to a house where there was smallpox, and purchase pustules full of matter. These were rubbed onto the skin between the thumb and fore-finger, and caused a milder form of the infection which was not fatal. The practice was thought to be very old and thought at that time to have been invented by the Arabs, although the practice had also been common in India and China for centuries. Reports from Bengal described it as having been in use for a very long time and performed by pricking the skin between some of the fingers with two needles, then rubbing some of the matter over the spots: 'a circle is made by means of several punctures, of the bigness of a common pustule, and matter is again rubbed over it. The wound is then dressed with lint, a fever ensues, and after some days the eruption, which if the fever has been strong is observed not to be very copious'. As this method was painful another had been used by 'people of quality and substance. A little of the matter is mixed with sugar, and swallowed by the child in any sweet and pleasant liquid. The same effect is produced but the first method is thought to be the best'.[19]

The Russell brothers also reported on inoculation in Aleppo in 1768, where the practice of 'buying the smallpox' was again described as common amongst Arabs and Bedouin, and as being 'as ancient as the disease itself'. It was reported also to be common in Baghdad and Mosul and that, since time immemorial, it had been a practice among the different Arab tribes across the desert to present day Iraq. It was also reported from Georgia, Armenia, Damascus, Syria, Palestine, Mecca, all of which performed it in the same manner, although some Georgians inoculated on the fore-arm, and Armenians on the thigh. Dr Russell stated:

> It is probable that the practice of inoculation in these countries was originally derived from the same source, and that it is of considerable antiquity can hardly be doubted, if we consider the large extent of country over which is must have spread, and the obstacles it must have met with in a progress through various nations, some of which are separated by polity as well as religion, while other, peculiarly tenacious of their own customs,

are little disposed to admit those of strangers.

Inoculation was not performed by Jews and rarely by Turks. Russell found it strange that the custom had up until then escaped the attention of those Europeans who lived and travelled in the Middle East and north Africa, and reflected that 'customs the most common in distant countries, are often or all others the least apt to attract the observation of travellers who, engaged in other pursuits, must be indebted to accident for the knowledge of such things, as the natives seldom talk of, from the belief that they are known to all the world'.[20]

By 1798 Edward Jenner was developing a new smallpox vaccine derived from cowpox, following the observation, made some years before, that milkmaids who had contracted cowpox seemed immune to smallpox. It is possible that the Middle Eastern form of inoculation was used,[21] but news of the new smallpox vaccine was brought to South Africa by a Mr Woody in 1800 while discussing the smallpox epidemics in England. The Governor, Sir George Yonge, wrote to the Secretary for the Colonies stating that the Cape inhabitants were anxious to try it and later a Dr Tyler arrived to start using it. A series of articles were published in the Cape Town Gazette on the vaccine and the experiences with it in Europe.[22] Vaccination first arrived in the Cape from Mozambique on the Portuguese vessel Belasario on 26 November 1803, having been carried by arm-to-arm vaccination of 342 slaves, none of whom developed smallpox.[23] From 1803 to 1806 the Cape was under the administration of the Batavian Government under the terms of the Peace of Amiens and became a province of the Netherlands. Part of the Cape's hospital, known as the 'Groot Hospitaal te Cabo de Goede Hoop', was set aside for a Health Bureau which set up a Vaccination Committee of 12 doctors. This Committee, after experimentation with arm-to-arm vaccination which kept the vaccine alive, recommended that a system of voluntary vaccination against smallpox should be introduced which was published on 12 December 1803.[24]

A smaller epidemic of smallpox occurred in 1807, which was controlled by a vaccination campaign[25] and again in 1812. The latter was more severe although was relatively quickly controlled through the application of public health measures - quarantine, street-by-street vaccinations and emergency isolation hospitals. Again slaves who had previously had the disease and were immune, as well as those who were immunised, were used as nurses. Vaccine was transferred to distant towns by arm from the vaccine centre at Paarden Island. The impact of vaccination was so great that thanksgiving services were held in churches in Stellenbosch.[26] Smallpox was also brought out to South Africa by the 1820 settlers, with cases aboard the ships Alliance and the Northampton. Many corpses were thrown overboard, sewn inside their contaminated bedding.[27] In 1836 the ship Lord William Bentinck arrived with smallpox on board. Chlorine gas was used for the first time to fumigate rooms and mail, and clothing and other items were destroyed. A military cordon was set up and cats and dogs in the area put down.[28]

Further small epidemics occurred in 1839 and 1858 by which time the authorities had some experience in how to control the disease. However, in areas where people were resistant to vaccination the disease still took its toll. Dr J.P. Fitzgerald reported from the King Williams Town area that the disease raged with great violence amongst the Fingoes and that the Fingo doctors were opposed to vaccination: 'they stuck forked wooden pegs in the grounds before the kraals, but the smallpox visited those locations and swept the people away including many doctors'. However later they accepted vaccination and those 'who eagerly availed themselves of the benefits offered escaped the disease to a great extent'.[29] By this time there were no longer slaves and paid attendants were used to do the nursing. Bedding and clothing were burnt after use, including in private homes, and houses were required to be fumigated with pots of tar kept boiling within the premises for four days. Washing of linen had to be undertaken by persons who were immune, and the dead had to be buried within an hour during the day or at daybreak if they died overnight. At the end of the epidemic instructions were given to whitewash and fumigate the whole of the premises which had been occupied by smallpox cases.[30]

The virulent epidemic of 1881, brought in December by the steamer the Garonne, spread far inland with high mortality among the unvaccinated. Despite the quarantining of its passengers in Saldanha Bay it continued to carry smallpox on to Australia in 1882.[31] Natal, which enforced strict quarantine measures on ships arriving at Durban from the Cape, was kept free of the disease. On the 19th of April the ship the Coldstream from India, carrying indentured Indian labourers, arrived with smallpox and 322 people were quarantined for four weeks, which effectively prevented spread to the Province.[32] The disease was again brought to the Cape by the steamship Drummond Castle in May 1882, spreading throughout the peninsula.[33] Despite implementing the measures which had proven helpful in past epidemics the effects were severe, particular amongst the Cape Malay population which had consistently refused vaccination, such that it was said to have 'practically exterminated them'. By November 1,146 had died.[34] It was as a result of this that vaccination was made compulsory by the Parliament of Cape Colony. The epidemic also drew attention to the conditions of squalor and overcrowding inhabited by the poor, and brought about cries for a degree of segregation between the Europeans and the poorer Malay and African populations.[35]

In Kimberley, worried about the wagons bringing people from Cape Town to the mines, a quarantine station had been established in anticipation at the junction of the Modder and the Riet Rivers some 30 miles south of the mines. Police diverted travellers to the quarantine station where all passengers from wagons coming up from Cape Town were fumigated for three minutes with sulphur before they were permitted to enter the town. Seven cases were detected and detained for treatment, with all those in the same wagon quarantined for 21 days. These measures apparently kept the disease from the town until 1883, although it was alleged that in 1882, due to fears of the mine-owners that if smallpox were mentioned the farmers would take fright and not bring in fuel and food, it was deliberately mislabelled chicken pox. The diagnosis continued to cause disagreement with some doctors denying that it was smallpox, instead labelling it 'Felstead's disease' after the farm on which the original sufferers died, or alternatively 'Kaffir pox' or, less objectionably the 'Transvaal disease'. The doctor in charge was later prosecuted for admitting a contagious disease into a general hospital and fined £10.

In 1883 it was finally admitted to have reached the town from a group of Africans coming from Klerksdorp. The outbreak lasted from November 1883 to December 1884, and cost the town and mines the sum of £37,503 in paying for medical services, iron hospitals, fumigating houses, dispensaries, ambulance wagons horses and officials. Some 2,311 cases were reported and the deaths numbered 700, or 32%. Patrols were stationed on the road from Kimberley to the Free State at which they established fumigation stations, fumigating everyone who passed along. [36] Following its spread to Durban, where it affected Africans working at the Point area of the docks, wood and iron huts were erected at the Back Beach for use as an infectious diseases hospital with guards and a security fence to isolate the patients.[37] The epidemic of 1882/83, in which over 4,000 people died, lead to the Public Health Act of 1883 which gave authorities the power to frame regulations for vaccination and quarantining.[38] It also empowered the local authority to order the cleaning or disinfection of any house or article. It made notification to the local authority compulsory, and gave them the power to establish hospitals. From this date no unvaccinated person was eligible for employment in the Public Service.

Vaccination became more acceptable through the 1880's and reports from the Eastern Cape indicated that, while smallpox continued to be present in pockets, it was rapidly stamped out with widespread vaccination efforts and restrictions on movements of people. The King Williams Town area experienced a further outbreak in 1884, which killed around 200, but was contained.[39] Welsh, reporting from the Aliwal North area in 1886 stated 'it is manifest that a free issue of passes to people to visit these areas [the Free State, Lesotho and the Transkei] would have increased the risk of introducing the epidemic for a second time into this Division a hundredfold. It was therefore solely in the interests of the people themselves that the restriction on the issue of passes was enforced'. A village where a case of smallpox occurred was put in quarantine for four months to prevent spread.[40] By 1885 control measures were deemed to be quite successful in stamping out epidemics and it was considered that it would be 'absurd, cruel and wrong' to quarantine ships arriving at Cape ports with cases of smallpox on board. It was thought that if vaccination were compulsorily enforced it would soon be eradicated from the country, although mortality was still high among non-vaccinating 'Mohammedans' who, despite warnings and cautions, continued to fail to vaccinate,[41] an attitude which was quite curious in light of the prevalence of vaccination amongst Arabs in north Africa and Arabia. Landsberg, the Vaccine Officer, in 1885 similarly reported that Cape Town was ripe for further epidemics unless the law requiring vaccination was enforced, 'especially among the Mohammedan population, who, notwithstanding all warning and caution, persistently neglect vaccination'.[42]

Towards the end of the nineteenth century it was reported that smallpox was present in the Transvaal amongst Africans, although there was some debate as to whether it was really smallpox. However the Natal Witness newspaper noted that the alarm prevailing was 'not so much attributable to any fear of infection as to the consequences to mining should labour become scarce'. It commented further in respect of the government's control measures 'It is not so much any fear of the disease which makes people uneasy as of a compulsory law and heavy penalties being put in force'. A Royal Commission had been sitting for the last four years investigating vaccination, and half its time was spent listening to the arguments of anti-vaccinators. A Bill before Parliament would render the action of the law in respect of compulsory vaccination more limited and would enable a parent to prevent his children from being vaccinated.[43]

At the end of January 1893 a case of smallpox arrived at the goldfields. The man was isolated in a tent on ground behind the jail, and finally allowed to leave when it was thought safe. However in April 1893 more cases started, affecting Africans on the mines. Drastic measures were taken to limit their movements with Africans attempting to leave being flogged and, following the posting of armed guards, shot. The epidemic worsened and a Smallpox Committee was established, with an isolation camp established at Hospital hill. Vaccination was provided, and often compulsory, with those objecting fined. In an effort to prevent its spread Pretoria guarded all roads entering and all passengers arriving by train or cart were fumigated. Altogether in 12 months around Johannesburg there were 2,000 cases and 94 deaths. Gradually during 1894 the epidemic died out.[44]

Hay reported on a smallpox-like disease which he saw affecting the BaVenda people in northern Transvaal from around 1903, which was locally called Amaas. Many of the Africans carried pock marks resulting from the disease. It was thought they had known of if for a long time as they had learned how to vaccinate against it, doing this for Chiefs on the forehead midway between the top of the nose and the hairline. Lesser leaders were vaccinated on the left wrist. The disease resembled a mild case of smallpox, with similar rash but less prone to complications and less fatal. It was thought to have originated in Mozambique and was controllable by vaccination.[45] It was later described as Variola minor, (although also known by the vulgar name of Kaffir-pox) and during 1940 occurred in an outbreak in the Eastern Transvaal, around the town of Piet Retief, later becoming endemic in the area. While the mortality was less than 1% the disease had a similar horrific appearance with a rash distributed over the face, scalp, torso, arms and legs. Although mortality was low the illness was quite severe, often complicated by pneumonia.

Smallpox was a regular concern at the beginning of the 20th century. Reports of District Surgeons from many parts of the country described cases and small outbreaks, particularly in the early years after the Anglo-Boer war. They were usually responded to rapidly with isolation, quarantine and vaccination of several thousand people in the vicinity. Cases were removed to Lazarettos and red flags distributed to indicate infected households. 1902, while there were still large movements of populations related to the war, was a particularly bad year in the Cape towns with most reporting cases. The District Surgeon of Colesberg reported an outbreak in 1902 affecting 34 people with three deaths in those previously unvaccinated. The vaccinated were also affected but with a minor form. Patients were housed in a tented camp away from the location.[46] Cradock had an outbreak affecting 210 people which then spread to Queenstown, Glen Grey had an epidemic of 443 cases and 32 deaths and similarly in De Aar an outbreak arose in the same year, brought by a soldier from Bloemfontein, which lead to 141 cases and eight deaths. Again the victims were isolated and a special camp set up where contacts were detained for three weeks.[47] In 1904 there was an outbreak of smallpox in Pietermaritzburg in Natal, with 60 European cases and 115 Indian and African cases. In 1905 there were another 17 cases in the surrounding areas. A similar outbreak occurred in Johannesburg in 1905 with 50 deaths. The outbreak started in the Malay Location and circulars were immediately sent to all the mine managers to alert them. A thorough inspection was made of all Africans to check their vaccination status with six officers stationed at the Pass Office. 20,273 workers were vaccinated. The high level of control over African vaccination meant that they suffered proportionately less from the epidemic that the Europeans, Indians and Cape Coloured communities.[48]

Smallpox continued to be a problem across the country throughout the early years of the 20th century with sporadic outbreaks reported in towns across the Cape and Transvaal down to the Transkei. Vaccination programmes were in place with reasonable effect in controlling the outbreaks, but with varying attendance by people after the disease died down. In January 1919 the Public Health Act was presented in Parliament which gave the Government power to undertake compulsory vaccination throughout the Union. The 'conscientious objector' clause present in the Natal and the Free State, enabling parents to avoid vaccination, was also abolished as it had lead to large numbers of children not being vaccinated.[49] That same year outbreaks of smallpox were reported across various parts of the country, including the Cape, southern Natal, and Transvaal. These continued through 1920, from the Waterberg in the Transvaal to Orange Free State and the Transkei.

In 1926 there was a severe outbreak in Durban during October and November, resulting in 57 cases with 16 deaths. It was almost entirely limited to Asians with the first six cases were found in a large and densely populated Indian Barracks. The original cases had been hidden by their friends. Many subsequent cases were also hidden, with mothers hiding sick children in cupboards, under their skirts and smuggled out of the barracks, by which means it spread north to Tongaat. It also contributed to the high mortality rate as patients were only discovered late into the disease 'after receiving most inadequate attention, under miserable housing conditions, during the critical stages of their illness'. The outbreak was controlled by widespread, compulsory vaccination of some 200,000 people to which few people objected, despite the fact that 'Durban was the chief stronghold of conscientious objectors in the Union'.[50] Provision for compulsory vaccination had come into force with the Public Health Act at the beginning of 1920 and strenuous opposition was offered by these objectors, particularly in Durban. During 1921 prosecutions had taken place for non-compliance and convictions obtained, but in 1922 the prosecutions were discontinued while the matter was considered in Parliament. The result of this had been a falling off in the number of persons vaccinated and the rapid accumulation of an unvaccinated population, with increasing risk of smallpox epidemics. Following the Durban outbreak there was the worry that other cities were at risk of epidemics, such as on the Cape Peninsula.[51]

The risk of smallpox arriving at South African ports continued with cases often arriving on ships from India, although these were usually dropped at other East African ports such as Zanzibar or Lourenço Marques (now Maputo) before arriving at Durban. On the 3rd of October 1929 the ship Umvuma arrived from London with five cases amongst Indian crew members. In each of the ships the passengers and crew were examined, vaccinated and the contacts isolated until the expiration of the incubation period after the last exposure to infection. 72 cases occurred in South Africa during the year and one death. The largest outbreak was at the Natal town of Kokstad where 20 cases occurred. Vaccination and isolation were very effective and the active enforcement of the law making vaccination compulsory made the campaigns more successful. 548,000 people were vaccinated during the 1929-1930 period and there were only 504 conscientious objections.[52] Regulations were in place that all passengers from Indian ports had to have been vaccinated not less than twelve days prior to embarkation, although some problems arose around crews on ships which docked only briefly at Indian ports. Altogether in 1935 there were 29 cases in the country, although these were of the mild from known as Amaas with no deaths. However this milder form still had the potential to develop into virulent smallpox in an unvaccinated person.

Smallpox in 1938 was still widespread in Transvaal and other provinces, with some cases in northern Natal, mainly among Africans and mainly of the milder type. Altogether 653 cases were reported, followed by 408 in 1939 and 681 in 1940, predominantly in the Transvaal. The compulsory vaccination of infants and unvaccinated persons was considered one of the most dramatic achievements of preventive medicine in reducing the incidence of any single disease in the country, but the disease still remained common.[53] In addition to the local infections the country was still at risk of the introduction of smallpox from the East, which risk had increased greatly because of the Second World War. Six cases of smallpox arrived from India in 1941 as members of the crews of ships who developed the disease within a few days of landing, and who then went on to infect three local people. The incidence rate at that time was increasing, with 1,023 cases notified in that year. The increase was blamed also on a failure of employers of Non-European labour to ensure their employees were vaccinated and the migratory wanderings of Africans in search of work, together with it being misdiagnosed by doctors as chickenpox. The threat continued to grow with 1,781 cases in 1942.

Outbreaks of a more virulent type increased in urban areas with 80 districts affected in 1944 and it appeared that the more virulent Variola major was displacing the milder Variola minor which had predominated before. The theory was that the large African reserves in Natal and Transvaal were being searched for recruits for the War effort with a resulting influx of unvaccinated Africans into the industrial areas, one such area being Pietermaritzburg in Natal. Five people had been diagnosed with smallpox from Edendale Township outside Pietermaritzburg in 1943, and four more were admitted to hospital in January 1944. Another patient, who appeared to have been infected by other patients while in the Epidemic Hospital, presented in February. Three months later an epidemic had exploded with arriving by bus, train, rickshaw, on foot and in taxis, into the crowded outpatients' department of the city's Grey's Hospital.

A public mass vaccination campaign was undertaken by the Local Authority reaching almost 25,000 people.[54] In the neighbouring Zwartkop African location smallpox was also introduced in June 1944 by a visitor from Durban. It was found that only 54.4% of the population had vaccination scars and mass vaccinations were conducted at various centres. By the end of July there were 36 cases and 12 deaths. In October a team undertook a six week vaccination programme, followed by home visits, which was found to be more effective in tracing people who had not been previously vaccinated. Altogether there were 65 cases in the surrounding area outside Pietermaritzburg in 1944, of which 21 died, giving a case-mortality rate of 32.3%.[55] By 1945 the situation regarding smallpox had worsened and another epidemic broke out in the city. Altogether 113 cases of smallpox were treated in municipal hospitals: of these 34 died, giving a case fatality rate of 30.1%. The use of sulphonamide antibiotics was found to make no difference. The Medical Officer of Health, Dr Maister, ascribed the disease to air-borne contagion suggested to him by the fact that all the Europeans affected, except one who was a direct contact, lived in the suburb of Scottsville close to the Isolation Hospital. Outbreaks were known to occur within the vicinity of smallpox hospitals. In this case, the prevailing winds were monitored and found to be blowing in a direction from the hospital to the affected residents. The possibility of fly-borne spread was also considered and stringent precautions against flies were enforced. Other measures taken included hospitalisation of all cases, disinfection of bedrooms with formalin, disinfection of clothing and bedding with steam, and vaccination and quarantine of all contacts for fourteen days unless recently successfully vaccinated. The entire area was visited house-to-house and surveyed for vaccination status, and almost 80,000 doses of vaccine were administered.[56]

While nationally in 1945 there were 3,317 cases and 305 deaths altogether, Natal alone accounted for 2,203 cases and 284 deaths. The high incidence in Natal, affecting the entire province, was considered due a combination of tribal customs and religious objections to vaccination having given rise to a population largely unprotected from the disease. It was said that the Zionist faith, practiced by many of the African population there, combined anti-vaccination with itinerant local preaching. In addition the large Asian population was prone to concealing cases, thus contributing to the spread. Vaccination was made compulsory to combat the epidemic and lay vaccinators employed to go from kraal to kraal. Outside of Natal an outbreak also occurred in the predominantly African and densely populated Alexandra Township just outside Johannesburg with 193 cases admitted of which 78 died – a case fatality rate of over 40%, which rose to almost 50% in those who had never been vaccinated at all. Vaccination was given at birth and thereafter recommended every five years. Alexandra had been long described in government reports as 'a menace to public health' and had been subject to investigations by several Commissions of Enquiry. It had been recommended that their Health Committee be abolished and that it be placed under the Peri-urban Areas Health Board back in 1940, but this had not occurred by 1945 and the situation was as bad as ever.[57]

Smallpox declined a little the following year with 1,271 cases and 60 deaths across the country. The majority of cases in Natal were in the Umzinto and Utrecht areas where most of the victims were said to be of 'Native religious sects opposed to vaccination'. Over 5.2 million doses of vaccine were issued by the Government Vaccine Institute.[58] In 1947 it dropped to just under a thousand cases with 27 deaths split equally between the Transvaal, Natal and the Transkei. At the end of 1949 and during 1950 there was a major outbreak again, affecting mainly the Transvaal province but also spreading around the country. Johannesburg reported 191 cases with 71 deaths. However, following this outbreak the figures for 1952 were the lowest ever recorded by the Department of Health with only 35 cases, which occurred to the west of Johannesburg around Klerksdorp. The Department, recording only 14 cases in 1953 stated 'the history of smallpox constitutes an example illustrating pre-eminently the triumph of public health measures in preventing the occurrence of an infective disease which, not so very long ago, claimed hundreds of victims every year'. However yearly vaccination campaigns were still critical as there was an ever present risk of the disease being introduced from outside the country.[59] Cape Town in 1955 had its first case in 10 years in an unvaccinated, European man in Rondebosch who, having been taken ill but then recovered slightly, had proceeded to expose 89 of his friends to the disease. 1,350 co-workers at his factory were vaccinated and a public appeal was made for people to come forward if not vaccinated within the previous three years. One million doses of vaccine were issued in one of the biggest mass vaccinations in the county's history and the spread was arrested. The initial case was traced back to a woman who had travelled back from Kitwe in Zambia carrying the disease, and then infecting two people in Rondebosch.[60]

From 1952 the Variola minor form of the disease again displaced Variola major with few cases occurring and a low case-fatality rate. For the period 1956 to 1959 there was not a single case of smallpox in the country, but the triumphal announcements were premature as, true to the Health Department's note of caution, a case of smallpox entered the country in 1960 and restarted the disease. 65 other people contracted it and from 1961 it was decided to require a vaccination certificate for all people entering the Republic. Initially this excluded Western Europe, the Americas and New Zealand but the following year the requirement was extended to all countries, as well as South Africans returning from overseas visits. 103 cases occurred in 1962 and 254 in 1963, most of which occurred in the Eastern Transvaal and Northern Natal.[61]

In March 1964 a family with cases of smallpox, but still in the incubation period, entered the country from Malawi and caused a smallpox outbreak in Port Elizabeth which led to more than 60 cases of whom eleven people died. Port Elizabeth had been free of smallpox since 1947, but on the 7th February 1964 a woman and her six unvaccinated children arrived from Blantyre in Malawi, one of them having a rash thought to be chicken pox. Other cases arose and were diagnosed as smallpox on the 4th March, following which an isolation centre and emergency hospital were established in a hall and tents in Walmer location. An immediate and extensive vaccination campaign commenced, and a massive publicity drive accompanied it such that by the 24th March over 300,000 people had been vaccinated or re-vaccinated in the city. Altogether 750,000 doses were given in the Eastern Cape. By the 16th March there were over 30 suspected cases filling the Walmer Location Isolation Centre and the facility was relocated to the Bomb Stores, which were re-fitted as an emergency hospital. By the end of March six patients cases had died and there were 39 cases in the emergency hospital from around Port Elizabeth and Uitenhage, all of which were Africans and several of whom were prisoners. Contacts were placed under 21 days quarantine with food supplied to them at home. A recommended drug, marboran, which was tried in order to prevent cases in suspects was found to be ineffective, but the widespread implementation of vaccination measures was thought be effective. The Medical Officer of Health of Port Elizabeth reported that 'Following a bonfire of mattresses the yellow flag of the Bomb Store Smallpox Hospital was lowered with the closing of the hospital on 21st August 1964'.[62] 301 cases occurred across the whole country that year. Stricter measures were introduced with effect from 1st January 1965 to try and get the disease back under control. Education campaigns were held, vaccination tours scheduled and local authorities enlisted to support the statutory requirements and over 14,500,000 doses of vaccine were given out. Vaccine production had been moved to the new State Vaccine Institute at Pinelands, Cape Town, with the capacity to produce 20 million doses a year, much of which was exported.

South Africa reported only 43 cases to the World Health Organisation (WHO) in 1967 and 81 in 1968, increasing suddenly to 246 in 1969, mostly in the Transvaal. This increase was queried by the WHO with the South African Secretary for Health and a letter was returned by the Director of Medical Services who, according to Fenner, displayed 'a dismaying lack of understanding of the epidemiology of smallpox'.[63] A subsequent report prepared by the WHO chided South Africa for being, along with Ethiopia, the only countries which had not initiated eradication programmes and stating that the continuing reservoir of infection in these two places was of increasing concern to neighbouring countries which were becoming smallpox-free. It also criticised the continuing use of the liquid form of vaccine when the others had changed to freeze-dried. Fenner states that the South African health officials were angered by the report claiming that their Variola minor form of the disease was of less importance in the transmission of smallpox, that their vaccination programme was effective and defending their liquid vaccine. In 1970 however the South African health authorities, in order to avoid expected criticism from other independent African countries, decided to take additional measures to control smallpox and changed to the freeze-dried vaccine. An intensified systematic campaign was started in the northern Transvaal where most cases were reported. Fenner stated that until 1972 little information regarding smallpox and the control programme in South Africa was available to the World Health Organisation, with that information provided focusing more on month and race rather than the geographical location of the disease, which would have been more useful to WHO as it engaged in a global programme to eradicate the disease. They commented 'as country after country in Africa became free of smallpox South Africa's dubious reputation as one of only a few endemic countries became politically intolerable to its authorities'.[64] This apparently spurred the country on to undergo intensive vaccination campaigns in the endemic areas from and the control of smallpox advanced rapidly from this point, with only ten cases notified in 1971. These were the last indigenous cases and were of the milder form Variola minor, rather than the more severe form which had lingered in other southern African countries until around the same time. Most of the last cases had been acquired at a hospital about 100km north of Pretoria in the Transvaal when smallpox in some children spread to the tuberculosis ward.

In June 1972, when Henderson of the WHO visited the country, he found a well-organized campaign although under-reporting of cases and it was found that while only ten cases and one death were notified in 1972 there had actually been at least 20 cases, mainly linked to the hospital outbreak. The last laboratory isolation of the virus in South Africa was made in 1972, imported from Botswana, and the disease was finally eradicated from South Africa some eight years before it was finally declared globally eradicated by the WHO.[65] It remains to this day probably the greatest global triumph of public health over one of the most disfiguring, lethal and frightening diseases in history.

ENDNOTES

1. Liebbrandt H.C.V. 'Journal of Governor Willem Adriaan van der Stel 1713' *Precis of the Archives of the Cape of Good Hope, Journal 1699-1732;* Cape Town 1896
2. Laidler P.W. and Gelfand M. *South Africa its Medical History, 1652-1898: A medical and social study*; Struik, Cape Town, 1971:40

3. Liebbrandt H.V. 'Journal of Governor Willem Adriaan van der Stel 1713' *Precis of the Archives of the Cape of Good Hope, Journal 1699-1732* Cape Town 1896
4. Laidler P.W. and Gelfand M. *South Africa its Medical History, 1652-1898: A medical and social study*; Struik, Cape Town, 197:40
5. Smith Andrew B. 'The Origins and Demise of the Khoikhoi, The Debate' *South African Historical Journal* 23, December 1990: 13.
6. Cory G.E. *The Rise of South Africa; Volume I*; Longmans, Green and Co; 1910:40
7. Chais Rev M. translated by Maty MDSRS; 'A short account of the manner of inoculating the smallpox on the coast of Barbary and at Bengal in the East Indies' *The Annual Register for the year 1769*; J. Dodsley 1770. 80
8. Mead, Richard; 'A discourse on the Small Pox and Measles, John Brindley 1748'; cited in *South African Medical Journal*, 25(1) 1951:10
9. Brockleby, Dr; 'Surprising instance of the great infectiousness of some diseases, where a free current of air is wanting, even in the most temperate climates' *The Annual Register*, v8 1765, J Dodsley, 1793:89
10. Searle C. *The History of the Development of Nursing in South Africa 1652-1960*; The South African Nursing Association; 1980:59
11. Scully W.C. *A History of South Africa*; Longmans, Green and Co; 1922:66.
12. Viljoen, Russel; 'Disease and Society: VOC Cape Town, its people and the smallpox epidemics of 1713, 1755 and 1767' *Kleio* 27; 1995:22-45
13. Laidler P.W. and Gelfand M. *South Africa its Medical History, 1652-1898: A medical and social study*; Struik, Cape Town, 1971:55
14. Bekker A.E. *The History of False Bay up to 1795*; Simon's Town Historical Society 1990:101;
15. Viljoen, Russel; 'Disease and Society: VOC Cape Town, its people and the smallpox epidemics of 1713, 1355 and 1767' *Kleio* 27; 1995:22-45.
16. Searle C; *The History of the Development of Nursing in South Africa 1652-1960*;' The South African Nursing Association; 1980:59.
17. Mentzel O.F. *A Geographical and Topographical description of the Cape of Good Hope; 1787*; Translated by Marais G.V. and Hoge J.; Edited by Mandelbrote HJ; The Van Riebeeck Society, Cape Town, 1944.
18. Russell P. 'An account of Inoculation in Arabia, in a letter from Dr Patrick Russell at Aleppo to Dr Alexander Russell'; *The Annual Register for the year 1769*; J Dodsley 1770:2
19. Chais Rev M, translated by Maty MDSRS; 'A short account of the manner of inoculating the smallpox on the coast of Barbary and at Bengal in the East Indies' *The Annual Register for the year 1769*; J Dodsley 1770:80
20. Russell P. 'An account of Inoculation in Arabia, in a letter from Dr Patrick Russell at Aleppo to Dr Alexander Russell', *The Annual Register for the year 1769*; J Dodsley 1770: 82
21. Hopkins D.R. *Princes and Peasants: Smallpox in History*; Chicago, 1983:180
22. *Cape Town Gazette* 25 September 1802 – 30 October 1802.
23. Laidler P.W. and Gelfand M.; *South Africa its medical history, 1652-1898: A medical and social study* Struik Cape Town, 1971:57
24. Searle C; *The History of the Development of Nursing in South Africa 1652-1960*;' The South African Nursing Association; 1980:60.
25. *Cape Town Gazette*; 25 April 1807
26. Smuts F. *Stellenbosch: Three Centuries*, The Town Council of Stellenbosch; 1979:242
27. Bryer L. and Hunt K.S. *The 1820 Settlers*; Don Nelson, Cape Town 1984:26.

28. Laidler P.W. 'Medical Establishments and Institutions at the Cape: Somerset Hospital, The Slave hospital and the First Pauper Establishment', *South African Medical Journal* 11(18) 1937:641-649
29. Fitzgerald J.P. *Report on the King William's Town Hospital 1882*, WA Richards, 1883:4
30. Searle C. *The History of the Development of Nursing in South Africa 1652-1960;*' The South African Nursing Association; 1980:68.
31. Van Heyningen E. 'Epidemics and Disease: Historical writing on Health in South Africa' *South African Historical Journal* 23; 1990:122-133
32. Finnemore R.I. 'Report of the Resident Magistrate', *Colony of Natal Blue Book 1883*, Vause Slatter and Co 1884; pGG43
33. Matthews J.W. *Incwadi Yami or Twenty Years Personal Experience in South Africa; 1887;* Africana Book Society; Johannesburg; 1976:108
34. Theal George McCall; *History of South Africa from 1873 to 1884: twelve eventful years*; George Allen and Unwin Ltd, London; 1919:200.
35. Bickford-Smith, Vivian, *Ethnic Pride and Racial Prejudice in Victorian Cape Town*, Witwatersrand University Press, Johannesburg 1995:100-105
36. Matthews J.W. *Incwadi Yami or Twenty Years Personal Experience in South Africa; 1887;* Africana Book Society; Johannesburg; 1976:108
37. O'Reagan M. *The Hospital Services of Natal*, Natal Regional Survey No 8, University of Natal, Durban, Robinson and Co, 1970:18
38. Swanson M.W, 'The Sanitation Syndrome: Bubonic Plague and Urban Native Policy in the Cape Colony 1900-1909'; *Journal of African History*; 18 1977:392
39. Dick R.J. 'Report of the Civil Commissioner', *Cape of Good Hope Blue Book on Native Affairs*; WA Richards, Cape Town, 1886:30
40. Welsh Alex R. 'Report of the Civil Commissioner' *Cape of Good Hope Blue Book on Native Affairs*; WA Richards, Cape Town, 1886:25
41. Ebden Henry; *Report of the Colonial Medical Committee, 1885*; WA Richards and Sons, Cape Town G2/1886:3
42. Landsberg P. *Report of the Vaccine Surgeon, 1885*, WA Richards and Sons, Cape Town G2/1886:4
43. *Natal Witness*, 7 June 1893.
44. Neame L.E. *City Built on Gold*, Central News Agency, Cape Town, 1960:49-51.
45. Hay, George Gray, 'Amaas' *South African Medical Journal* 12(17) 1938: 639-641.
46. Tait K.R. 'Report of the District Surgeon of Colesberg 1902' *Cape of Good Hope Reports on the Public Health 1902*; Cape Times Ltd; G66-1903; 1903:42
47. Fitzgerald N.C. 'Report of the Additional District Surgeon, Sub-District of De Aar, 1902; *Cape of Good Hope Reports on the Public Health 1902*, Cape Times Ltd, G66-1903; 1903:28-29
48. Lagden G.Y. *Annual Report of the Commissioner for Native Affairs 1905-06*, Government Printing and Stationary office, Pretoria, 1906 pA6
49. Watt, Thomas, 'Public Health of the Union' *Cape Times* 30th January 1919:24.
50. *Annual Report of the Department of Public Health, Union of South Africa, 1927*, Government Printing and Stationery Office Pretoria, UG 35-'27, p41
51. Ibid, 43
52. *Annual Report of the Department of Public Health, Union of South Africa, 1930*, The Government Printer Office Pretoria, UG 40-'30,p17,41
53. *Annual Report of the Department of Public Health, 1940*, Government Printer Pretoria, UG No 8-'40, p40.
54. Maister M. 'Annual Report of the Medical Officer of Health' *Pietermaritzburg Corporation Yearbook* 1944: 74.

55. Harding Le Riche, Smallpox control in the Swartkop Native Location; *The Medical Officer* No 4; 1945:280.
56. Maister M. 'Annual Report of the Medical Officer of Health', *Pietermaritzburg Corporation Yearbook* 1945: 75-81.
57. *Annual Report of the Department of Public Health, Union of South Africa 1945*, Government Printer Pretoria, UG No 6-'1946:22.
58. *Annual Report of the Department of Public Health, 1946*, Government Printer Pretoria, UG No 18-'47, p25.
59. *Annual Report of the Department of Health, Union of South Africa, 1953*, The Government Printer Pretoria, UG 23-'1956:12
60. *Annual Report of the Medical Officer of Health*, City of Cape Town, 1956:38.
61. *Annual Report of the Department of Health for the Five Years ended 31st December 1964*, The Government Printer Pretoria RP 11/1966
62. Saville Lewis J. *Annual Report of the Medical Officer of Health for Port Elizabeth, 1964*, Waltons, Port Elizabeth, 1964:40
63. Fenner F. Henderson D.A. Arita I, Ježek Z, Ladnyi I.D. 'Smallpox and its eradication'; World Health Organisation; *History of International Public Health* No 6, Geneva, p984
64. Ibid, p985
65. Ibid, p982-988

PLAGUE: THE ORIGINS OF APARTHEID SEGREGATION

Few diseases have had the ability to strike terror into people as much as the Plague, which has caused the deaths of millions through the ages. Caused by the bacteria Yersinia pestis, it occurs primarily in wild rodents and is transmitted from them to man by the bite of an infected flea. The fleas generally prefer their rodent hosts, but once the rodents have died they will leave them to attack people. Person-to-person transmission of the disease occurs either from the movement of fleas or from the inhalation of droplets spread by the cough of a patient with plague with pulmonary (lung) lesions, giving rise to primary pneumonic plague. All forms have a very high fatality rate if untreated – 60% for the bubonic form (characterised by the bubo - an inflamed, tender swelling in the joint areas, groin, armpit or neck) and a virtually 100% death rate for the pneumonic form.

The link between rats and plague was first made by the ancient Phoenicians and the inhabitants of Hindustan who, more than 900 years ago, warned residents to leave their dwellings immediately if they saw rats dying in large numbers. In ancient Syria also a high mortality among rats was well known to accompany plague. The deaths of rodents from plague is often a warning sign for a plague epidemic in humans as, having killed their rodent hosts, the fleas carrying the disease abandon the dead animals and then look for other hosts such as people. However in ancient times the fact that it was spread by fleas was not known – only that there was a link with rodents. In Canton, China in 1894 22,000 dead rats were buried by officials before an epidemic which went on to kill 80,000 people. The fact that both rats and people were infected by the plague bacteria which caused the disease was discovered in Hong Kong in the same year.[1] It then appeared in Bombay (Mumbai) India in 1896 and thereafter spread to Europe, Australia, America and Africa.

Shortly after the rise of plague in Asia in the 1890's it was first introduced to southern Africa during the Anglo-Boer War (South African War) by rats from vessels with cargoes of horse forage from infected South American ports, which was being brought into the country in increasing amounts to cater for military needs. The first small outbreak was reported in 1899 in Delagoa Bay.[2] A single case was found in

Durban in 1900 in someone recently arrived from Mauritius. Plague hit Cape Town, a major port, in 1901 with the first case being reported on the 1st of February. The patient had started being ill on 27th January but the cause was not diagnosed correctly for several days. As a response to the plague in Cape Town an emergency Cape Peninsular Plague Advisory Board was set up, which had its first meeting on 14th February 1901, by which time 11 cases had been reported. The cases and people who had been in contact were removed to a Quarantine Camp established at Uitvlugt, initially in tents until a wood and iron house could be built. Dead rats had been noticed in the area around the docks for some months previously but had not been properly investigated, and it was only after the initial human case that enquiries were followed up about the dead rats. It was found that there had been large numbers dying around the Army stores at the docks over the previous couple of months - as many as 20 a day had been appearing, described as staggering around in a dazed state before dying and over 200 had been found dead in a haystack. In 1901 the precise way in which the disease went from rat to human was still not known although the spread by fleas was one of the modes being considered, along with the possibility of infection through wounds or scratches on the hands. It was recognised that dead rats should not be touched while the bodies were still warm without pouring carbolic acid, boiling water or a corrosive substance over them. The diagnosis of plague was confirmed in the dead rats and rat catchers were sent to the docks who within a week had killed a further 2,000. While controls were put in place around the docks, with labourers prevented from leaving, the disease still spread to the town appearing next in the Malay quarter. There were concerns that Africans in particular would panic and flee out of the city, and the railway and shipping authorities were requested to refuse to convey them. They were also requested to ensure that they did not convey rats around the country in their freight.

Concern was raised in meetings about the insanitary state of the city and its surrounding villages and inspectors were sent out to assess the situation. Attention focussed heavily on the presence of Africans, whom they associated with the social and sanitary conditions linked to plague in areas such as the Rondebosch Extension. The towns were to be cleared of litter, refuse and insanitary housing and owners of industrial furnaces were requested to render assistance by accepting refuse delivered for burning by the authorities. Concerns were also raised about the dreadful state of certain dairies and slaughterhouses, and the Masonic Hotel was said to have been in a worse state than any place previously inspected. A notice was drawn up to householders by Cape Town Council asking them to kill and burn rats immediately with paraffin and to keep their houses clean and well ventilated, with detailed advice given as to how to clean their houses with carbolic acid, whitewash and disinfectant.

The surrounding small towns and villages took extensive measures to try and control the outbreak. In the Green Point and Sea Point Municipality, between Table Mountain and the Bay, a reward of two pennies was offered for killed rats. At Woodstock the Municipality distributed 10,000 handbills, conducted extensive inspections and cleansing of dairies, butcheries, and bakeries, drains and gutters were disinfected; horse droppings were picked up and landlords were asked not to let their premises to African tenants as they were being provided for in a new location. In Rondebosch dogs had to be chained up to stop them from killing rats and stray dogs were destroyed. Pigs were banned from the municipality and three pence per rat offered. In Simon's Town 20 convicts were used to collect and destroy all street rubbish. At Kalk Bay several houses were completely destroyed by fire. A report on the state of Yzerplaat beyond Maitland by the Engineer Alex Shand described horrifically dirty conditions in the dairy, dwelling houses, and slaughter-house: 'decomposing heads and feet of oxen and portions of entrails lie indiscriminately about the place, and on these the pigs are feeding', and 'to convey any idea of the state of the quarters is beyond my powers. The stench emanating from the locality is absolutely sickening and enough to poison the immediate neighbourhood'. Another – 'the structure is built of corrugated iron and is extremely filthy inside, all the utensils belonging to the slaughter house are likewise disgustingly dirty'. Shand urged that action be taken to clean up the premises and the accompanying squalid shacks where people lived.[3]

By the 13th March 1901 137 cases had been reported: 24 European, 46 Coloured and 67 African. The total deaths up until then were 27. Locations for African workers (referred to as 'Aborigines') were initiated at the Docks to take them out of their insanitary homes and limit their movements. There were some 1,000 people at the quarantine camp in Uitvlugt including patients, contacts and staff. One patient, quite delirious, escaped and ran naked into Rondebosch before being captured some hours later, following which the camp was then fenced in. Residents ejected from insanitary dwellings were placed in tents and Africans were starting to be ejected to the location on the Cape Flats.[4] The suggestion was made that the removal of Africans to the new location would release many buildings which could then be cleansed and given to the Coloured population. During March 1901 some 6,000 to 7,000 Africans were moved to a hastily constructed settlement, later renamed Ndabeni, on the Cape Flats and their slum homes destroyed. The removals were effected in terms of the Public Health Act of 1883, which had been inspired by the smallpox epidemic in Cape Town in 1882 when over 4,000 people had died.[5] 1,500 African dock workers were evicted from their homes to a Dock Location, 27 huts established at the harbour, fenced in and controlled. Africans were forced to choose between life in the dock location or Ndabeni, the latter being at a great distance from their work.[6] Africans continued to be stopped from leaving the Cape by train or ship and their movement on tramcars was also prohibited. A Mr Withenshawe proposed a resolution that prevented 'Aboriginal Natives from walking on the side-walks and from travelling in any vehicle not specially set aside for that purpose'.[7] Mr Bradford representing Sea Point said that they had urged for the complete removal of Africans from the Municipality and Mr Hansen of Kalk Bay proposed that Africans should be prohibited from entering another Municipality without a pass. Mr Withenshawe's proposal was not passed, but the suggestions had echoes of future controls on Africans that would later come into being. The reasons for turning the proposals down were not always humanitarian either – three gentlemen said that 'the low class Coloured population were in many ways more objectionable than the Kaffirs, and that it was unjust to impose restrictions on the latter unless they were extended to the former, which was impracticable'.[8] In the face of the terror of plague attitudes of the White population towards Africans and other 'races' were hardening rapidly.

The cases had jumped to 246 by 25th March with 85 deaths. Many corpses had been found concealed by the Cape Malays. One European was found dead on the top of Table Mountain. In order to stop it spreading beyond the Cape Peninsula measures were put in place to medically examine all people travelling on the two main roads to the interior of the country. It was noted that the appalling state of housing in the Cape, which contributed to the spread of plague, was in great measure exacerbated by the refugees who had come to Cape Town to escape the War in the Transvaal and Orange River Colonies over the previous eighteen months.

As the epidemic progressed the cases were noted to be progressively more severe and more rapidly fatal. Many unidentified corpses were found in the streets. By 10th April there had been 366 cases with 139 deaths. Between 40 and 60 cases were reported each week with no sign yet of it slackening off. Inoculations were being undertaken with Haffkine's Prophylactic, which was said to be 80% effective, some 12,000 having been inoculated in Cape Town by that time. However it could not be used on the very young, old or sick people and was of limited use. The fact that some people who were inoculated still got the disease deterred people from coming forward for the inoculation. The state of the cemeteries was also disastrous with them being used for the deposit of trash and with crumbling vaults housing rats. Many of these cemeteries had been closed for years and lay neglected and decayed, being used as latrines and refuse dumps. It was recommended that several of them be completely done away with and the bones removed by relatives, if they wished, to be buried elsewhere. The cemeteries could then be transformed into parks or recreation areas: 'no good reason can be adduced why all these cemeteries should not now be completely done away with and their site be appropriated for a more sanitary purpose'. The neglect by the Trustees and the families of the graves and the state that the cemeteries were in 'should preclude the possibility of anyone opposing such a change on sentimental grounds. Sentiments which have been so long dead, as far as practical expression is concerned, cannot be very deep, and should now receive no consideration when the interests of the health of the living are concerned'.[9]

The toll of disease by 1st May had risen to 537 cases with 236 deaths: 44 European, 132 Coloured and 60 Africans. An increasing number of corpses were being found due partly to the reluctance of people to report sickness and partly to the disease becoming virulent and progressing so rapidly that people died within a few hours of onset. Great efforts were being made to clean up the municipalities and kill the rats, but the descriptions of some of the premises inspected were so dreadful that it makes one wonder why and how things had ever been allowed to deteriorate into that state. Pressure continued to remove Africans out of the towns with an additional location to Maitland sought on the Cape Flats for those Africans living in Wynberg, Claremont and other villages. A resolution was taken on 24th April that

> a Location be established somewhere on the Cape Flats which would provide a centre for Native labour supply for the suburbs; and that no Natives be allowed to wander about the suburbs without passes.[10]

This decision was to mark a seminal moment in the development of the country, setting the tone for future separate residential areas for different 'races'. In a Report from the Cape Divisional Council dated 15th May 1901 concern was expressed over the conditions on the Cape Flats, at which it was said that 'with regard to the Coloured people squatting all over the Flats, and whose hovels are mostly kept in a filthy state, great difficulty is experienced in trying to remove them from their present quarters'. They were not able to move into the African location and there were worries that driving them out would simply force them to settle elsewhere, also in squalor. The movement of Africans out of Wynberg appears have been successful with a later comment being made on 6th June that they were now at the location and their goods were being forwarded to them. By this time the plague at Cape Town was starting to diminish with fewer new cases being reported, and less than one a day by July. The camp at Maitland was used to accommodate those whose houses had been destroyed for being unsanitary. By the time the Board started to wind down at their meeting of 10th July 1901 some 35,630 rats had been destroyed and there had been 727 cases in the Cape Peninsula.

Forced removals of Africans as a response to plague, similar to the removals in Cape Town in 1901, would go on to be also carried out in Johannesburg in 1902–1903 and the related health legislation started the movement towards segregated urban housing in the country.[11] Serious outbreaks occurred soon after the Cape Peninsula outbreak in Port Elizabeth, East London, and other places in the Cape. The movement of grain and people across the country facilitated the spread along with the movement of ships through the ports, together with the unsanitary, overcrowded states of the towns and cities which had been exacerbated by the movements of people in the war. A case of plague broke out in Gubbs location, Port Elizabeth in April 1901, contracted while working at the harbour and carried by a ship from Buenos Aires, and dead rats were found on the harbour property near the forage dump. The fears of the white population were aroused and a cordon was placed around the location where some 5,000 Africans lived. The Port Elizabeth Council also created a Plague Board comprised of local representatives and public health experts which was empowered to take action regarding the control of the disease. Suspected cases or patients who had contracted the disease were placed in quarantine at the lazaretto and restrictions placed on the movement of Africans. Altogether the outbreak caused 183 deaths and 343 cases of plague in Port Elizabeth, 69 of which were among Whites. Rat-infested stores were fumigated, while homes in the locations were destroyed. By September 1902 over 600 dwellings had been condemned and burned down. The Board became a driving force in a plague eradication campaign, which turned into an anti-black health crusade, which forced many Africans out of the town.[12] The authorities drove the occupants out of the town carrying what they could of their dwellings on their heads. Some 7,000 Africans out of a total population of nearly 10,000 were removed in 1904, giving rise to the large townships of New Brighton and Korsten.[13] The original New Brighton accommodation was in a converted old Boer military camp and known as Red Location, later to degenerate into a slum giving rise to other diseases and health problems.

In Durban the Natal Government erected a Plague Hospital on Salisbury Island in the harbour in anticipation of the epidemic spreading across the country, and the wood and iron huts previously erected at the Back Beach during the smallpox outbreak were taken over by the Plague Administration Committee for the compulsory isolation of Africans and Indians.[14] Plague infected rats were reported from East London and Orange River by mid-1901. In 1902 a similar plague outbreak started in Durban and spread to Pietermaritzburg, and further outbreaks occurred in King Williamstown and Queenstown in 1903.

The first case in Durban was on 4th December 1902, the day after infected rats had been found, and during a period when the city was described as grossly insanitary, particularly in the back yards and servants' quarters. Hill described the conditions as ready for the plague to attack the city –'the numerous buildings of wood and iron provide easy harbourage for vermin, to the numbers of which accessions are made on the arrival of every ship'.[15] In the first week the disease was found to be causing a heavy mortality among rats around the Point area and it was thought most likely to have come from a load of Lucerne hay on the ship the S.S. Kassala from Argentina. The Town Councils of both Durban and Pietermaritzburg, which suffered far less than Durban from the plague, were considered to have neglected to have maintained their Boroughs in a satisfactory sanitary condition. The first cases had been limited to Durban's Point area by the harbour, where it was the responsibility of the Colonial Government, until 10th January when it had clearly moved to the centre of the town. At that point a Plague Committee was established by the Town Council with the Medical Officer of Health in charge of disinfection, sanitary measures and destruction of vermin. Circulars were issued to medical practitioners and the public and cases were removed to the ready-prepared Plague Hospital on Salisbury Island, which had twenty eight beds in four wards. When the first case occurred in a Muslim the community were given permission to erect separate accommodation for Muslims on the Island, but it was never completed. While the Island was considered well suited in terms of isolation the disadvantage was the transfer of the patient from the ambulance, across the wharf to a boat and then again by stretcher to the hospital. Those who died in the hospital were at first buried at sea to avoid the funerals passing through the town, but when this proved too expensive and difficult they changed to burning them on an open pyre in the way of the Hindus, except for Muslims who were allowed to remove them in lead-lined coffins.

The outbreak caused only minor panic, mainly in mid January when the African population started to leave in large numbers – partly because the White population started to prevent them from sharing lodgings with their employees and many were then rendered homeless, and partly due to a degree of panic after the open cremations commenced. In the eight months of the outbreak 221 cases were found, of which 164 had buboes. Of these bubonic cases 59 recovered and 105 died. Altogether out of the 221 cases 162 died, or 73%. The disease spread out from the centre to the Berea, Malvern, and other places outside the Borough as far as Pietermaritzburg where there was a small outbreak which started at the Brewery with nine cases and six deaths. Altogether only 20 of the cases were European, 83 being African and 92 Indian, with the vast majority being male due to their greater exposure at work – 22% were found to have worked in stores or stables. Some cases were thought to have been concealed due to the fear of the authorities. The Report of Hill stated that the outbreak fell:

> with greatest severity where-on persons living in those parts of the town which are maintained least in accord with the principles of sanitary science. Where the dwellings are of the worst construction and most dilapidated, where ventilation is most deficient, where overcrowding and filth are greatest, where scavenging [street litter collection] is least attended to, there plague most prevailed among the residents.[16]

While the disease was known to be spread by rats and other rodents the matter of the flea as a vector was still being debated – it was certainly recognised by then that it could be spread by fleas, but spread through rat droppings or other methods was still under consideration. In pneumonic plague spread via the nose, mouth, in the air or food was considered. Every case was investigated carefully and detailed discussion made on the cases in the Report on the Natal Plague of Ernest Hill of 1904.

The control measures employed included the destruction of vermin by phosphorus and arsenic. In Pietermaritzburg the Council had been paying the public for some time to bring in dead rats as a preventive measure, which possibly contributed to the low numbers of plague there. Some 24,000 rats were brought in between February and August 1903 at a cost to the Council of £500, but this was rejected in Durban as encouraging people to carry dead plague-infected rats about with them.

However the measure in Pietermaritzburg was thought very effective by Hill and considered money well spent. At the Pietermaritzburg Brewery where the few cases originated the premises were rapidly fenced with corrugated iron, the floors disinfected and vermin destroyed. No infected rats or mice were subsequently found in the town. In Durban particular attention was paid to stores, granaries, stables, houses where plague had occurred and particularly dirty or dilapidated buildings. Evacuation was undertaken in the areas of Bamboo Square, Brickhill Road and the Indian Immigration Depot. Numbers of wood and iron shacks and hovels were pulled down and inhabitants moved to the outskirts and suburbs. Haffkine's inoculation was used as treatment, as was Yersin's serum which was found to be ineffective. Where cases occurred in African Kraals (family homesteads) the whole kraal was placed under quarantine, but generally segregation of those who had been exposed was not undertaken for fear it may cause concealment and flight of people, thus spreading it further.

Precautionary measures were taken to try and stop rats boarding ships at the harbour, using structures attached to the cables and hawsers and raising the gangways at night, but it was thought fumigation before sailing would be more effective had they had the correct apparatus. No special measures were taken to examine people travelling by road or rail, save to watch carefully at stations for people who looked sick. However Special Regulations were passed by the Governor of the Colony under the Natal Public Health Act of 1901 in January. This included the compulsion by all owners of stores in which grain, bran, flour, hay and fodder were stored to block all rodent holes with cement, and the storage or movements of such produce was strictly controlled. The Medical Officer of Health was empowered to destroy any stores or produce that was suspect, and to remove suspect patients to the plague hospital. He was also empowered to close any building, dispose of any body, demolish any structure and remove the occupants of any house which posed a threat. All employers of Coloured labour in Durban had to report any sickness absenteeism to a Medical Practitioner and suspect cases had to be reported to the Plague Administration Department at the Point. Concealing any sickness became an offence. After eight months the epidemic eventually wound down, with the last Natal cases being in August 1903.[17] As a comment in the Plague Report of Ernest Hill, the then Medical Officer of Health of Durban, Dr P. Murison, described the city thus 'The housing of servants was in many cases of a most wretched description, and many houses occupied by Europeans were quite unfit for such a purpose'. He continued

> With an Indian or Kaffir population constant supervision is essential, for their ideas of sanitation are not sufficient, in my opinion, to allow them to live in any area where Europeans reside; but while such is the order of things they will have to conform to the habits of the White man. Durban has benefitted very much regarding sanitary matters by the incidence of plague.[18]

While mass African removals outside the city were not recommended in the Report of Hill, it is clear that this was starting to occur in the thinking of the Medical Officer of Health. In the early years of the twentieth century epidemic plague started to present an opportunity for those who were promoting segregationist policies, by equating black urban settlement, labour and living conditions – which actually resulted from underpay and neglect - with threats to public health, described by Swanson as 'the Sanitation Syndrome'. As with Cape Town and Port Elizabeth beforehand, segregation due to the plague at the start of the twentieth century was also noted in other colonized countries, including what was then the colonial city of Salisbury in Rhodesia (now Harare in Zimbabwe) and Dakar in Senegal.[19]

In 1904 a considerable outbreak occurred in Johannesburg which persisted up until 1905. It broke out in the area of Brickfields, which was at that time an 'insanitary area', considered a giant slum, of some 5,000 to 6,000 people of whom 2,000 were European. The plague occurred in what was known as the 'Coolie Location' on the edge of the area, where both Indians and Africans lived, with the first case occurring on 20th March 1904. Those affected had been moved to one hut, where it was found that seven people had died. A police cordon was set up but within two days 42 people had died. Measures to combat the disease included the offering of three pence per tail for dead rats, the removal of the entire population to an isolation camp and the burning of the entire location by the Fire Department on 3rd April 1904. 1,600 houses and shops and one Indian temple in six blocks were surrounded with sheet-iron fencing, doused in paraffin and destroyed. In May dead rats were found in the Market buildings and thousands of people watched a huge bonfire on 18th May of the fixtures which were removed from the building, and the building was cleansed. A Rand Plague Committee was established to deal with the outbreak and its aftermath. After the outbreak the Market, which had been closed for eight months, was bought out by the Johannesburg Town Council, and the cleared area of Brickfields was re-designated Newtown and stands sold to Europeans.[20] Altogether the outbreak had caused 147 cases by mid 1904 and 96 deaths – the Asian population suffering particularly severely with 55 deaths. An isolation camp was formed at Klipspruit to which 1,500 inhabitants were removed before their homes were destroyed. A depot was formed at the Pass Office in Johannesburg to receive them and to allow them to claim back their property. All Africans wanting to travel were examined at the Pass Offices beforehand – over 47,000 being examined by the end of June.[21]

The insanitary area that formed parts of the Burgersdorp and Fordsburg townships was laid out, with 646 new stands and provision for an abattoir. The cleared residents were re-settled nine miles from the centre of town in the location of Kliptown, later known as Pimville, where the Town Engineer's department had erected iron barracks and huts. Others put up shacks for themselves.[22] The Native Affairs Department assisted with the removal of some 7,000 people and compensation was offered to them for their 866 wood and iron buildings. The Department considered the new arrangement and the new location a model which other towns could adopt, based on the 'liberal treatment and consideration' which the town council had extended to the people. Water had been laid on and buildings could be acquired by lease for 33 years. Others were encouraged to erect their own dwellings and facilities established for schools, churches and public buildings. A cheap and regular train service was laid on. The Native Affairs Commissioner for the Transvaal commented:

> In these and other ways the Johannesburg Town Council has used its best endeavours to study the interests and provide for the requirements of the Natives. I trust that in course of time the conditions which prevail in other township locations may be improved in a similar manner, for it is quite certain that the better they are made the more prospect there will be of securing a permanent supply of town labour and of inducing a respectable class of native to settle in such locations.[23]

However it was not long before Pimville deteriorated into a slum.

The total cases reported nationally up until 1905 was 1,694 with 947 deaths.[24] These outbreaks were associated with a plague amongst the local rodents, mainly black and brown rats and ordinary domestic mice. During the outbreaks in Knysna, Mossel Bay and Graaff Reinet wild striped mice were found dead of the plague around the towns. Small outbreaks occurred in King William's Town in 1903, 1905 and 1907 with 33, 11 and 25 cases respectively, thought to have been brought up from East London in trains by infected rats. In 1903 the rats were found in a dilapidated and insanitary building known as the Market Building and belonging to the King William's Town Council, which was subsequently condemned and demolished, for which the Council claimed £1,286 compensation from the Government. In the 1907 outbreak a government Medical Officer was despatched to investigate and found after extensive enquiry how the disease had travelled between family members, kraals, and villages due to the various meanderings of infected individuals, spreading the disease as pneumonic plague across the district.

During the period up to 1912 no human plague was found in the country, but in 1912 an outbreak occurred in Durban with 32 cases and 26 deaths, presumed to be introduced by infected rats from vessels from Eastern ports. In 1914 a virulent outbreak of pneumonic plague occurred in the Tarka District of the Eastern Cape, which then spread to Queenstown, Middelburg, Glen Grey and Uitenhage. In 1914 there were 35 cases with 31 deaths, in 1915 45 cases with 26 deaths, and in 1916 24 cases with 13 deaths. It then began to appear on scattered farms of the Free State, moving on the following year to the Transvaal district of Potchefstroom where 15 cases, 14 fatal, occurred. In March 1920 an outbreak came again in Kroonstad. In most of these cases the source of the infection remained a mystery as the ordinary species of domestic rodents were practically non-existent in these rural districts. Extensive searches and research were undertaken to try and ascertain the responsible rodents, with rodent trackers and trappers employed across the areas. Samples of fleas on various wild rodents were examined, including gerbils (Tatera lobengulae), the large-eared mouse (Malocothrix typicus) and the multi-mammate mouse(Matomys coucha), and it was noted that the rodent populations of the Free State had increased due to the almost complete eradication of jackals, lynxes and wild cats. Following the death of a farmer near Bothaville from plague in February 1921 an extensive search was undertaken of the area where he had been ploughing, which unearthed eight dead gerbils and 150 dead multi-mammate mice later found to be plague-infested. This ended a long and painstaking investigation, and it was concluded that the two types of rodents were the connecting link between the infected fleas and man.[25] The plague had moved from the classic rat-borne urban type of plague to a sylvatic rural-rodent type.

By the mid 1920's plague was described as smouldering or active in rural rodents throughout the greater part of the Orange Free State and considerable areas of the Cape Province and Transvaal. While outbreaks were usually fairly quickly stamped out, the greatest danger was a delay in diagnosis and notification. The National Health Department expected local authorities to take all possible and practicable measures to meet the danger and to prepare for emergencies. Guidelines were issued on how to make the initial diagnosis, and how to take and dispatch specimens for laboratory analysis to the government laboratories in Johannesburg, Cape Town and Durban. Rodents were to be searched for and carcasses dipped in petrol or paraffin to destroy the fleas before sending for analysis. Where specimens were expected to take two days or more to arrive it was recommended to 'sew up in a thick towel or cloth the fruit or jam jar containing the specimens...and place it in a pail or milk can two thirds full of ice, and cover with a lid or towel'. Those undertaking post-mortems were advised to wear rubber gloves and at all times to beware of fleas, which left the body soon after death: 'the examination should even be made in the open (on farms etc) in preference to a hut or room in which there may be infected fleas'. Under the Public Health Act and Regulations every case or suspected death from plague, or any unusual mortality in rodents, cats, dogs or other susceptible animals, had to be reported to the Local Authority along with the Magistrate, a Justice of the Peace or the Police. Confinement of cases and contacts was enforced, and the disinfection of contacts, bedding, clothing, houses, storage sheds etc described. Cyanide fumigation was recommended or soaking in disinfectant and the soaking of African huts with perchloride of mercury solution followed by re-plastering. The property and boundaries were to be marked with yellow flags or paint and quarantine measures enforced.

There was no specific treatment for the plague, although anti-plague vaccine was thought to have considerable protective value. Treatment was of the symptoms, using adrenaline, strychnine, oil of camphor and brandy as cardiac stimulants to prevent heart failure. Dealing with the rodents in outbreaks was difficult. In a badly rat-infested town once the infection was introduced amongst the rodents the limitation of spread was almost impossible and a severe outbreak in man was almost inevitable. The rats died of plague in under-floor spaces and the fleas then made their way up through the cracks in the floors and onto the legs of the residents.[26]

By 1925 natural plague infection had been recorded in other animals, including the striped mouse, the ground squirrel, the Eastern Karoo rat, the spring hare, the suricat and the yellow mongoose. Every rodent tested had been found to be sensitive to infection and all veld rodents appeared to be more sensitive than the common black rat, which made them all potential agents in the spread of plague. The suricat and mongoose were thought to get plague by feeding on infected rodents.

The spread in gerbils was thought to be exacerbated by their habit of feeding cannibalistically upon sick gerbils. Continuous catching and testing of rodents was occurring but few infected fleas were found. Their burrows however were found to be infected for a period of at least six months after the inhabitants had died of plague.[27] A rodent survey of the Union had been completed and it was being found that the ploughing and cultivation of land formerly hard and unsuitable for burrowing rodents were improving the conditions for their multiplication. Occasional cases of human plague were still reported from around the country but not in epidemic form. By 1927 the plague infested areas were increasing northwest-ward and was expected to shortly reach the coast. Attempts were made to create rodent-free belts of veld one to two miles wide, but there was a risk that hares, which could travel considerable distances overnight, could spread the fleas across the belt. Gerbils and hares were exterminated by either by gassing or by burning their nests and killing with sticks or dogs. The disease was also spreading in the Eastern Cape and Transvaal through drought, which increased the migration of rodents and hares, through ploughing and through the destruction of natural rodent enemies such as mongoose, wild cats and owls.[28]

In 1930 there were 145 cases with 89 deaths, mostly traceable to local veld rodent infection. 107 of the cases were in the Free State and adjacent Transvaal of which 84 were bubonic, 16 septicaemic and nine pneumonic-type plague.[29] Cases remained low during the early 1930's although the risk remained. The Department of Health was concerned that local authorities in the Cape were not taking it seriously enough, except for Cape Town, although the South African Railways and Harbours administration were putting more effective anti-rodent measures into place with rat-proofing of structures and gassing taking place.[30] An increase was experienced in 1934 with possibly the worst outbreak and mortality amongst rodents yet seen, following weather conditions which had been favourable for the growth of the grasses, the seed of which fed the gerbils. The National Department had issued a warning in November 1934 that spread could occur from the gerbils to domestic rodents and then humans, In the predicted outbreak which ensued urban areas were largely spared, due to the authorities having enforced rodent proofing of buildings and stores where previously rodents had been harboured. However in some local authorities the National Department ascribed their avoidance of a worse epidemic to 'good luck rather than to good management', particularly in the case of Bloemfontein where the local authority had 'always systematically ignored the requirements of the rat-proofing regulations and repeatedly shelved the recommendation of its own Medical Officer of Health in regard to their enforcement'. This had given rise to an extreme infestation of rodents, which lead to 35 cases and 29 deaths from plague in humans in Bloemfontein District in an outbreak which began in January 1935. Altogether that year in the Orange Free State, neighbouring Cape areas and western Transvaal there were 290 cases and 184 deaths. In the Marico District of the Transvaal the plague spread rapidly through a densely populated African location. 850 huts were dealt with by dusting the floors with cyano-dust and subsequent flaming with a blow-lamp, one of several methods under investigation for the control of rats and fleas.[31.] A similar number of cases occurred in 1936 but then started to decrease. In the Port Elizabeth-Uitenhage area of the Cape outbreaks were experienced between 1930 and 1934, and then again in 1938 when there were 26 cases with 17 deaths. Analysis found that in urban areas the flea bites were more likely to be on the legs, leading to buboes in the inguinal (groin) area, and in rural areas the bites were more likely on the arms causing axillary (armpit) buboes. It was suggested that the arm bites came while collecting firewood with fleas in mice nests, handling animal carcasses, or eating rats in the case of young boys.[32]

As a major area of risk for the spread of rodents and plague the railways had specific programmes in place in the affected areas to try and prevent the movement of rats by rail, with rat-proofing taking place on their premises. They were 'building the rat out of railway premises' by preventing access to guttering, roof ridging and hollow walls with wire netting and sheet iron, planting them to a depth of 60 centimetres to prevent access to the foundations. This applied to goods sheds, stations and grain stores. Cracks and loose stones in drains and channels were cemented smooth and canalised.

The Health Department employed a Plague Consultant in 1939 to survey the plague situation in the country with specific reference to urban areas. The most prevalent area for human plague was the Glen Grey area of the Transkei, where heavy mortality also occurred in domestic rodents. Continuous and extensive analysis of the various types of rodents, breeding sites and fleas took place across the country and across a broad spectrum of locations, from floor sweepings of African huts to farmhouses and burrows in open veld. In 1940 there was an outbreak of pneumonic plague in the Bothaville district of northern Free State where the rural rodents were first identified. Eight Europeans had died, and it was traced back to the handling by a child of an infected dead or dying rodent found outside the homestead. Bothaville was an important maize growing area where the large areas of cultivated land and abundant grain were favourable factors for rodent infestation and the sandy soil favoured the gerbils which infested the area. An increase in plague was marked by a decrease in visible rodent activity due to their deaths, which caused the fleas to move on to humans. Plague was also reported to the north of Vereeniging, which was considered unnervingly close to Johannesburg. The following year it occurred in an African reserve called Morokwen, a remote place in the Kalahari Desert where an investigation was undertaken with 'a most arduous search amid the waterless and almost trackless wastes of the Kalahari, along all possible further avenues of spread'. 1,000 people were vaccinated with a new live plague vaccine, but altogether 36 people died of pneumonic plague.[33] The onset of World War 2 increased the risk of plague arriving at the ports due to the greatly increased number of ships arriving, owing partly to ships having to be diverted away from the Mediterranean and passing around Africa and the Cape instead on their way to the East. It was difficult to tell if these ships had come from plague-infested ports so there were strict controls with 'rat shields' and inspections undertaken both on arrival and before the discharge of cargo.

The Bothaville area was again visited by plague in 1942, the first case being an elderly African woman, from whom it spread through the community after her death. The affected houses were quarantined, but it was thought to be too late as many people had visited the sick. Altogether there were 11 cases of pneumonic plague, all middle aged or elderly Africans, of whom 10 died – no children were affected, even those in close contact with victims. The one recovery was considered quite remarkable, as the pneumonic form of the disease was usually 100% fatal. The entire location was vaccinated and quarantined until 12 days after the last case, to prevent the spread to the nearby European population. Food and fuel was delivered to their houses.[34] The only specific treatments available at that time were the sulphonamides, although their effectiveness was only proven in animals.

Experiments with the insecticide DDT started from 1945, following its remarkable success with typhus control during the Second World War, and its use was being suggested as a possible means to control the plague by pumping it into gerbil and other rodent burrows. This would address the fear that killing the rodents released the fleas which then jumped onto human hosts instead. The residual effect of DDT meant that its impact lasted for long periods and there was reason to hope that the vigorous quarantine measures employed would be able to be relaxed, except in the case of pneumonic plague. The distribution of plague in animals remained mainly in a wide swath from the northern Orange Free State down through most of the Province, through the Transkei to Port Elizabeth, with some scattered cases throughout the Karoo. A rodent-free belt was maintained between the small towns of Citrusdal and Elandsbay in the Cape which was 65 miles long and between one and four miles wide to attempt to prevent the movement of plague-carrying rodents. A team was employed to keep it clear and destroy domestic rodents living in farm buildings in the belt. Rodents were killed using strychnine, cyano-gas dust and by hand and over 10,000 were killed in 1946 alone. Cape Town itself, although being infested with gerbils on the Cape Flats, did not have another serious outbreak after the 1901 epidemic – possibly from having since pursued energetic rodent and plague control measures. In 1948 the addition of streptomycin to sulphonamides in the treatment of plague was being considered helpful, with another case of pneumonic plague – contracted through a laboratory – surviving.

The incidence of plague continued to remain low through the 1950's due to stringent rodent surveillance and control measures. The advent of the chemical warfarin as a rat poison made a huge difference to the fight against the rodent population. Extensive experiments had resulted in the production of bait which was both acceptable to the rodents and very effective in destroying them. Some 6,000kg were used in Cape Town in 1954 and the beaches and other rodent infested areas were almost completely cleared.[35]

While ever hovering in the background, plague made its appearance only sporadically in small outbreaks such as one in the Uitenhage district in October 1959 with ten cases and four deaths, all African. It was commented that at least one of the patients was a 'rat-eater' – said to be a common practice amongst children in that area.[36] Flea destruction was commenced at the New Brighton location and surrounding areas just four days later but in November plague infected fleas were found just outside the Port Elizabeth boundary. Intensive gassing with cyanide gas was undertaken in the area and in the Zwartkops village, with further destruction of fleas and rodents in the African villages nearby. The treatment regimes were said to be quite effective if commenced within a day or two of onset, using streptomycin, aureomycin and other antibiotics, but some patients still presented to medical authorities too late which meant that the overall mortality was still much the same as in the pre-antibiotic era, and it was hard to show that antibiotic treatment had yet made any difference. Still it was anticipated that prompt treatment would save 90%, the main problem being making an early diagnosis, particularly of the first cases. As a response to the outbreak an

Eastern Province Plague and Health Committee was established, which first met on 2nd February 1960 after the Uitenhage outbreak and included representatives of the Department of Health and Local Authority. The main hosts of the fleas in the area were Namaqua gerbils (Desmodillus) and attention was focussed on eradicating the rodents and fleas, similar to the programme in the Orange Free State and the Transkei. The programme aimed at dusting all rodent burrows for a radius of 200 yards around farmsteads and African kraals with DDT 10% or malathion 5% dusting powder, followed three to four days later with laying poisoned wheat in the burrows.[37] In town the predominant rodents were rats and the municipality proceeded to inspect 3,410 dwellings and 156 rodents in the following year.

Similar odd cases continued to occur through the 1960's and an epidemic occurred in neighbouring Lesotho in 1968 which killed 50 people. It still smouldered in wild rodents in the eastern Cape, the Orange Free State and the northern Cape, and still occurred in neighbouring countries, but there were no significant outbreaks reported in South Africa. Only one human case was reported in the period 1972-1981 due to the extensive control measures in place, until an outbreak occurred in 1982. In this year record rodent increases were found in the dense natural bush near Port Elizabeth, Uitenhage, Dispatch and Kirkwood. Two cases of plague in man were reported in February 1982 in Coega, a small village of 15 mud and wood huts around a church mission near Port Elizabeth, and a further 13 cases occurred shortly after. The 100 inhabitants of Coega were examined daily and suspect cases admitted to hospital. Extensive capture and examination of rodents and their fleas was undertaken with residents reporting that both had been abundant in and around the huts before the outbreak. The striped mouse Rhabdomys pumilio was found to be positive for plague, as were all eight cats and dogs tested at the mission who also died of the disease. At least one of the human cases had eaten a cat which had died with a swollen head, indicating plague infection. Altogether some 93 dogs and cats and 139 small mammals were caught and tested within a 5km radius of the village. An extensive response was organised including quarantine, preventive treatment, rodent and flea control involving multiple government departments and the outbreak was contained with only one death. Plague remained a potential problem in the area as plague-positive dogs and rodents were traced over a wide area, and because the plague bacteria could remain alive for a year in deserted rat tunnels. Follow-up surveys were done of the entire Eastern Cape, testing some 1132 small mammals and almost 6,000 dogs. Of these 6 of the mammals, 21 of the dogs and 2 out of 6 cats tested positive for the plague.[38,39] However no cases in man were reported in the years that followed, and there is no mention in subsequent Department of Health Reports.

Across South Africa, while plague may remain a lingering threat, the continuing rodent control measures and surveillance hopefully mean that the disease is largely in the past. However as rodent numbers increase in uncontrolled peri-urban settlements, and local government refuse removal services are often unable to cope, it could perhaps reappear – the disease still exists in other parts of the world from which it could be brought to South Africa, especially considering the vast amount of shipping calling at the ports. However any future outbreaks would probably be rapidly brought under control due to the long experience in implementing remedial measures, and the disease itself is now treatable, with a much lower mortality than in the pre-antibiotic era.

ENDNOTES

1. Simpson W.J. *Memorandum dated 10 February 1901 to the Cape Peninsular Plague Advisory Board*, WA Richards, Cape Town, G61- '1901, 1901: 30-36
2. Cluver E.H. *Public Health in South Africa*, Central News Agency Ltd, Fifth Edition (no date given) p194.
3. *Report and Proceedings of the Cape Peninsular Plague Advisory Board*, WA Richards, Cape Town, 1901, G61-'1901
4. 'Minutes of the Meeting of 13th March 1901' *Cape Peninsular Plague Advisory Board*, WA Richards Cape Town, 1901, G61-'1901: 39-42
5. Swanson, M.W. 'The Sanitation Syndrome: Bubonic Plague and Urban Native Policy in the Cape Colony 1900-1909'; *Journal of African History* 18 1977:392.
6. Bickford-Smith, *Vivian, Ethnic Pride and Racial Prejudice in Victorian Cape Town*, Witwatersrand University Press, Johannesburg 1995:183,205
7. 'Minutes of the Meeting of 13th March 1901', *Cape Peninsular Plague Advisory Board*, WA Richards Cape Town, 1901, G61-'1901: 39-42
8. 'Minutes of the Meeting of 20th March 1901', *Cape Peninsular Plague Advisory Board*, WA Richards, Cape Town 1901, G61-'1901: 57
9. 'Medical Officer's Report on Disused Cemeteries, Dated 18th April 1901,' *Cape Peninsular Plague Advisory Board*, WA Richards and Sons, Cape Town 1901, G61-'1901: 191
10. 'Minutes of the Meeting of 24th April 1901', *Cape Peninsular Plague Advisory Board*, WA Richards Cape Town 1901, G61-'1901: 122
11. Packard, R.M. *White Plague, Black Labour: Tuberculosis and the Political Economy of Health and Disease in South Africa,*: University of Natal Press, Pietermaritzburg 1989: 53
12. Holland, E.M. An Experiment in Slum Clearance Housing in Urban Native Areas, *Race Relations* 7(4) 1940: 70.

13 Baines Gary; 'The Control and Administration of Port Elizabeth's African Population circa. 1834-1923'; *Contree* 26 1989:16
14 O'Reagan M. *The Hospital Services of Natal*, Natal Regional Survey No 8, University of Natal, Durban, Robinson and Co, 1970:19
15 Hill Ernest, *Report on the Plague in Natal, 1902-1903*, Cassell and Company, London 1904:10
16 Ibid, 29
17 Ibid, 79-86
18 Murison P. cited in Hill Ernest, *Report on the Plague in Natal, 1902-1903*, Cassell and Company, London 1904:
19 Swanson, M.W. 'The Sanitation Syndrome: Bubonic Plague and Urban Native Policy in the Cape Colony 1900-1909' *Journal of African History*; 18 1977:410.
20 Neame L.E, *City Built on Gold*, Central News Agency, Cape Town, 1960:158-160.
21 Lagden G.Y. *Report by the Commissioner for Native Affairs, Transvaal, for the year ended 30th June 1904*, Pretoria, Government Printing and Stationery office, 1904, pA6.
22 Shorten J.R, *The Johannesburg Saga*, John R Shorten for the Johannesburg City Council, 1970:240-241
23 Lagden G.Y. *Report by the Commissioner for Native Affairs, Transvaal, for the year ended 30th June 1906*, Pretoria, Government Printing and Stationery office, 1906 p A24.
24 Cluver E.H. Public Health in South Africa, Central News Agency, Fifth Edition (no date given), p194.
25 Mitchell J.A. 'Plague in South Africa: perpetuation and spread of infection by wild rodents'. *South African Medical Record*, 19(24) 1921:475-477
26 'Plague: Control Eradication and Prevention', Extract from a Union Public Health Memorandum published *in South African Medical Record*, 23(7) 1925:146-150
27 Ingram A. Harvey Pirie J.H, 'Report on Bacteriological Research carried out in connection with Plague during 1925', *South African Medical Record*, 24(11) 1926:252-257
28 *Annual Report of the Department of Public Health, Union of South Africa, 1927*, Government Printing and Stationery Office Pretoria, UG 35-'27, 1927:36-39
29 *Annual Report of the Department of Public Health, Union of South Africa, 1930*, Government Printer Pretoria, UG 40-'30, p39.
30 *Annual Report of the Department of Public Health, Union of South Africa, 1933*, Government Printer Pretoria, UG 30-'33, p31
31 *Annual Report of the Department of Public Health, Union of South Africa, 1935*, Government Printer Pretoria, UG 43-'35, p32-34
32 Prinsloo A.J. Address given by Mr AJ Prinsloo, Medical Ecology Centre, Johannesburg to meeting of the Eastern Province Plague and Health Committee at Town Hall, Walmer, on Thursday the 2nd March 1961 – 'The Eradication of the Namaqua Gerbille and fleas' in: *Annual Report of the Medical Officer of Health for Port Elizabeth, 1960*, Longs, 1961:50-53
33 *Annual Report of the Department of Public Health, Union of South Africa, 1941*, Government Printer Pretoria, UG 46-'41, p27
34 Maule Clark B. 'Pneumonic Plague: Recovery in a Proved Case', *South African Medical Journal*, 17(4), 1943:57-60
35 *Annual Report of the Medical Officer of Health, City of Cape Town, 1954*, Cape Times, Parow, 1954:64
36 *Annual Report of the Department of Health, Republic of South Africa, 1959*, Government Printer 1962, RP 28/1962 p2

37 Prinsloo A.J. Address given by Mr AJ Prinsloo, Medical Ecology Centre, Johannesburg to meeting of the Eastern Province Plague and Health Committee at Town Hall, Walmer, on Thursday the 2nd March 1961 – 'The Eradication of the Namaqua Gerbille and fleas' in: *Annual Report of the Medical Officer of Health for Port Elizabeth, 1960,* Longs, 1961:50-53

38 Retief F.P. *Report of the Director-General for Health and Welfare for the year 1982*; Department of Health and Welfare Pretoria; 1982:1-3

39 Shepherd A.J. Hummitzsch D.E. Leman P.A, Hartwig E.K. 'Studies on Plague in the eastern Cape Province of South Africa', *Transactions of the Royal Society of Tropical Medicine and Hygiene,* 77(6) 1983:800-808

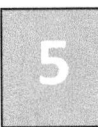

TYPHOID: A PROBLEM RELOCATED

The origins of typhoid (caused by the bacteria Salmonella typhi) in South Africa are not entirely clear, owing probably to it having been hard to distinguish from other causes of high fever and generalised illness before microbiological diagnoses were made. Certainly fever is mentioned frequently and it is possible that it started with the very first settlers. Just one month after the surgeon Johann van Riebeeck's arrival at the Cape to set up a station for the Dutch East India Company in April 1652, the ships the Walvis and the Oliphant arrived with large numbers of sick men. Although their sicknesses were mainly dysentery – or the 'red flux' – there may also have been typhoid, as the severity of the disease and the high fever which lasted around six weeks, indicated that some of the men may have suffered from it. It also appeared to occur at the start of the rainy season at the same time of the year, which was very suggestive of typhoid. One of the main reasons for the establishment of a settlement at the Cape was to provide care for the many sailors who got sick on the long voyages, particularly from scurvy. The ship Walvis had lost 45 men and the Oliphant 85 by the time the ships landed at the port. Again in February 1653 Van Riebeeck reports much illness: 'one after the other is being laid up with weakness, dysentery, dropsy and fever to such an extent that this week between 30 and 40 have fallen ill, unable altogether to work'.[1] The first hospital was established in tents, followed by a permanent structure in 1656. This was a year in which a great deal of sickness was reported in the winter, which the council considered to be 'beyond doubt a punishment inflicted upon them for their sins'.[2] However the vast majority of sickness seems to have been due to scurvy rather than infectious disease as once on land most of the sick recovered. The toll from scurvy continued to be severe – the ship Amersfoort in 1665 arrived with 39 dead, and more than 80 sick sailors were taken to the hospital. The De Walcharen had lost 62 men since leaving Holland, and '120 were prostrate, and the others so stiff with scurvy that they could hardly move hand or foot'.[3]

Instructions for general hygiene on ships were issued in 1696, including the recording of illness and separation of the sick, and instructions for Surgeons were added in December. Should any 'stench or impurity' be observed the ships were to be washed, cleansed and purified, 'removing the stench and dirt from which also much sickness springs'. The keeping of medical records was stressed, along with treatment given 'in order so to find out the cause of the disease, and the great mortality raging for some time on the ships'.[4] It is not easy to determine the nature of some of these early diseases: for example in 1700 it was recorded that 'a contagious disease having broken out among the slaves, so that within six months about 220 slaves have died, and the mortality has not yet ceased'.[5] One can probably assume, however, that it was not smallpox or the plague as they would have been easily recognisable.

A further hospital was built in 1759 to cater for the large number of sick arriving at Simon's Bay and policies for the separation of patients with infectious diseases, for the reporting by Captains of sick crew members and the cleanliness of the facility were introduced in 1765. By 1787 health control measures in Simon's Bay laid down that a ship with sick sailors, possibly suffering from infectious diseases, would not be allowed to anchor in the normal anchorage and must fly a red flag while at anchor.[6]

While we are uncertain of the extent of typhoid at the Cape in the early years it was certainly a feature in Europe - in the Franco-Prussian War of 1870-1871 there were 73,000 cases of typhoid in the German Army with 6,900 deaths.[7] Prior to this period it remains difficult to accurately assess as it was not identified and recorded as a separate disease until the mid 1800's. Following this the sanitary reform movement in Europe promoted the construction of piped waters supplies and water-carriage of sewage to abolish the open-draining, foul and insanitary latrines. The spread of these interventions in water and sanitation resulted in a fall in typhoid in England and Wales by 50% up to 1900 and by a further 46% over the next 25 years. However, while Europe was actively cleaning itself up, South Africa was rapidly becoming worse in many urban areas due to the rush into mining and industrialising cities, with inadequate provision for the arrivals.

Following the gold rush to the Witwatersrand towards the end of the nineteenth century the insanitary conditions created by the early arrivals created perfect conditions for the spread of typhoid. Just four years after the commencement of the town in 1886 an epidemic raged and, although the climate was considered healthy, the water supply was described as 'thick and muddy'. Wells were shallow, just a few feet deep, and received drainage from the surrounding cesspools and garbage such that the water sometimes resembled diluted sewage. Other wells were contaminated by cattle kraals. Sanitary provision was primitive and there was no proper provision for refuse removal. In the suburb of Doornfontein in May when night soil removal ceased it was followed shortly thereafter by an outbreak of typhoid.[8] Typhoid was then widespread across the country, with an epidemic in the George area on the south coast which, in the space of three months, affected 100 people and caused 20 deaths in the nearby village of Pacaltsdorp. The school was used as an isolation hospital and cash donations came from Cape Town, Port Elizabeth and George to help the needy. By the time the outbreak was over in September 30 people had died.[9] Typhoid continued to rage across Johannesburg for the first 20 years of its existence due largely to the uncontrolled and over-rapid urbanisation for which little sanitary provision had been made. The Johannesburg hospital was opened in 1890 and approximately 40% of the admissions were typhoid sufferers.[10] 196 Europeans died in 1896 in the city from the disease, although after piped water was installed, around 1897, the incidence started to decline. Still tests showed that only half of the water supplied was fit for drinking and the state of water in the wells was even worse.[11]

The most devastating typhoid epidemics in South Africa occurred during the Anglo-Boer War (South African War) of 1899-1902, when the British Army alone had nearly 58,000 cases out of 556,653 men who served in the war. Of these 8,225 died – more than the 7,792 reported as killed in action. When the war started on 11th October 1899 the disease was already endemic across the country and was reported as present in Kimberley at the end of November 1899. The disease then arose early in the War, largely after the battle of Magersfontein just south of Kimberley in the Orange Free State in December 1899, when for a long period some 30,000 troops were static on the banks of the Modder River. They started to drink water straight from the river which was heavily polluted and the result was a massive outbreak of typhoid fever with the first cases reported on 23rd December. By January 1900, 97 cases with 17 deaths had been reported which had risen to 156 cases and 27 deaths by 6th February. When the army started to march on to Kimberley and Bloemfontein at the end of the month the disease went with them, with increasing numbers of soldiers becoming ill and the men enduring great suffering having been on half-rations for most of the march.

While camped in Bloemfontein, within one month of their arrival on 13th March 1900, between 4,000 and 6,000 out of some 25,000 British soldiers were taken ill with typhoid. The military field hospitals were unable to cope and every available space in the city had to be taken for typhoid hospitals, including the town hall, churches and school buildings.[12] The epidemic was said to have been exacerbated by the

Boers having cut the water supply to Bloemfontein, leading to the drinking of polluted water out of old wells. Mr. W. Burdett Coutts, a British Member of Parliament, described the situation in April: 'hundreds of men...were lying in the worst stages of typhoid with only a thin blanket and a thin waterproof sheet between their aching bodies and the hard ground, with no milk and hardly any medicines, without beds, stretchers, mattresses ... without a single nurse amongst them'. He continued 'in many of these tents there were ten typhoid cases lying closely packed together, the dying against the convalescent, the man in his crisis pressed against the man hastening to it'.[13] Yet the details of the epidemic were being hidden by the military with the disease statistics describing it as 'Simple Continued Fever' rather than typhoid. While Burdett Coutts wrote letters to The Times newspaper in England, detailing his observations in Bloemfontein, they were not published due to press censorship until the letter outlined above finally appeared on 27th June. It caused much outrage and debate as the British public had been lead to believe that medical management and sanitary conditions for the army in South Africa were near perfect, but it finally culminated in a Commission of Inquiry appointed to investigate the case of the sick and wounded in South Africa.[14]

Similarly to Bloemfontein, at Ladysmith - where a British defending force of some 13,500 men was besieged for four months from November 1899 to February 1900 - some 10,668 men were admitted to hospital and 551 died, of which 393 of these were from typhoid.[15] There had already been an epidemic of typhoid in Ladysmith the year before the war.

The British had been aware of the risks their troops would face from typhoid in South Africa. It was known to occur after the first rains of the summer season and also that the disease was spread by pollution of the soil, but their preparations were nevertheless inadequate for what they would encounter. The importance of adequate sanitary provisions was not appreciated before the war, so that only after the troops had been decimated were sanitary officers appointed. Drinking water was obtained from dams and rivers and there was insufficient fuel to boil the water before drinking. The lack of control over latrines and refuse led to excessive fly breeding which spread the disease still further. The toll of typhoid on the British troops throughout the war was extremely high. On January 12th 1900 there were 120 in hospitals with typhoid, but by 25 May 1900 that had risen to 6,084, or 7.4% of total army strength.[16] It was particularly devastating on the British troops because of them being massed in a slow-moving army with a greater risk of contamination of food and water supplies, whereas the Boer Commandoes were constantly on the move and relatively less affected. However the Boer soldiers were also affected with Cronjé's laager at Paardeberg, also on the river Modder, described as having a raging epidemic in January 1900. The soldiers were said to be drinking the river water without boiling it.[17] This typhoid amongst the troops and commandoes spread across the country to the other towns and cities. From Bloemfontein the British marched via Kroonstad to Pretoria, and at Kroonstad many more fell victim to the disease where it had become known as 'Cronjé's fever'. By the time they reached Pretoria it was still serious but things were starting to improve with increased hospital provision and improving sanitary conditions.[18]

In Cape Town there was a marked increase in typhoid in 1900 with 166 cases admitted to the Somerset Hospital and 31 deaths, and large numbers amongst the Boer prisoners in Simon's Town. Many of the cases were brought to hospital almost moribund which lead to the high mortality rate. Similar increases were experienced in other towns across South Africa with 88 cases treated in King Williams Town's Grey Hospital. A number of these cases came from the War Front and arrived in a hopeless condition. 55 cases were admitted to the newly opened Queens Central Hospital in Cradock of which 11 died, the greatest cause of death that year. The Frontier Hospital in Queen's Town received 101 cases with 17 deaths, which seems to reflect a fairly consistent case-fatality rate of around 17-20%. Kimberley Hospital had over 500 cases that year although it was thought that many cases among Africans did not come to the hospital or were misdiagnosed.[19] In addition to the soldiers many of the nurses and medical officers were also killed by the disease.

In the later stages of the war the British had established camps for the containment of Boer women and children as they enforced their policy of burning the Afrikaaner farms to deny the Boer soldiers food and shelter. The camps also were to cater for refugees from the war, for those leaving unprotected farms with all their men at war, for those unable to travel across the country with the Boer Commandoes and for those with nowhere else to go. With so much typhoid in the country it was inevitably taken into the camps where it spread rapidly. The inmates of the camps were devastated by diseases, much of which was typhoid, with some 27,000 women and children dying there – far more than the men who died in the war. While the infants died of measles the adolescent and adult women died of typhoid.[20] Measles accompanied by bronchitis and pneumonia accounted possibly for 80% of the deaths, particularly in the latter half of 1901, but the conditions in the camps also lead to the spread of enteric fever, as it was then known, due to overcrowding, inadequate and often contaminated water supplies and poor sanitation. Some of this was blamed on the inmates themselves as the Ladies Commission, appointed by the British War Office in July 1901 to investigate the camps after the reports of Emily Hobhouse, reported:

> It is necessary to put on record the insanitary habits of the people. However numerous, suitable and well-kept may be the latrines provided, the fouling of the ground, including river banks, and slopes and trenches leading to the water supply, goes on to such an extent which would probably not be credited except by those who have seen it ... the extensive fouling of the floors of tents and the ground of camps by it has been the direct cause of a devastating attack of enteric in more than one camp – their inability to see that what may be comparatively harmless on their farms becomes criminally dangerous in camp.[21]

Others reported similarly that urine and faeces were thrown close around the tent openings, and that the mortality was at least in part due to the behaviour of the residents not changing from an open veld life to a densely populated, settlement life. The causes of the great mortality in the camps became a hotly debated political issue between the British and the Boers with the latter making great use of it for anti-British propaganda. However it would appear that it was at least in part multi-factorial – as pointed out by some commentators typhoid was a regular feature of wars around the world in that period, as the mechanisms for containment were poorly understood. It was then virtually inevitable that it would spread to areas in a war zone where any large groups – whether soldiers, prisoners of war or refugees - were living in dense settlements with make-shift sanitation and water supplies, with inadequate food and poor medical care. There is also evidence that many of the women were already in a very poor state of health when arriving at the camps. The extent to which the British forcibly brought the women and children into the camps, and to what extent the Boer men sent them to the camps to stop them travelling with the commandoes and slowing them down, was also hotly debated. However, regardless of causality, there is no denying that there were large numbers of deaths from the disease and that the Boer women and children suffered greatly. The politicisation of the problem between British and Boer also appeared to distract attention away from the conditions of others in the camps, in particular the Africans and Coloureds, and less investigation of the conditions and statistics of these groups was undertaken.

Just two years prior to the War work was being undertaken on the development of a typhoid vaccine by Sir Almroth Wright and colleagues at the Royal Army Medical Corps laboratories in Netley, England. Some of this was tried on the British Army going to India and those going to South Africa had been offered the vaccine but it was not compulsory. About 20,000 were inoculated. It was found that there was a reduction by half of the number of cases in those immunised, sometimes higher, and a decrease in case mortality. One of those assisting Wright was a Medical Officer, Captain Hughes, who was shortly after sent to the front on active service where he died at the battle of Colenso during an attempt at the relief of Ladysmith. At his tomb is engraved '...he was a pioneer in the field of bacteriology. If it had been possible for him to continue his research instead of to serve as a front line soldier typhoid vaccine, crude but promising as it then was, might largely by his efforts have been perfected in time to save the lives of thousands of soldiers and civilians'.[22] The vaccine was subsequently refined and used to better effect in the First World War, along with improvements in the hygiene and sanitation provisions in the army and during warfare.

The typhoid remained throughout the country, no doubt exacerbated by the poor sanitary conditions already existing in towns and rural areas. Many towns operated on the pail system of sewage disposal, with the tubs being emptied into stinking, tank carts doing their noisy, rattling rounds at night. Often the buckets were described as leaky, were not properly cleaned or disinfected, and without lids. The stench from the carts doing their rounds was often described in graphic and colourful terms by District Surgeons of the times. From the carts they were emptied into pits. The District Surgeon of Albert stated in his report of 1902

> The disposal of night-soil has in the past year been conducted during one of its stages in a most objectionable way, the tubs being emptied into a tank cart as the latter goes its rounds at night. Who on earth devised such a system I do not know, and it is a matter for wonder that any Municipality in the world could be got to adopt it. The explanation of why the plan has not been sooner abolished is probably that most or all of the Councillors are in the happy position of being able to spend each and every night in comfortable beds, and therefore their nostrils are not assailed by the horrible odour that sickens one.[23]

Yet over a century later, in 2012, this 'bucket system' was still in use in some parts of South Africa's African townships. Other domestic waste water was generally thrown into the streets or back yards. The District

Surgeon for Barkley East reported on the troops having brought typhoid to the town in October 1901, which lead to an epidemic with 36 cases and four deaths. Water supplies were generally still unprotected wells or streams and were easily contaminated, either in the well or while being conveyed in open furrows accessible to animals, or in barrels which were often dirty and full of leaves, twigs and other contaminants. African locations had no sanitary controls and were in a worse situation.

The high levels of typhoid in South African towns and cities in the early 1900's were gradually brought under control by the expansion of piped water schemes and improving sanitation. Johannesburg suffered 795 cases in 1903 after the Anglo-Boer War, for which additional tents had to be erected in the grounds of the hospital. The incidence amongst Europeans in Pretoria dropped from 5.6 per 1,000 in the period 1904-1909 to 1.35 per 1,000 twenty years later, attributed to the provision of a pure water supply and the general improvement in sanitary conditions. In Cape Town the levels declined but still by 1916-1920 the death rate was 34 per 100,000 – only a little less than England and Wales *before* they had undergone the implementation of sanitary improvements back in the 1860's. At that time the whole municipality of Cape Town had piped drinking water, but only the central part had water-borne sewerage, the remainder using the pail or 'bucket' system. The real drop in typhoid death rate in Cape Town came in the period up to the 1930's when it fell by about 90% due mainly to the extension of the water-borne sewerage system to the whole municipality.[24] In Pietermaritzburg, which had suffered regular outbreaks from the late 1890's, the number of cases fell from a high of 231 in 1904 to between 10 and 20 a year by the early 1930's, again linked to dramatic improvements in hygiene, drainage and sanitation in the city. However these declines in incidence of typhoid in cities from the early 1900's were also linked to the policies of removal of the poor Indian and African populations from the central city areas, where their slum dwellings with poor sanitation and drainage were contributing to disease spread, to new areas outside the local government boundaries. In some cities like Pietermaritzburg typhoid was the excuse for the forced removals, in others such as Johannesburg and Port Elizabeth it was plague. Much of the decrease in diseases of insanitation seen in the city centres over this period was as a result of pushing poverty and sanitation problems out of sight, and out of city statistics.

Between 1927 and 1932 the number of reported typhoid cases hovered at between 3,800 and 5,800 per year across the country, although the true number was probably much greater, with an incidence in the larger urban areas of around 1 per 1,000. Often the disease was not diagnosed and in rural areas without adequate laboratories it would probably have gone unrecognized. The difficulties in making further reductions were attributed mainly to the problem of carriers.[25] There were still problems in addressing inadequate sanitation with only pit latrines in rural areas and many urban areas, particularly African townships, still operating on the disgusting 'bucket system', in which households collected urine and faeces in metal buckets which were then emptied periodically by a municipal collection truck. These trucks then disposed of the sewage in locations and ways which were not always sanitary. The factors adversely affecting the survival of the bacteria outside the human body were high temperature and desiccation. Humidity and low temperatures favoured the survival, with bacilli having been isolated from frozen faeces up to four months after excretion. If they were washed into water they could survive five to six days, which increased to several weeks if the water was close to freezing point. Although they did not increase greatly in number it was found that the purer the water, the greater the chance of survival of the bacteria. They were able to multiply rapidly in milk, which made milk a potent and dangerous source of spread of infections. Up to 10% of all cases of typhoid ultimately became carriers, either urinary or intestinal.

In urban areas, where there was some reasonable control over sanitation and water supplies, the incidence of the disease usually remained low but with occasional outbreaks. The low endemic prevalence related to the presence of carriers, which usually spread through the contamination of food supply, in particular the milk supply. Having moved the sanitary and sewerage causes of typhoid spread outside the city boundaries into the un-serviced, peri-urban townships, the control of typhoid in South African urban areas therefore turned to the elimination of the carrier and his removal from all trades concerned in the handling of milk and foodstuffs. It followed that this necessitated a careful investigation of each case of typhoid and the use of the complement fixation test, which was found to be more reliable than the Widal test, to identify the carriers. The carrier would then be excluded from trades such as restaurants, boarding houses, hotels, tea-rooms, groceries, butcheries etc. In the case of milk however, it was fraught with many administrative difficulties due to the large number of people involved in the trade. In Pretoria alone there were estimated to be 2,000 Africans (deemed to be a greater threat than Europeans) involved in the dairy trade, with frequent changes in employees. The approach was therefore aimed at the source of the milk and its pasteurisation at depots which should be under the control of the municipalities. Laing recommended that, as 'the native carrier, even when discovered, is practically impossible to control ... what is required is some form of national registration of carriers over whom constant supervision could be exercised through the medium of the Native Affairs Department'.[26] It was the practice in Pretoria to have the passes of African typhoid carriers stamped with the phrase 'not to be employed in the handling of foodstuffs.' However this was thought to be largely ineffective. The national registration of carriers was felt to be preferable as it would enable the 'repatriation of African carriers and their control on lines similar to those employed in the case of home-segregated lepers'.[27]

Laing estimated that around 50% of the African population had had typhoid and that around 4% were considered chronic carriers. The link of carriers with milk-borne outbreaks was repeatedly proven, with such outbreaks occurring almost every year in the 1920's and early 1930s in Pretoria, with between 10 and 25 cases occurring in each instance. The majority of carriers were found to be female, which was unexplained, although in the past it had been blamed on 'the effect of corsets on the gall bladder'.[28] It was suggested by the Department of Public Health that the only really effective method of treatment of a carrier was by operative removal or the gall bladder or kidney, although they acknowledged that 'it is hardly to be expected that affected persons will agree to such a procedure'.[29] Following the ineffectiveness of repatriation on the Africans out of Pretoria a scheme was devised where they were removed from their work with foodstuffs and taken into the employ of the Municipality and given alternative work. The idea of extending pure water and water-borne sanitation systems into African townships to reduce the number of carriers does not seem to have been discussed as a possible solution at that time.

In rural areas, where the population was scattered and there was no local government, the problem of typhoid control differed. While it was recognised that as the sanitation of a given area improved so its typhoid rate diminished, there was little sanitation provision in the rural areas and what there was generally catered only for the European population. As Cluver noted 'it is an axiom that in regard to public health there is no colour bar, but in actual practice this principle is very often lost sight of'.[30] While the incidence in the large towns which had public health and sanitary departments and Medical Officers of Health was, by 1933, generally less than 1 per 1,000, in the rural villages the rates were often as high as 20 per 1,000, rising in some cases up to 60 per 1,000. The factors responsible for its spread in rural areas were mainly fly-borne infection; uncontrolled disposal of human waste, pollution of drinking water supplies, milk-borne infection and carrier-spread infection. The majority of rural communities were said to be plagued with flies with no precautions to prevent them in both animal and human manure. This was thought to be the cause of most rural outbreaks, and particularly related to the lack of sanitation facilities for African workers on farms.

The pollution of drinking water had been found to be the cause of an outbreak in February 1932 where 50 Africans had been affected of whom 14 died. The outbreak had only been reported once it started to affect Europeans in the area, when it was found that the streams from which the Africans obtained drinking water were grossly polluted. In rural areas trees and large bushes were often only found adjacent to water courses, which were then used as latrines for privacy. The faeces were then washed into streams by the rains. The spread through milk was similar to the urban areas where most milkmen were usually not Europeans and 'whose illnesses are not generally a matter of much concern to his European employer. Should such an individual suffer from an undiagnosed attack of typhoid fever the danger of a milk-borne epidemic is obvious'.[31] Milk was also contaminated through flies or contact with contaminated water. The prevention of typhoid in rural areas was therefore based upon prevention of fly-breeding by treating animal manure; the fly-screening of milk-rooms and dairies and promoting an high standard of cleanliness; the isolation of patients with enteric fever and safe disposal of waste and soiled linen etc; the inoculation of contacts; the protection of water sources and the provision of toilet facilities. At that time both pit latrines and the bucket system were in use which needed to be rendered fly proof. The need to improve notification of non-European illness was noted, and the prevention of carriers working with milk and foodstuffs.

In the treatment of typhoid the diet of the patient was thought to play an important role with particular concern being the risk of intestinal perforation. In early years a starvation diet had been favoured, which later moved to patients being often fed exclusively on milk diets to reduce this risk, although it was also found that a more liberal diet improved resistance to the disease, including such items as broth, jelly, eggs, chocolate, strained porridge and sugar.[32] Immunisation for typhoid was done either by immunisation with a TAB vaccine (Typhoid, Para A and Para B), or by administration of the Besredka pill, an oral vaccine which was given to typhoid contacts and to sufferers during convalescence to prevent them becoming carriers, although this was not completely effective.[33] It was also used on the mines for the immunisation of African labourers, and in prisons. The first widespread use on Europeans was at the Vaal-Hartz development scheme north of Kimberley in 1934, where all labourers and most women and children were vaccinated with the new typhoid endotoxoid vaccine. There were few reactions apart from local pain and stiffness at the injection site. Altogether 5,664 people were immunised and no cases of typhoid were encountered over the following two year period, although it was noted that the sanitation facilities were excellent which would have contributed to the absence of cases. In the Rand gold mines trials of the endotoxoid were also undertaken. In an outbreak in 1934 almost 14,000 Africans were vaccinated and it was found that both the endotoxoid and the Besredka pill gave reasonable protection, but those who had had the endotoxoid suffered lower mortality and fewer complications. Mass inoculation of some 5,700 Africans on the Durban Deep mine (on the Witwatersrand, not near the city of Durban) was undertaken, resulting in very few cases occurring. It was also found out in a study that mines still using the bucket system of sanitation had a 50% higher incidence of typhoid than those with water-borne sewage.[34] Typhoid remained a regular visitor to the mines in the 1930s with the incidence peaking during the summer months from October to April. Inoculation with endotoxoid became a regular occurrence and where instituted, such as at the Van Ryn Deep Gold Mine, had a clear impact in reducing the typhoid cases, which occurred mainly in those who had not been inoculated.[35]

In the rural areas most cases of typhoid probably continued to go undiagnosed. It was generally agreed that the incidence of typhoid was directly proportional to the degree of insanitation in the community. In rural areas the incidence often rose as high as 35 per 1,000, whereas in the developed large urban areas it was generally less than 2 per 1,000 by 1935. The Union Health Department devoted its attention to the rural areas and the levels of hygiene but found that the main challenge was the lack of rural local authorities outside of the Cape Province. It noted that the actual incidence in rural areas had to be vastly greater than the figures suggested, with the Department commenting:

> Since it punishes gross un-cleanliness it is most prevalent among the lowest strata of our society, namely the least civilised of the Bantus. Among them notification of disease and death is extremely faulty. Among the Bantu too the causative bacillus not infrequently produces a condition which is not recognisable as typhoid apart from special laboratory tests.[36]

The survival of the bacteria outside the body was being found to be increasingly long, being up to two years in ice cream and having been found several months after an epidemic in sewage effluent. Fly breeding was associated with outbreaks in rural areas along with polluted water. The water-borne outbreaks were more explosive in character, with many cases occurring simultaneously. This was often followed by a series of sporadic infections spreading from one house to another through flies and it was 'a well-known fact that if there are flies in a neighbourhood they will make a bee-line towards the enteric sufferer'. Similarly the milk-related outbreaks were of the explosive type.[37]

In 1937 an outbreak occurred in the Caledon area in an isolated village, where the sanitation was by means of the pail or bucket system, in which the faeces were unprotected from flies and close to houses. 27 cases occurred and three deaths out of a population of 190 and attributed to 'fingers, flies and filth'. The first case was possibly acquired through a party at which people from other areas were present. Within a week 18 cases had occurred and a temporary hospital had to be established in the school. The poor sanitary conditions at this rural location which had given rise to the rapid spread were highlighted as an example of conditions in 'the majority of the locations attached to our smaller towns and villages' and, were they close to the towns, 'spread to the European community would have been almost inevitable'. A further outbreak at the Great Brak River affected 23 people, nearly all Europeans, and highlighted the dangers associated with dairies which operated under the 'very primitive conditions which prevail in many or our rural areas'. Three boys who first contracted typhoid were nursed by the dairy owner in her living room, following which she threw their excrement into the kraal where the cows were kept and milked the cows there by hand. The clothes and bedding were washed in the same irrigation furrow as provided the drinking water. Within the next two weeks all the families who used her milk had caught typhoid, including the lady herself who subsequently died.[38]

The sanitary and health conditions of peri-urban areas near to the larger cities and towns, which contained mainly poor Black, Indian and Coloured residents along with some poor Whites, were a major issue by the late 1930's. These areas had arisen outside the control of local authorities, often deliberately created by them by forced removals earlier in the century, and were largely ignored by them. The housing was described as very primitive with either pit latrines or else a rough contraption over a bucket or empty tin to serve as a toilet, both of which were exposed to fly breeding. The faeces from the latter were often buried on the plot. Household and other refuse such as animal manure were left lying around with flies breeding and spreading disease to household food and milk, in particular gastro-enteritis and typhoid. Water supplies were equally primitive using shallow wells, irrigation furrows and streams, and milk and meat supplies were similarly contaminated. Some settlements had grown from the drift of poor European rural inhabitants towards towns for fixed waged jobs, combined with their desire for cheap accommodation and the avoidance of municipal rates. These residents were often opposed to local authority control of any kind as the imposition of municipal charges increased their expenses. African peri-urban settlements were also generally in a poor sanitary state, with 'notorious examples of such black belts' being Edendale outside Pietermaritzburg and Kliptown near Johannesburg. Kliptown had arisen due to the forced movement of people to the outskirts of the city at the turn of the century as a result of the fears of the white population about plague. Similarly the Edendale area, which originally was a prosperous agricultural community, had degenerated into a slum due to the removal of people from the centre of Pietermaritzburg in the same period because of fears about typhoid.

The living conditions in these 'black belt' areas were described by the Health Department as grossly overcrowded, with sanitation 'of the most primitive and disgusting type' and water coming from grossly polluted shallow wells. Typhoid was said to be common but not accurately measured and, together with other related diseases, lead to extremely high mortality and morbidity rates. The National Department of Public Health pointed out that this was not just a risk to the African population, but also to the neighbouring European communities in the towns as nearly all the African wage earners were engaged in the towns, many as domestic workers or food handlers. The Department of Public Health was of the view that these areas should be incorporated into the neighbouring local authorities, but at that time in 1939 the Thornton Commission was examining the situation. Where local authorities were looking after urban locations the disposal of excreta remained unsatisfactory with the bucket system extensive. The Department commented:

> 'few local authorities seem able to escape from the delusion that the total number of pails required for the receipt of the excreta of a given population is less if the pails are placed in communal latrines than if they are placed in individual household privies.

It was common that, under the communal systems, there was less than one pail for 30 persons, sometimes as low as one per 100 persons. The

Department continued:

> by the inexorable law of the non-compressibility of solids and liquids insufficient provision can have only one result – the overflow of pail contents on to floors and seats, and the use, by those Natives who are revolted by this spectacle, of any convenient cover they can find in the vicinity: fences, hedges, trees, dongas [gullies], river-beds and even the open streets.[39]

It was estimated that more than 50% of the faecal output of some of these locations was deposited on an open surface and well within fly range of European towns. They recommended individual household privies and added that a well constructed pit privy was undoubtedly superior to any type of pail privy. At this time in 1939 the annual reported cases of typhoid were 3,558. The Urbanised Areas Administration Committee recommended that many of these peri-urban areas be placed under some kind of health control, which in Natal resulted in the creation of the Local Health Commission which took over the administration of Edendale along with many other peri-urban areas and rapidly growing European settlements in the Province.

Smaller settlements in rural areas and on European farms, while somewhat better placed than the densely populated and insanitary peri-urban locations, were still at risk. These settlements were completely outside of control aside from the Divisional Councils in the Cape. Where Africans lived on premises directly controlled by their employers the National Department of Health commented that it was only occasionally that the Europeans set a very high standard or provided their employees with adequate washing facilities and hygienic latrine accommodation. Kark reported on some 13 outbreaks occurring in the vicinity of his Polela Health Unit in rural southern Natal. One of these was estimated to have resulted in over 100 deaths. In a study of the area it was noted that there was a complete absence of toilet facilities, that the disposal of refuse and faeces were ideal for the spread of disease, that water supplies were liable to faecal contamination and that flies were a great pest in nearly all homes.[40] On farms, irrigation settlements and some villages domestic water was often drawn from streams, irrigation furrows and wells which were frequently grossly polluted by faecal matter washing in from the surrounding areas.

Outbreaks were reported in the early 1940s in cities across the country. In Kimberley between 1939 and 1940 there was an outbreak involving 60 people traced back to milk. Milk was a major culprit in cities in the spread of typhoid, and yet there was still little enforcement of pasteurisation. While pasteurization plants existed in the major cities the efficiency of these was uncertain. Milk-borne outbreaks had occurred in Durban in 1941, Johannesburg in 1942, Cape Town in 1943, Pretoria and Germiston in 1944 and in Pietermaritzburg in 1946. The outbreak in Cape Town had involved 104 people, and was traced back to a dairy employee who was found to be a typhoid carrier. A survey of 400 African milkers in Cape Town found that 1% was carrying typhoid. Tuberculosis also was said to be present in 3-4% of Cape Town milk samples and bovine tuberculosis was causing the deaths of some 2,500 people annually in Britain, mostly children.

The control of milk production and distribution generally across the country was still inadequate. The first serious attempt to control pasteurisation was made in Port Elizabeth where the local authority was able to achieve an increase in successful pasteurisation, using the phosphatase test, from 74.3% in 1941 to 95% in 1943. Within Johannesburg efficiency of pasteurisation varied from over 99.5% to as low as 35%. The military were also engaged in testing the efficiency of pasteurisation and similarly found a wide variation in results, although it was shown that with close supervision and guidance a level of around 95% could be reached fairly easily, although this did not improve the quality of the milk from the producer, but only rendered it safe. It was considered of paramount importance that entire chain of milk production from the farm to the market be improved.[41]

In 1945 the Medical Officer of Health for Cape Town, Dr F.O. Fehrsen, submitted a report to the City Council proposing compulsory pasteurisation for the City, which he said was a subject regarded with so much prejudice by lay people that no reasoned scientific opinion was listened to. He noted that this attitude was no new experience in preventive medicine, as 'each new step in public health legislation throughout the world has involved a fight against the forces of ignorance and prejudice'. Yet the lack of precautionary measures necessary to ensure a safe supply of milk was one of the factors limiting the intake of one of the most valuable foodstuffs. Milk was particularly associated with the spread of typhoid, along with other gastro-intestinal diseases, streptococcal infection, scarlet fever and diphtheria, much of which was introduced at the milking stage, along with bovine tuberculosis, undulant fever, salmonella, gastro-enteritis and dysentery. Numerous outbreaks of these diseases in England, America and Europe affecting hundreds of people and with many fatalities had been traced back to contaminated milk supplies during the early decades of the twentieth century. A study of milk-borne outbreaks in America between 1908 and 1926 had covered 612 outbreaks of various of these diseases, affecting a total of 42,327 people and causing at least 410 deaths. An outbreak of salmonella had occurred in Johannesburg and Germiston in 1944 which affected 100 people and was traced back to a milk producer and the distribution of raw milk. Regardless of hygiene efforts at the milking and distribution phase of the milk industry it was said that no amount of care in the production of raw milk could prevent its being a danger to the consumer – clean raw milk was not necessarily safe and pasteurisation was also required. Dr Fehrsen cited numerous examples and various distinguished academics and authorities on the subject and stated that compulsory pasteurisation had been accepted by 'the great bulk of enlightened countries', including Sweden, France and Ontario, Canada. Yet he faced vehement opposition groups within the city with people citing concerns about change in taste, loss of nutritional value (although disproven in numerous studies), and 'digestibility'.[42] Others asserted that it caused reduced fertility in rats, and that there may be a fertility vitamin in milk which would be destroyed by pasteurisation, which was of importance in the post-war situation as 'as a race we are within the shadow of depopulation'.[43] Given the great increases in global population since the war this theory would appear to have been subsequently disproven.

While the large cities were battling to bring in milk controls the situation in smaller towns and rural areas was worse, with the Department of Health commenting that they lagged behind and were mainly responsible for the unsatisfactory situation of the country in regard to typhoid with the 'almost invariable practice of keeping cattle …giving rise to gross insanitary nuisance' and which it described as opposed to civilized standards of health. The lack of supervision and haphazard disposal of dung were causing fly breeding and the Department recommended the establishment of communal stables outside the towns for which local authorities could charge rental. As the Africans moved into urban areas it was noted that they still faced insanitary conditions as the sanitation 'in these human 'hives' has not improved *pari passu* with that in European urban areas. Latrine facilities, often of the insanitary communal type, are usually woefully deficient thereby leading to the evils of overfull pails and promiscuous defaecation in the environs'.[44] The practice of 'rationing' the supply of sanitary services and water supplies in these areas by local authorities was deplored by the Department.

The position of the typhoid vaccine had always been questionable, with its efficacy debatable as to whether it was simply reducing mortality coincidentally to improvements in water supplies, chlorination and public hygiene. The old phenolized vaccine had been replaced by a newer alcoholised vaccine between the wars, but was still of doubtful effectiveness. After the Second World War further doubts arose when vaccinated inmates of prisoner-of-war camps in North Africa experienced high levels of typhoid in the face of gross overcrowding and poor hygienic conditions. It was suggested that the vaccine was only of value in reducing mortality not morbidity. Overall opinion suggested that it could reduce both mortality and morbidity but only with relative immunity and that it could not withstand a heavy assault of exposure to unsanitary conditions and high bacterial loads.

By 1946 experiments with the new antibiotics were being undertaken in the treatment of typhoid, although it was still declared that it did not respond decisively to any presently known drug therapy. Streptomycin, which, as with penicillin post-war, was still only available in limited amounts to civilian hospitals, was found to be somewhat effective, but thought to be of more use in the treatment of tuberculosis, urinary tract infections and meningitis. Typhoid was still a significant cause of illness and death in South Africa, with an incidence rate around 40 per 100,000 in the European population (around eight times that in England and Wales) of whom around 12% died. The problem of carriers remained, exacerbated by their excretion of the organisms being highly intermittent. One working in a dairy farm started an outbreak in Brakpan near Johannesburg which caused 300 cases, many of which were children. The epidemic was so explosive that the town hall had to be converted into an emergency hospital staffed by the Department of Defence. A Committee of Enquiry set up after the event made several recommendations regarding the control of dairy workers and milk supplies including pasteurisation wherever practicable. However there was still a large body of public opinion who were considerably opposed to it.[45]

In Pretoria treatment of carriers was along racial lines - European carriers were given written instructions on the methods of prevention of spread of the disease and were periodically visited by a health visitor; Coloured females (mixed race or African) were similarly dealt with but visited more frequently. Coloured or African males were taken into the employ of the City Council and accommodated in a compound known as the 'Typhoid Fever Carrier Camp' and kept under supervision day and night, being allowed to visit their families occasionally. 'They are so comfortably accommodated and well fed that there is rarely any discontent, and although a small percentage abscond, in many cases where convalescent or temporary carriers have lost their bacilli, these have been loath to leave the camp'[46] Several case histories are given of men aged up to 35 years (all of whom were referred to as 'boys') who had been admitted to the camp for many months after testing positive and caused outbreaks. There was no known way to treat the carriers, although cholecystectomy (removal of the gall bladder) was around 75% effective in intestinal carriers. Although the Pretoria system of a Typhoid Camp seemed to them to work well it was not copied by other municipalities. The suggestion that African Passes be endorsed to the effect that they were typhoid carriers was also not adopted as the Native Affairs Department thought it would prejudice them in trying to obtain employment of any kind.

Regulations compelling the pasteurisation of milk in Cape Town were published in January 1950, to come into effect in January 1953, although notifications were at an all time low with just 46 notified in the city in 1950. While there were still cases occurring – 101 in 1953 – it was noted with some gratification that none were related to milk. However the implementation of compulsory pasteurisation was not without problems - originally it was planned that there would be a municipal pasteurising plant to pasteurise all the milk entering the city, but this was opposed by representatives of the milk trade. Then the private plants were unable to cope, with one machine handling 25% of the city's milk breaking down completely and an acute shortage of milk bottles occurring. The backlog of milk awaiting pasteurisation which was rapidly deteriorating in a particularly hot summer, the mistaken belief by some producers that pasteurisation would render poor milk good, and the continued agitation by people opposed to it on principle, caused major problems for some time until eventually coming under control.[47] A later similar attempt to compel pasteurisation by the Medical Officer of Health of Port Elizabeth in 1972 was rejected by his Council.

From the end of the 1940's new antibiotics were being discovered with some speed. Chloramphenicol, related to streptomycin, was found to be effective in typhoid with dramatic results and, when combined with anti-typhoid-paratyphoid vaccine, gave striking results. Unfortunately it did not eliminate the carrier state, and it appeared that relapses were more common than in those not treated with it, although it shortened the length of stay in hospital. Still, in the early 1950's it was the treatment of choice and generally gave an excellent response. Chloramphenicol was said to have reduced the case-fatality rate to less than 1% by the late fifties and to have revolutionized the outlook. But while the number of deaths from the disease started to decline there was very little decline in prevalence, with 4,230 cases in 1956 – very similar to that of 30 years earlier. The Department of Health commented that it was disappointing that year after year there were still large numbers of notifications, with 3,599 cases in 1958 mainly in Africans – 'incontrovertible proof that the hygienic and sanitary practices of this section of the population leave much to be desired'.[48] Localised outbreaks continued to occur linked to milk distribution or institutions, one such being in the Johannesburg Gaol in May 1959 which lead to great public alarm. Some 22,000 Europeans and over 130,000 non-Europeans were vaccinated.[49] A gaol in Cape Town suffered a similar outbreak in 1961 with fourteen cases.

Investigations and large-scale trials held in Yugoslavia into the vaccine in the mid 1950's found that the older phenolized vaccine, which was replaced before the War, actually gave a better response at 70% protection, whereas the newer alcoholized vaccine was of poor and doubtful value. The South Africans were producing their own endotoxoid vaccine at the South African Institute for Medical Research which was not assessed in trials similar to those in Yugoslavia, but it was thought to be about as effective as the TAB vaccine used by British and American troops in the War. It was clear however that none of the vaccines in use were highly effective and that community hygiene, sanitary improvements and carrier tracing remained the mainstay of typhoid control around the world.[50] Carriers were identified by testing of stool and urine samples to see if they were excreting the organism. In addition the Vi agglutination test was used to identify chronic carriers. However, the test was considered unreliable and frequently misapplied by local health authorities, some of which required all food handlers to be subjected to them, with those who tested positive removed from their jobs. This was patently unfair as it did not specifically indicate that the person was actively excreting the bacteria. It was recommended rather that the tracing of chronic carriers depended 'upon 'police' epidemiological investigations to find the suspects and secondly on bacteriological tests to prove which suspect is guilty. Whenever a case of typhoid fever occurs every effort should be made by the local health authority to trace the responsible carrier".[51] These carriers would then be treated to try and erase the bacteria, failing which they would be given instructions regarding their danger to others, the need to wash their hands after visiting the toilet and the need to disinfect their pails after use if they had no water-borne sewerage. They were forbidden to handle food at work or at home, and could not go on holiday, change address or enter hospital without notifying the local authority.

The numbers of cases hovered at around 2,000-3,000 during the late

1950's and early 1960's and were attributed to the poor hygienic conditions in rural areas. While the larger cities and a few of the smaller towns had implemented water-borne sewerage, outside these it was not generally available in the South Africa and water supplies were of varying degrees of quality. In smaller towns and villages the pail system remained in use, as well as in many peri-urban and rural areas. In many areas there were still no latrines at all and the bush was used for both urination and defecation. These rural and peri-urban hinterlands continued to pose a risk to cities for typhoid, for 'so long as uncontrolled migration is taking place into a city from parts of the country, near or far, where typhoid is endemic, especially of non-European servants and labourers, typhoid carriers will be introduced into the city'.[52]

The Red Location at Port Elizabeth, originally created in 1902 for Africans as a response to plague, started an outbreak of typhoid in 1965. The Medical Officer of Health described the conditions in the location some 60 years after its creation in his Report:

> During the period 1902 to date, with the exception of re-roofing in 1964, very little has been done to the buildings by way of repair or improvement, or to the environs by way of road-making. They lack provision of individual sanitary accommodation or water supply, drainage or adequate refuse removal. The conditions pertaining in regard to faecal, urine and refuse disposal are, to say the least, primitive. Fly-breeding is encouraged in the filth which is ever-present in the mixture of faeces, urine, rubbish, foul and stagnant water found in the vicinity of the communal latrines and water standpipes in this area. Overcrowding and poor living conditions are indescribable.[53]

He had reported these conditions annually prior to the typhoid outbreak and warned that they would be the cause of a major infectious disease outbreak, even reminding the Council that many of the domestic servants and food handlers working in the city came from that area. He recommended the location be completely rebuilt. Still nothing had happened and the conditions gave rise to 23 cases of typhoid in the city with two deaths.

Typhoid increased in the mid 1960's to a maximum of 5,791 cases in 1966, due largely to drought in the Northern Transvaal and parts of Natal which lead to inadequate and polluted water sources. These figures were undoubtedly still underestimates of the extent of the disease as, particularly in rural areas, many cases would have gone undiagnosed and, even if diagnosed, would not be notified. In the latter half of 1968 for example, typhoid was rampant in the Transkei following during the prolonged drought. As Transkei was nominally independent the epidemic did not draw attention until cases started coming into the city of East London. By December the local hospitals in Transkei were unable to cope with the number of patients pouring in and many had to be transferred to the East London hospitals. By January the disease had spread to East London and 79 patients had been admitted to hospitals there. The tuberculosis ward was evacuated and turned into a typhoid ward. The Medical Officer of Health, J.R. van Heerden, reported on the reaction of the citizens of the city: 'The public of East London went berserk ... people seemed petrified to visit even the larger centres in the Transkei. Calls flooded in from telephone workmen, drivers of railway vehicles, commercial travellers and people who intended taking their annual fishing holidays on the Transkei coast'. The local Health Department was forced by public demand to provide mass immunisation. It commenced on the 20th of February and by the 24th the Traffic department had to be called to control the crowd. Additional nurses were recruited to man mass inoculation sites across the municipality. Over 135,000 doses of vaccine were given, and Van Heerden described the public panic as an exaggerated reaction to a disease which did not pose a great threat to those city dwellers with good water and sanitation.[54]

During the late 1960's, 70's and 80's the annual number of cases notified remained remarkably constant at between 2,000 and 5,000 per year with a peak of 5,648 in 1985, although the increasing population size meant this was a decrease in incidence. However the actual figures were clearly much larger than this, as under-notification continued during this period of divided and fragmented health services and political upheaval. Fortunately the disease was fairly easily treatable with antibiotics, such that in the 1990's the case-fatality was only around 1.5%. The annual incidence rate had dropped to just 2 per 100,000 people by the time the new Government came into office in 1994, although the changes in administration and political turmoil may have reduced the accuracy of the figures. At that time the highest incidence was in the northern and eastern areas of the former Transvaal, possibly due to the extreme poverty in the densely populated homeland areas of that region, but the figures were declining. Still the incidence was far higher in the Black population with rates between five and ten times higher than in other groups, and with 97% of cases between 1985 and 1994 being reported in Africans. In an extensive review by the Department of Health in 1995 typhoid 'hotspots' were identified, the worst being the area of Mkomazi in the Eastern Transvaal – being interestingly also where cholera first took hold in 1980 – along with several areas of the northern Transvaal. The main age group affected was between 5 and 29 years.[55]

Sporadic outbreaks and seemingly unrelated cases continued to occur, although after 1994 the widespread implementation of public water schemes and sanitation projects in rural areas and townships under the national Reconstruction and Development Programme started to improve the sanitary conditions of the poorer parts of the population. However an outbreak in Delmas in Mpumulanga (formerly in the Eastern Transvaal) between August and October 2005, which affected 596 people with five deaths, indicated that there were still problems in certain areas around the country – in this case found to be the continued use of the bucket sanitation system. The disease is likely to remain in existence at a low level in the country as the problems of typhoid carriers remains. However the heavy toll of the early outbreaks is less likely to occur as water and sanitation schemes continue to be implemented, and effective antibiotic treatment of cases keeps the death toll from the disease down.

ENDNOTES

1. Leibbrandt H.C.V. Journal of Jan van Riebeeck, *Precis of the Archives of the Cape of Good Hope*, Cape Town 1885:31
2. McCall Theal G. *History of South Africa 1486-1691*; Swan Sonnenschein, Lowrey, 1888:85
3. Liebbrandt H.C.V. 'Journal of Zacharias Wagenaer', *Precis of the Archives of the Cape of Good Hope, 1662-1670*, Cape Town 1901:144,
4. Liebbrandt H.C.V.' Letters Received 1695-1708' *Precis of the Archives of the Cape of Good Hope*, Cape Town 1896.
5. Liebbrandt H.C.V. 'Letters Despatched 1696-1708' *Precis of the Archives of the Cape of Good Hope*, Cape Town 1896:170
6. Bekker A.E. *The History of False Bay up to 1795*; Simon's Town Historical Society 1990:104
7. Cluver F.W.P. 'The Urban and RuralAspects of Enteric Fever Control', *South African Medical Journal*, 11(11) 1937:402-409
8. Neame L.E. *City Built on Gold,* Central New Agency, Cape Town, 1960:41-44
9. Du Preez I.F. *From Mission Station to Municipality*; Municipality of Pacaltsdorp, 1987:111
10. Searle C. *The history of the development of nursing in South Africa 1652-1960*; The South African Nursing Association; 1980:25
11. Shorten J.R. *The Johannesburg Saga*, John R Shorten,, for Johannesburg City Council, Johannesburg 1970:490
12. De Villiers J.C. 'The Medical Aspect of the Anglo-Boer War 1899-1902, Part II' *Military History Journal* 6(3) June 1984:102-105

13. Burdett Coutts cited in Martin A.C. *The Concentration Camps 1900-1902: Facts, Figures and Fables;* Howard Timmins Cape Town 1957:25
14. De Villiers J.C. 'The Military Significance of Typhoid in the Anglo-Boer War' *Jagger Journal*; University of Cape Town Libraries, 2, 1981:34-41
15. Gear J.H.S. 'The Anglo-Boer War of 1899-1902: Enteric Fever and Captain Maxwell Louis Hughes' *Adler Museum Bulletin*, 7 (1) March 1981:10-13
16. Searle C. *The history of the development of nursing in South Africa 1652-1960*; The South African Nursing Association; 1980:25
17. De Villiers J.C. 'The Military Significance of Typhoid in the Anglo-Boer War' *Jagger Journal* University of Cape Town Libraries, No 2 1981:36
18. Ibid, 39
19. Collins V.E 'Report of the Resident Surgeon Somerset Hospital' *Reports on the Government and Aided Hospitals and Asylums, 1900,* W.A. Richards, Cape Town, , G41-'1901 1901:3
20. Gear J.H.S. 'The Anglo-Boer War of 1899-1902: Enteric Fever and Captain Maxwell Louis Hughes' *Adler Museum Bulletin,* 7(1) March 1981:10-13
21. 'The Report of the Ladies Commission' cited in Martin A.C. *The Concentration Camps 1900-1902: Facts, Figures and Fables;* Howard Timmins Cape Town 1957:41
22. Gear J.H.S 'The Anglo-Boer War of 1899-1902: Enteric Fever and Captain Maxwell Louis Hughes' *Adler Museum Bulletin,* 7 (1) March 1981:10-13
23. Bolger James T. 'Report of the District Surgeon for 1902; Cape of Good Hope' *Reports on the Public Health 1902;* Cape Times Ltd 1903, G66-1903; 10-11
24. Editorial, 'Typhoid: The Outlook in South Africa' *South African Medical Journal* 33(31) 1 August 1959:641-642
25. Laing G.D. 'The Public Health Aspect of Typhoid Fever' *South African Medical Journal,* 8 (21) 1934:793-796.
26. Laing G.D. 'The Public Health Aspect of Typhoid Fever in Urban Areas', *South African Medical Journal,* 7 (9) 1933:288-289
27. Laing G.D. 'The Public Health Aspect of Typhoid Fever' *South African Medical Journal,* 8(21) 1934:793-796.
28. Donnolly F.A. and Nelson H. 'Some Observations on the Control of Infectious Disease', *South African Medical Journal,* 9 (18) 1935:629-641
29. *Annual Report of the Department of Public Health, Union of South Africa, 1933,* Government Printer Pretoria, UG 30-'33:21,
30. Cluver F.W.P.' Enteric Fever Prevention in Rural Areas' *South African Medical Journal,* 7(9) 1933:290
31. Ibid, 290
32. Seeff Harry, 'The Dietetic Treatment of Typhoid Fever' *South African Medical Journal,* 7(9) 1933:291-292.
33. Donnolly F.A. and Nelson H. 'Some Observations on the Control of Infectious Disease' *South African Medical Journal,* 9(18) 1935:629-641
34. Orenstein A.J. 'Enteric Fever in the Rand Mines' *South African Medical Journal,* 11(11) 1937:401-402
35. *Annual Report of the Department of Public Health 1935,* Government Printer Pretoria, UG 43- '35, 1935:24.
36. Grasset E. et al, 'Immunisation against Typhoid Fever by means of a single injection of Typhoid Endotoxoid Vaccine' *South African Medical Journal* 11(18) 1937:660-662.
37. Cluver F.W.P. 'The Urban and Rural Aspects of Enteric Fever Control', *South African Medical Journal* 11(11) 1937:402-409

38. *Annual Report of the Department of Public Health, Union of South Africa, 1939*, The Government Printer Pretoria, UG 57-'39 1939:21-26
39. Maule Clark B. 'Two interesting South African Typhoid Outbreaks' *South African Medical Journal* 13(24) 1939:806-808
40. Kark S.L. 'The management of an enteric fever outbreak in a "Native Territory"', *South African Medical Journal*, 17(6) 1943:87-88
41. Pullinger E.J. 'Pasteurisation of Milk in South Africa' *South African Medical Journal* 19(4) 1945:50-55
42. Fehrsen F.O. 'Pasteurisation of Milk, Report submitted to the City Council of Cape Town', in *South African Medical Journal* 19(17) 1945:302-305
43. Erasmus Ellis L, 'A case against the general pasteurization of milk' *South African Medical Journal*, 21(12) 1947:432-433.
44. *Annual Report of the Department of Public Health, 1945*, Government Printer Pretoria, UG No 6-'46, p24.
45. *Annual Report of the Department of Public Health, 1946*, Government Printer Pretoria, UG No 18-'47, p31
46. Nelson H. 'The Carrier in Enteric Fever' *South African Medical Journal*, 21(14) 1947:506-520
47. *Annual Report of the Medical Officer of Health, City of Cape Town, 1954*, Cape Times Ltd, Parow, 1954:66
48. *Annual Report of the Department of Health, Union of South Africa, 1958*, The Government Printer Pretoria, UG 33/1960,:48
49. Scott Millar J.W. *Report of the Medical Officer of Health on the Public Health and Sanitary Circumstances and Housing in Johannesburg during the period 1st January to 31st December 1959;* City of Johannesburg. 1959:10
50. Turner R. 'Vaccination Against Typhoid Fever' *South African Medical Journal* 33(31) 1 August 1959: 639-640
51. Turner R. 'The Role of the Laboratory in the diagnosis and control of typhoid fever' *South African Medical Journal*, 33(31) 1 August 1959:647
52. Editorial, 'Typhoid: The Outlook in South Africa' *South African Medical Journal* 33(31) 1 August 1959: 641-642
53. Saville Lewis J. *Annual Report of the Medical Officer of Health for Port Elizabeth, 1965*, Longs, Port Elizabeth, 1965:30.
54. Van Heerden J.R. *Annual Report of the Medical Officer of Health for East London January 1968 to December 1971*, Griff-Stan, East London, December 1976.
55. Küstner H.G.V. 'Typhoid Fever in South Africa, 1919–1994' *Epidemiological Comments*, Department of Health Pretoria, 22 (2) February 1995:24-38

6   TYPHUS: 'DEVERMINATION' AND DDT

Typhus is another disease which is fading from memory and common knowledge, yet it was one of the earliest mentioned infectious diseases to be brought to South Africa and was devastating to both the local and immigrant population. Caused by Rickettsiae, which are intracellular organisms resembling viruses and bacteria, it occurs in several strains. Transmission to humans is by an insect or arthropod vector such as lice, fleas or ticks. The most dramatic epidemic form is caused by Rickettsia prowazekii and is transmitted by body lice through their faeces – when a bite is scratched the organisms from nearby louse droppings can make their way into the wound, and into the blood stream. This mechanism was only recognised in the early 1900's however, with a widely quoted experiment by a Serbian doctor who placed typhus patients, after a thorough delousing process, into one bed with healthy people and found that no transmission of infection took place.

    The lice spread from person-to-person in unhygienic and overcrowded conditions – amongst the poor in slums, soldiers in war time, prisoners in overcrowded jails and refugees in camps. After seven to fourteen days fever and headache occur, with very high temperatures, severe headaches and a widespread rash. Collapse of the circulatory system, kidneys and pneumonia can occur, followed by death, particularly in older people if untreated. The disease was introduced by Dutch sailors arriving at the Cape, probably on the ship Medemblick which arrived in 1665, during which year over 12% of crew members died.[1] 1666 was the year with the highest mortality in the Cape up until 1670 and four-fifths of the 'Hottentots' (Khoikhoi) died from an epidemic, thought to be typhus. Theal McCall, writing in 1888, stated that 'the Hottentots suffered very severely from a disease which broke out among them. What its nature was is not stated, but as the Europeans were not attacked by it, it is not probable that it was introduced by them. It was certainly not smallpox'. However that reasoning was probably flawed – that Europeans were not fatally affected is more suggestive of the fact that they had been previously exposed and acquired immunity.

He goes on 'Mr Wagenaar [Commander of the Cape 1662-1666] computed the loss of the Goringhaiquas and Gorachouquas at one-fifth of their original number ... the Cochoquas suffered even more'.[2] As a louse-borne disease it was probably aided by the fact that, at that time, the only bath in South Africa was for the treatment of venereal-diseased patients and there was apparently minimal washing of people or clothes.[3] In October 1671 the Journal of C. van Breitenbach reported 'the hot fevers, accompanied with wild delirium, have for some time occupied some persons here, and though mostly all have recovered towards evening our chief surgeon, Jan Hol of Harderwyck died'. Specifically what these infections were is uncertain – they were put down to the wind, which was 'considered to cause much sickness by throwing up the vile and stinking sea vapours'.[4]

In April 1687 an epidemic attacked the indigenous inhabitants, thought again to be typhus. Half of the 'Hottentots' died and the remaining survivors were all left sick. The European population was also reduced by half, from 612 to 309. At that time the authorities thought that it was spread through the burning of grass and bush by the 'Hottentots'.[5]

Typhus continued to be endemic at the Cape through the 18th century and appeared on almost every vessel which called at Table Bay, from which they were taken to the hospital buildings. Many of the recruits had previously served in the military, and the conditions on board ship were ideal for harbouring lice. As many as 300 men were on board, and their quarters were cramped and airless. While the English East India Company checked all who were embarking for the voyage to the East, in Holland it was usual to insist on vessels sailing, regardless of however many sick were on board. When it was realised that there was some connection between filth and disease efforts were made to keep the ship clean, by washing it down twice a week, but the lice infestation of the men was not addressed. The disease was attributed to 'malignant vapours' as were many others at the time, rather than louse-born spread.[6] An epidemic of typhus broke out in Malmesbury in April 1824. By this time it was endemic amongst the Khoikhoi population, although it did not appear to be prominent in the Cape Town prison, unlike in England where it was known as 'gaol fever'.

The next major reference to the disease comes with the severe outbreak of typhus which occurred in the Eastern Cape in the early 1900's. In 1909 – 1910 Drs W. and R.L. Girdwood submitted reports to the Cape Department of Health of a disease they described as typhus in the Kentani District of the Transkei. The diagnosis was not accepted by the Department of Health and the doctors were told that they were dealing with malignant influenza.[7] It was only some years later that the Assistant Medical Officer of Health for the Union, Dr Mitchell, reported that typhus had commenced probably in the Victoria District around 1900, and by 1908 there were some 200-300 cases in the Transkei. The disease was known locally as Fever Mnyama, or Black Fever, and had been known to local people for some 40-50 years or longer. It may have been around for longer as a low fever without rash and was possibly linked to the time when housing construction changed – when they stopped building reed huts which were periodically burned, as was still the case in Zululand at that time.

The Inspector of Native Locations at Glen Grey in 1910 reported a large number of deaths from what was then called Black Fever, which was described as a kind of low fever combined with a bad form of influenza, which the local population thought was being brought back by labourers on the mines. It was recommended that a delegation from the Health Department be sent to investigate it. A similar outbreak occurred in 1916 around Queenstown, at first thought to be typhoid, and then later found more likely to be typhus. It was thought that the majority of cases notified in the area as typhoid were really a form of typhus and estimated that in the Queenstown area and 15 surrounding districts, as far as Matatiele, there had been at least 50 cases of that form of typhus in Europeans and 1,000 or more African cases with a considerable mortality. They now called the disease Mbatalala meaning that the disease strikes and knocks one down, as the predominant feature was an acute and severe prostration.[8] Further symptoms included severe headache, pains in the back and limbs, neck stiffness, tremor, delirium, swelling of the face, and high temperature. The tongue became brown and cracked with a blackish crust, giving rise to the name Black Fever. Mortality was between 10 and 30% between the 6th and 14th day, usually from heart failure. Spread was thought up until 1909 to have been due to 'exhalations and emanations' from the patient and by 'fomites' in infected bedding, clothing etc.[9]

Typhus was by then endemic in the Eastern Cape and Transkei and had increased in virulence. Between 20 and 30% had the typical rash, starting on the chest and abdomen and excluding the face, palms and soles, although this was less easy to see in dark skin. In children the diseases was generally mild. In 1910 the discovery had been made by researchers in Mexico that the disease was transmitted by body lice and possible causative organisms identified. The causative organism, Rickettsia prowazeki, was first discovered in 1913 by Prowazek in experiments which cost him his life. However debate went on for some years thereafter as to whether this was in fact responsible for the disease. During the early 1900's, around 1917, the increasing recognition of typhus as a threat caused great confusion in diagnosis between typhoid and typhus. The tests available, the Widal and the Weil-Felix, were sometimes both positive, and the symptoms were so variable for each that accurate diagnosis was difficult.

It was postulated by Dr Mitchell that the wearing of old European clothing by Africans, along with the reduction in the habit of burning huts after disease or death, had contributed to the increase in the disease in the Eastern Cape and Transkei. It was also noticed that, as in Mexico, the disease was more prevalent in colder conditions – either the upland areas or in winter - due to the lice being less able to survive in hot weather.[10] Dr Mitchell proposed that the main methods of control related to the improvement of housing and a campaign against lice, as being the main conveyors of the disease. In the towns he recommended the construction of ferro-concrete huts for Africans with or without thatched roofs, adequate lighting and ventilation, a cleanliness campaign and the boiling, disinfection or destruction of the clothes of infected persons. He recommended also the restriction of movement of people between clean and infected areas, cleansing and disinfection of 'verminous persons', encouragement of outdoor sleeping and cyanide fumigation and cleansing of railway carriages and other public vehicles. Suspects were to be removed if possible to isolation hospitals and nursed as far as possible by 'immunes' – those who had recovered from an attack. Rubbish, rags and useless articles should be burned and if necessary infected dwellings should be closed or burned. Those involved in nursing or disinfection should protect themselves with suitable overalls, and rubber gloves.[11]

By the end of 1917 the disease was being reported from Paarl through to the Eastern Cape, and was extending northwards to the then Basutoland (Lesotho) with almost 3,500 cases reported by October and 700 deaths. A system of border guards was established on the border of the Orange Free State with Natal to try and prevent the spread of disease into the Free State, with a disinfecting station at Sterkstroom, and leaflets were distributed in local languages giving information about the disease, the need for cleanliness of dwellings and the destruction of lice and vermin. But by 1918 typhus was occurring widely across South Africa with outbreaks reported from the Eastern Cape, Natal, the Transvaal and the Orange Free State.[12] For travellers across country by train inspections were made of new arrivals from the Cape at the Sterkstroom Junction disinfection station to try and prevent the arrival of the disease. Any Africans, Coloureds or Asians who arrived by train in third class coaches had to be cleansed from head to toe in the presence of a European with their clothing boiled or disinfected. The carriages were emptied and the passengers had to undress, hand over their blankets and clothes to be fumigated and then proceed to wash themselves in a large concrete disinfecting bath with cold water. They were then sprayed with a chemical emulsion which had to be rubbed into the head and body, after which they were given a clean blanket and sent for medical inspection. Following this they would wait for their disinfected clothes to be returned before continuing on their journey. This process applied to all third class passengers, African, Coloured or Asian, and applied equally to African women, who were also subject to the humiliating cleansing and head-shaving process. While degrading for all, it was the more educated, better clothed and more affluent who raised the most vehement objections to the process.

After some public outcry the Sterkstroom junction was investigated by the Native Affairs Department with a view to exempting those more educated and westernised Africans from the process. Much debate ensued between those health professionals who insisted that the entire process should continue, and those who felt that there should be a preliminary assessment to exempt those who appeared clean and well attired.[13] The regulations were amended in 1918 to make it a requirement that every African, Coloured and Asian person coming from a typhus area carried a certificate that they were healthy and free of vermin.[14] The incidence of typhus peaked in 1920 when there were over 11,000 cases and almost 1,800 deaths, although it was thought this figures only represented a fraction of the total cases as many in the rural areas went unreported. The Ndabeni location in Cape Town, created by the forced removal of the poor following the plague, was particularly badly hit. The Typhus Regulations were in force across the Union and required farmers, mining companies and other employers and local authorities to provide their employees and residents with reasonable means and facilities for cleansing themselves and keeping themselves free from vermin. It was suggested that these be attached to the municipal beer-halls so that access to beer could be an incentive for the 'dirty or verminous' to get cleansed. By 1922 the Department of Health was estimating that some 2,500 Africans per year were dying of the disease.

In 1923 there was an outbreak of epidemic typhus at one of the African compounds in the dock area at Durban with 99 cases. Many of these had initially been misdiagnosed as paratyphoid and influenza. From

1924 to 1928 about 200 cases were seen in the Durban municipal area and surrounds. The earlier cases were in the low-lying part of town and the dock area, where a large percentage were railway workers, later spreading to higher grounds. The cleansing procedures put into place by the Durban Municipality to tackle the outbreak were similar to those of the Sterkstroom disinfection centre and by the mid-1920's some 50,000 black men were regularly put through these 'deverminisation' processes. To the Africans who endured them they were known as 'dipping', in line with the process used on cattle to prevent bovine diseases. The humiliation of the system lead to a major campaign by the Industrial and Commercial Workers Union, who complained of its embarrassment and indignity, in which men of all ages were stripped and disinfected together. However after a temporary respite the Durban municipality resumed the procedures in the 1930's.[15] Other forms of typhus existing in the country were tick-borne typhus, which did not cause mortality or epidemics, and endemic or flea-borne typhus (murine) which tended to affect 'better class Europeans' in coastal towns and also was less severe. Sometimes it was difficult to distinguish between flea-borne and louse-borne typhus.[16]

In 1930 there was a peak of 1,782 cases of typhus, in 88 different districts across the country, although mostly in the Cape with 1,530 cases. Altogether it caused 212 deaths. The increase was ascribed to the wearing-off of immunity, and a survey of the Eastern Cape suggested it was also due to increasing poverty of Africans resulting from prolonged and repeated droughts and over-population. Glen Grey was a particular case in point where there was a dense population and great poverty, with the children noted to be suffering from malnutrition. The Department of Public Health noted that the problem of typhus in the African territories was largely an economic one:

> The disease will tend to tail off and disappear with agricultural development and corresponding improved nutrition and better conditions of living. The impoverished native offers little resistance to the disease because of malnutrition, and the poorer he is the more infested in general is his body with the insect vector of the disease, the louse.[17]

This then caused concern about the increasing incidence in European areas adjoining Africa areas, with several typhus outbreaks in Queenstown traced back to Glen Grey, and a severe outbreak in the Maclear District being traced to the neighbouring African districts of Tsolo and Qumbu.

Outbreaks in 1931 occurred in the Ventersdorp and Lichtenburg areas due to the Africans living in squalid conditions on alluvial diamond diggings, where some 60-75% of dwellings were considered unfit and where the diet was often barely above starvation level. By 1934 epidemic typhus was still on the increase with mortality amongst Africans of up to 30%, frequently due to secondary pneumonia. Deaths in Europeans were less common, thought to be due to their increased resistance. The peak incidence was in the winter months with almost 7,000 cases reported in the 1934/35 season and a thousand deaths. Again it was noted to be related to the increasing acute economic stress along with the wearing-off of immunity acquired during the earlier epidemic periods of the previous decade. Much of the increase was in the Orange Free State, where the economic stress was said to be severe. Outbreaks occurred in 30 districts introduced from the then Basutoland (now Lesotho).

> Natives suffering from the effects of extreme poverty, badly infested with lice have been streaming over the border from Basutoland to look for work in the Free State. Typhus is apparently rife in Basutoland since many of these Basutos brought infection with them and lit up the disease in the various districts to which they travelled[18]

Inspectors were stationed along the between Lesotho and the Free State border and temporary additional 'de-verminisers' employed. Other factors cited by the Department of Health in the spread of typhus were:

> The backwardness and poverty of the Bantu population of the Eastern Cape ... even if some notion of the desirability of cleanliness is impressed upon them, their customs often make reasonable cleanliness impracticable. According to tribal custom the native must take whatever piece of ground that is allotted to him. His allotment is generally far from water which has to be fetched in receptacles. Under these circumstances only the water absolutely necessary for drinking and cooking is conveyed to the huts. Washing of bodies, clothing or blankets is out of the question.[19]

Along with the fact that many of them were very poorly nourished, the traditional beliefs were also considered to be a contributing factor to the spread of typhus: 'The Xhosa is still very superstitious. When a severe sickness such as typhus attacks his family he consults the witch-doctor and readily believes that evil spirits have come among his family. He generally acts on the advice to leave the kraal with his stricken family. Verminous typhus patients and contacts scatter infection on their journey'. However the Department recognised that the problem was more complex than simply the customary behaviour of the African population. They continued in the same report: 'the imitation of [European] civilisation is also having harmful effects. The semi-civilised Xhosa will adopt European clothing without the cleanliness which should accompany the wearing of such clothing. The increased possibility of lousiness is evident'. This reflected one of the negative health impacts of the merging of two cultures that were occurring in South Africa at that time, although phrased in the colonial terminology used by White South Africa in that era. The control of typhus in this situation was seen as unlikely, and the Health Department was mainly responding to outbreaks when they were reported with deverminisation of patients and contacts by rubbing with naphthalene oil, and clothing and blankets being treated by means of a 'tent deverminizer' or 'barrel deverminizer'.

In 1935 at the request of the Council of Public Health an investigation of South African epidemic typhus strains was commenced with a view to eventually obtaining a vaccine for use against typhus in the union. It was discovered that the Zinsser-Castenada vaccine from Mexico produced immunity against South African murine and epidemic typhus in guinea pigs and felt that this must eventually lead to a consideration of the procedure as a means of combating typhus in the Union. While delousing was also considered important it was felt that a reliable vaccine would be more effective, given the large and far-flung population.[20] In 1935 and 1936 there were again many cases, with almost 13,000 cases reported and 1,600 deaths over the two year period. As with the 1920 epidemic the outbreak was linked to severe droughts which caused a failure of crops and a severe food shortage among the population. This led to under-nutrition, which contributed to the spread of disease. The shortage of water in the drought reduced the frequency of washing, and the poverty lead to concentrations of destitute people on the farms of the Free State who were in search of food and work once the drought broke.

The classifications of the different variants of typhus, or Rickettsioses, and their different hosts – lice (epidemic typhus), fleas (murine or sporadic) and ticks (tick-bite fever) - were a source of much debate and research in the 1930s. The three Rickettsioses in South Africa were often confused, and outbreaks responded to as they occurred. Tick bite fever could generally be distinguished by the presence of the tick bite site with its typical black centre and painful lymph glands. While the symptoms resembled typhus the course was milder and fatalities did not occur. Most cases were said to occur a week after an excursion such as visiting a farm, a picnic, a camping party or a country walk. Occasionally ticks were brought back into urban houses on blankets or clothing and most cases could be traced back to the veld. Domestic dogs were not thought to bring the diseases into the houses. Tick bite fever was found not to give immune protection against epidemic or murine typhus.[21]

Epidemic louse-borne typhus remained mainly among the African population, except for those Europeans living in 'exceptionally bad hygienic conditions, such as diamond diggings'. Infection was found to confer immunity against the other two types of typhus. Murine typhus was typically much milder than the epidemic form, although some became severely ill. The two diseases were often mistaken for each other. Murine typhus however typically appeared only sporadically, being an epidemic disease of rats and only occasionally being transmitted to man. Sporadic cases occurred every year in Pretoria and all over South Africa, mostly in summer, and many were probably misdiagnosed as typhoid, German measles (rubella) etc. It protected against tick bite fever but not epidemic typhus.[22]

By the late 1930s cases of epidemic typhus were averaging around 1,000 a year with a case-fatality rate of between 10 and 30%. While control focussed on 'deverminisation' the search for a vaccine continued. One method advocated by Weigl consisted of feeding lice on infected individuals for at least seven days after they were infected, and then making a suspension of infected louse intestines, which was perhaps accurately described as 'laborious'. The preferred vaccine in South Africa was the Zinsser-Castenada vaccine, which required three doses and had been found effective in animals.[23] Typhus remained common throughout the Transkei with the inland, higher areas more affected than the coastal areas. Again this was presumed to be related to the wearing of more clothes and less frequent washing in the cooler areas. While murine typhus was known to be present, the majority of cases were louse-borne epidemic typhus. The spread across the area was thought to be contributed to by the travelling of the people across the region where they were put up in huts in the villages they visited, thus aiding the spread of lice from kraal to kraal. Also during illness it was the custom for relatives and friends to come from all over and stay in the kraal to offer support. They would then return to their villages with the lice. Spread was also common at functions and ceremonies such as weddings and funerals, particularly the latter where mourners would gather in the deceased's hut, where the lice would leave the body of the dead person and migrate towards the visitors. If young married women became ill it was the custom to return to their home village, and other women might come to care for her children, all of which aided its spread. While children were rarely affected they also wandered from hut to hut.

Those Europeans affected were generally either nurses and doctors, or traders with close contact with the African population, others being less affected due to their lack of contact as they were 'in every sphere of life...separated by the colour bar'. The migratory labour system then spread the disease across the country. The case-fatality rate from the disease in the African population was less than 5% in children, but increased with age to be almost always fatal in the elderly. The diagnostic test remained the Weil-Felix test. There remained no specific treatment for the disease with the sulphonamides being ineffective except for the treatment of any associated pneumonia. Quinine was also tried as a treatment, but the control of the disease was considered to be best achieved through delousing of the population. There were three methods used – the application of heat, the application of insecticides to clothing, and the anointment of bodies with insecticidal oil. It was recommended that, rather than just attending to kraals with proven infection, centres should be established at borders to delouse every African leaving the territory as happened in the 1918 epidemic, although these had been closed down due to difficulties, including the complaints of the Africans. Gear recommended re-introducing them along with a vaccination campaign.[24] In the urban areas the provision of public showers and hot water was recommended.

The disease was again particularly prevalent in 1939, particularly in the Lusikisiki district, to the east of Lesotho, where 70 deaths were reported in just one week. The high mortality was thought to be a reflection of their malnourished stated and inadequate nursing services. At that period signs of extensive malnutrition were said to be everywhere with outbreaks of scurvy and pellagra occurring in African territories. The extent to which typhus and typhoid spread among Africans and indigent Europeans was attributed to malnutrition, resulting not from insufficiency of food so much as from a gross insufficiency of protective foods such as milk, vegetables, eggs, fruit, milk and fish. The staple maize meal was particularly poor in vitamins, minerals and protein.[25] Murine or flea-borne typhus continued to occur occasionally, with several cases being reported from the Port Elizabeth area in 1944 spread by rats. The Weil-Felix test could not differentiate between this and epidemic typhus. A Rickettsial complement-fixation test however became available with could distinguish between the two.

During the Second World War the use of the insecticide DDT

(dichlor-diphenyl-trichlorethane) had commenced in the fight against typhus. First synthesized in 1874, its insect-killing powers were not discovered until 1940. In early 1943 it had been concluded that the simplest and most effective method of delousing the hundreds of thousands of labourers in the army in the Middle East would be by dusting their clothing with an insecticide. A cyanogas dusting pump was tried, then replaced with a hand-dusting gun using the British Army anti-louse powder known as AL63. This was later replaced with DDT, first used in Naples in dealing with a typhus outbreak by the American Typhus Commission and Allied Military Government. During a single month 1,300,000 civilians were dusted with it and within three weeks the outbreak was completely brought under control. This made history as the first time ever that a typhus epidemic fever in Europe was arrested in midwinter. Shortly thereafter all troops in Europe were issued with DDT impregnated garments which protected against lice for at least two months, even after laundering.[26] Originally the formula was secret and it was only with some difficulty that the formula was obtained for South Africa and a small plant established to make it. By 1945 production had been increased and DDT was being recommended for use on Africans in rural areas as a 10% powder mixed with talcum powder, using a dust gun or air compressor. It was recommended that individuals pass along in a queue and be treated for a few seconds each without removing their clothing, using approximately 1.5-2 ounces of dust per person, blown into the hat, up each arm, between each layer of clothing, down the neck in front and back, and down the lower garments front and back. In that way thousands of people per day could be treated. Such methods were effective for around three weeks so that hatching lice were also killed.[27]

Typhus remained a problem into the 1940's, with there being 5,600 cases in 1944 and 2,600 deaths (only 3 of which were European), followed by 2,000 cases in 1945 and over 500 deaths. It was widespread among the rural African population and outbreaks occurred particularly in the Eastern Transvaal through the 1930's where Africans lived mainly in collections of huts on European-owned farms. The huts were mostly rodent-infested with numerous flies, cockroaches and fleas, and with shortages of water restricting hygiene. An outbreak occurred in the Middleburg district affecting four farms and 50 victims which spread to different places following attendance at the funerals of those who succumbed. In order to deal with the outbreak in January 1945 a supply of DDT was obtained from the Ministry of Supply Chemical Warfare Factory in Midrand and the epidemic was contained by spraying with DDT solution as well as with DDT dusting powder distributed by mechanical dusters. In October of that year another outbreak occurred in the Witbank area affecting several farms and 150 people. The disease spread from farm to farm across the African compounds, by the movement of people away from affected farms to new farms. Again DDT was used to control the epidemic, applied in the form of a dust mixed with talc to the clothes and blankets of all the inhabitants of the kraals, and as a 5% solution in paraffin to the floors, mats, walls and roofs of the huts.[28]

In addition to the use of DDT, noting the connection between famine and typhus, the authorities were urged to secure sufficient supplies of food, and 'Headmen' were urged by Magistrates to reduce wastage of maize meal through rodent damage and to avoid its waste through using it for beer-making. Drought and widespread crop failures had caused food shortages among Africans and relief measures were being put into place. In urban areas the Public Health Department noted that the eradication of the disease among the African population required the provision of hygienic homes with adequate ablution and sanitary facilities and the improvement of peoples' economic status. It said that:

> while some progressive urban local authorities are aware of the necessity for providing their non-European inhabitants with the essentials requisite to living healthy lives, it is regrettable that many others still do not measure up to their responsibilities. Consequently they still present the depressing picture of non-Europeans living in dreary, over-crowded insanitary hovels, deficient in light, water and sanitary facilities.[29]

Massive movements of people towards Cape Town in particular were causing concern about the introduction of typhus, as Africans who had arrived to work on major construction schemes remained and established new settlements. It was estimated 500 people a week were arriving from the eastern areas of Transkei and Ciskei. In respect of food it was said that Africans moving into town for work often moved to a worse dietary intake, with white bread, tea and sugar replacing the maize, milk, meat and vegetables of rural areas.

Despite all the poverty, shortage of soap and malnutrition however, the impact of DDT on the country's disease toll from epidemic typhus was dramatic. In the space of just two years of usage by 1947 the case load had dropped to 626 and the number of deaths was down to 32 – a tiny fraction of what had been occurring each year since the disease was first recorded back in 1917. There were still localised outbreaks with 130 cases and 31 deaths in the Barkley West district in 1947 and a small outbreak in the Orange Free State in 1949 with ten cases of which two died, although the newly discovered antibiotics of aureomycin and chloramphenicol were tried and found helpful if used early in the illness. These numbers continued to fall due to the extended use and increasing acceptability of DDT usage and the fact that cases were more rapidly reported to the Department so that the typhus inspectors could step in and control any outbreak. DDT was also available for purchase and use by Africans in rural stores. 1952 gave a low total of 98 cases and 8 deaths across the country.[30] By 1953 the Department stated 'with the remarkable decline in the incidence of this once 'formidable epidemic disease' the stage has now been reached where it can no longer be regarded as a menace to public health' – a considerable achievement for a disease which just nine years earlier had killed 2,600 people, and affected thousands of people annually since first fully recognised in the early 1900's.[31]

The extensive use of DDT powder for lice control started to raise fears of resistant lice by the mid 1950s, with lice in Queenstown showing the highest degree of resistance of any lice in the world. However if applied correctly 10% DDT powder in talc still gave a 100% kill of lice. Occasional cases were aggressively dealt with, as in Port Elizabeth where one notified case in December 1960 in the 'Red Location' lead to a programme of dusting some 8,000 people and the deverminisation of 1,300 houses over the next few weeks.[32] The decline in typhus continued through the 1960's with the notified numbers rarely exceeding 100, usually in the Eastern Cape area, and this fall was ascribed to the success of DDT measures. The Department of Health reported that 'the deverminisation of the population of the endemic area in Western Tembuland is carried out regularly and each year thousands of persons and huts are dusted with 10% DDT. All cases, suspected cases and contacts, as well as their dwellings, clothes and bedding are deverminised without delay and the process is repeated within 14 days'. In addition to educational measures it continued: 'in 1965 the routine deverminisation of all migrant Bantu labourers was commenced; this is done at Lady Frere before their departure'.[33]

The number of cases continued to fall and, after a small surge in 1968 to 192 cases, all in the Eastern Cape region, the last significant recording was 48 cases in 1972. The 1968 outbreak was ascribed to prolonged heat and drought which had created favourable conditions for the breeding of the body louse. The de-lousing measures were applied to their homes, clothing and bedding. The routine delousing of the population with 10% DDT in the endemic areas of the Ciskei and

Transkei continued through the 1960's. Following 1972 there were no cases except for the last notified, confirmed case of louse-borne typhus in 1981, although through the 1980's it was still present in other African countries including Ethiopia, Burundi, Nigeria and Rwanda.[34] It had effectively been eradicated from South Africa, the use of DDT for delousing and 'devermination' had ceased, and the disease appears at this stage to be unlikely to return.

ENDNOTES

1. Laidler P.W. and Gelfand M. *South Africa its Medical History, 1652-1898: A medical and social study*; C Struik, Cape Town, 1971:15
2. McCall Theal G. *History of South Africa 1486-1691* Swan Sonnenschen, Lowrey and Co, London, 1888:175
3. Laidler P.W. and Gelfand M. *South Africa its medical history, 1652-1898: A medical and social study*; C Struik, Cape Town, 1971:17
4. Liebbrandt H.C.V; 'Journal of C. van Breitenbach' *Precis of the Archives of the Cape of Good Hope 1671-1674 and 1676*; WA Richards, CapeTown 1902.
5. Laidler P.W. and Gelfand M. *South Africa its medical history, 1652-1898: A medical and social study*; C Struik Cape Town, 1971:21
6. Searle C. *The history of the development of nursing in South Africa 1652-1960*; The South African Nursing Association; 1980:17
7. Saville Lewis J. *Annual Report of the Medical Officer of Health of Port Elizabeth*, Longs Port Elizabeth 1962:63
8. Mitchell J.A. 'Address on Typhus Fever' *South African Medical Record*, 15(16) 1917:244-248
9. Mitchell J.A. 'Typhus Fever ("Black Fever" or "Mtetalala") in the Cape Province' *South African Medical Record*, 15(17) 1917:259-262
10. Mitchell J.A. 'Address on Typhus Fever' *South African Medical Record*, 15(16) 1917:244-248
11. Mitchell J.A. 'Typhus Fever ("Black Fever" or "Mtetalala") in the Cape Province' *South African Medical Record*, 15(17) 1917:259-262
12. Barrett E. *Report of the Department of Native Affairs for the years 1913-1918*, Cape Times Ltd UG 7-19, 1919:29
13. Marks S. and Anderson N. 'Typhus and Social Control: South Africa 1917-1950' in MacLeod R. and Lewis M. *Disease, Medicine and Empire, perspectives on Western Medicine and the experience of European Expansion*; Routledge, London, 1988:265-283
14. 'Public Health Bulletin: Typhus' *South African Medical Record*, 16(19) 12 October 1918:302
15. Marks S. and Anderson N. 'Typhus and Social Control: South Africa 1917-1950' in MacLeod R and Lewis M, *Disease, Medicine and Empire, perspectives on Western Medicine and the experience of European Expansion*; Routledge, London, 1988:275
16. Rhodes W.F. 'Typhus-like fevers in the Union of South Africa' *South African Medical Journal*, 8(21) 1934:797-799

17 *Annual Report of the Department of Public Health, Union of South Africa, 1935*, Government Printer Pretoria, UG 43-'35 p43
18 'Annual Report of the Department of Public Health, Union of South Africa, 1934', Government Printer Pretoria, cited in Küstner H.G.V. 'Louse-borne Typhus – an Overview', *Epidemiological Comments*, Department of National Health and Population Development, 16(5) May 1989:7.
19 *Annual Report of the Department of Public Health, Union of South Africa, 1930*, Government Printer Pretoria, UG 40-'30 p45
20 Finlayson M.H. and Grobler J.M. 'A study of South African Epidemic Typhus strains and the protection afforded by the Zinsser-Castenada vaccine against infection with these strains'. *South African Medical Journal* 14(7) 13 April 1940:129.
21 Pijper A. 'Rickettsioses of South Africa' *South African Medical Journal*, 12(17) 1938:613-630
22 Ibid, 630
23 Finlayson M.H. 'South African Typhus with special reference to the use of an Alum-Precipitated vaccine' *South African Medical Journal*, 14(12) 1940:247-249
24 *Annual Report of the Department of Public Health, Union of South Africa, 1939*, Government Printer Pretoria, UG 52-'39, p91-93
25 Gear James, 'Typhus Fever in the Transkei', *South African Medical Journal*, 18(8) 1944:144-148.
26 *Annual Report of the Department of Public Health, 1945*, Government Printer Pretoria, UG No 6-'1946, p49.
27 Gear J.H.S. 'A note on the use of DDT in Medical and Health Problems', *South African Medical Journal*, 19(16) 1945:290-292
28 Gear J.H.S, 'Typhus fever in the Eastern Transvaal, with Special Reference to an Epidemic occurring in 1945', *South African Medical Journal* 21(7) 1947: 214-218
29 *Annual Report of the Department of Public Health, 1945*, Government Printer Pretoria, UG No 6-'1946, p29
30 *Annual Report of the Department of Health, Union of South Africa, 1952*, Government Printer Pretoria, UG 40-'1954, p19
31 *Annual Report of the Department of Health, Union of South Africa, 1953*, Government Printer Pretoria, UG 23-'1956, p14
32 Saville Lewis J. *Annual Reports of the Medical Officer of Health for 1960, and 1962*, Longs, Port Elizabeth.1960:49 and 1962:51
33 *Report of the Department of Health for the years 1965, 1966 and 1967, Republic of South Africa*, Published by Authority 1969, RP 53/1969 p15
34 Küstner H.G.V. 'Louse-borne Typhus – an Overview' *Epidemiological Comments*, Department of National Health and Population Development, 16(5) May 1989:2-8.

7   MIGRANT LABOUR AND THE PANDEMIC OF INFLUENZA

Influenza was known to have existed from the 12th century, first being described in epidemic form in the year 1173. Its name came from the Italian word 'influenz', because in the 17th century the Italians ascribed it to astral or telluric influences. While epidemics raged in Italy, France and Germany in 1387, the first record of a pandemic was in 1510, which started in Malta and spread through most of Europe. A second pandemic occurred in 1580.[1]

Burchell mentions an outbreak of influenza in South Africa around 1815 which occurred at the Cape and which affected 6,000 people although comparatively few died. Mention was made of epidemics of influenza in Cape Town in November 1836, 1853 and 1854, and again in 1862, December 1871, 1892 and 1900. A mortality rate of 1 per 1,000 was given for 1862 and 1871, and a similar mortality rate of 1.04 per 1,000 was given in the Cape Colony for 1895/96.[2] Studies in the pandemic which started in 1889/90 found that the influenza was spread by human contact, not airborne. From around 1892 it became generally accepted that it was an infectious disease, not spread by 'miasmatic influence', with the causative organism thought to be a bacteria called Bacillus influenzae, described by Pfeiffer. This epidemic had started in Bucharest, from where it spread across Europe and then to South Africa. The South African epidemic in the early nineties was milder than the one in Europe of which it was an extension, attributed to the milder climate exposing the patients to less risk of pulmonary complications.[3] Known as the Russian influenza it first came ashore at Table Bay and primarily affected young adults.

The development of the mining industry around Kimberley and Johannesburg in the late 1800's was one of the factors contributing to the spread of infectious diseases generally in South Africa, as it brought together hundreds of thousands of men living in heavily overcrowded, insanitary conditions with inadequate nutrition. From there they were ideally placed to spread disease across the entire Southern African region when they returned to their homes. After the Anglo-Boer War in 1903 the shortage of labour to serve the mines and industrial areas was acute and it was estimated by a Commission sitting in the Transvaal that as many as 195,000 additional labourers would be required over the next five years. A Labour Importation Ordinance was passed to bring in additional labourers from other countries. Recruitment to the mines was intense and covered not only South Africa but also countries such as the then Rhodesia (now Zimbabwe), Portuguese East Africa (Mozambique), German South-West Africa (Namibia), and British Central Africa (Malawi).[4] In June of 1903 large numbers of men arrived from central Malawi and other countries to the north where they had enjoyed a hot, tropical climate, to find themselves in the Witwatersrand mines in the middle of a cold Highveld winter, where an influenza epidemic was raging. The desperate need for labour had also brought in additional South African labourers who, although used to cold winters, were of insufficient physique for mine work and also men who were undernourished due to the failure of the mealie crops in their own homesteads. Many of these men were quite unable to withstand the severe climate change and died shortly after arrival on the mines. The mortality rate soared to an annualised rate of over 80 per 1,000 from acute respiratory infections in the second half of 1903.[5]

The men who came from tropical Malawi faired particularly badly. Each had been given a sweater, shirt, suit of clothes, overcoat and two blankets, and were fed a diet of coffee, biscuits, meat and vegetable stew, rice, mealie meal and traditional sorghum beer. Still the death rate was the highest since mortality rates had been recorded, reaching 112.5 per thousand (annualised) in July 1903. Some 615 labourers on the mines died of disease in that month. An investigation of the influenza epidemic commenced which included daily inspections of the labourers, with the sick ones being admitted to hospital and others removed to a separate compound with proper shelter and heating. Instructions were issued to recruiters to exercise more care in their selection of men, to ensure they were physically strong enough to endure the tough conditions. The epidemic led to some changes in the treatment of miners with hot coffee provided when they emerged from the mine, along with improvements to their accommodation such as replacing the mud floors, inserting wooden bunk beds rather than the former concrete shelves, fitting proper stoves for heating, improving lighting, ventilation and sanitary arrangements. Supportive Coloured Labourers' Health Regulations were brought in. Still in the following years the mortality rate amongst those from central Africa was very high – up to 195 per 1,000 in the second half of 1905 – upon which it was concluded that, should the high rate continue 'it would be humanly indefensible to countenance further recruiting from tropical areas'.[6]

The next significant outbreak of influenza was the worst ever seen. The great influenza pandemic of 1918 appeared at the end of World War 1 commencing in a mild way in America, taken by American troops to Europe, and from there across the rest of the world. Germany and Austria were initially badly affected, but there were few fatalities. However it was said to have been sufficiently bad to have delayed the German offensive. It then appeared in Spain where it was reported as affecting over 8,000,000 people. It then became known as the Spanish flu, although only 700 died in Spain and it did not originate there. The disease began at the Western front among Allied French, English and American troops in May from Dunkirk, and then spread to Paris and London towards the end of June.[7]

Seven ships calling at Cape Town during the period between April and September 1918 carried influenza cases from overseas. Similarly ships reaching Durban also carried the disease. Evidence from the Port Health Officers indicated that ships arriving in the Union for some months prior to the outbreak had influenza cases on board, but the cases did not appear sufficiently unusual for special precautions to be taken. In particular three ships are associated with the outbreak in September 1918 – the SS Salamis arrived at Durban on 5th September with 187 soldiers from Dar-es-Salaam and Mozambique, and with some of the Chinese sailors and firemen suffering from influenza. The soldiers were placed in camp at Congella in Durban and within 10 days several hundred African in the harbour area were ill. By the 14th of September it had broken out in the City and had reached both Ladysmith and Pietermaritzburg by the 30th. Also arriving at Durban were the ships Borda from Australia on the 17th August with several cases among the troops and the Professor with four cases among the crew. Several ships had arrived in Cape Town from July with cases – the Essex from Liverpool on 5th July with 12 cases, the Iyomara also from Liverpool on 21st July with one death, and the Cawdor Castle from England which reported that most passengers had had 'Flu' during the voyage. The Marathon arrived from Australia on 21st August reporting four cases, and the Ebani came from the east coast with 37 cases on 11th September. The SS Jaroslav and the SS Veronej arrived at Cape Town on 13th and 18th September respectively, having stopped at Sierra Leone which was badly affected by the flu and had reported numerous deaths. This information was not timeously available to the South African authorities however and the full extent and severity of the disease there were not recognised. The Jaroslav reported 44 cases of which 13 landed, and the Veronej reported eight cases. The patients from the ships were taken to the military isolation hospital at Woodstock, and the healthier among them were quarantined at the Rosebank depot. After two days those who were not sick were permitted to proceed to their homes. Even had the severity been known at that time the law would not have allowed for quarantine of the ship as influenza was thought of as a mild disease, not included in Cape law as a disease for which the Port Medical Officer could enforce quarantine, although they did take the precaution of having the vessel fumigated. No official reports had been received from any other country warning them of the situation. By 23rd September influenza had broken out at Rosebank, with 30 out of 84 Africans at the Rosebank depot contracting influenza. The African labour contingent on these ships was destined to travel by train to almost every town in the country, and Lesotho.[8]

Influenza broke out on 18th September on the Transvaal mines and the Department of Health was advised by a phone call on 24th September. Kimberley was affected on 23rd September, and on 25th September it was in Cape Town and Johannesburg. The mines were particularly vulnerable due to the vast numbers of men living in densely overcrowded hostels with poor sanitary conditions and nutrition. By 1st October it had appeared in Germiston and Vereeniging. By 2nd October it had reached Volksrus and East London and the Magistrate of Kimberley sent a telegram to Pretoria: 'Natives in Location and Convict Station getting ill in very large numbers. Isolation cannot be carried out. Five deaths yesterday'. He continued in a second telegram that there had been nine deaths in the gaol, 630 were ill in the Convict station, and 900 in Wesselton compound. He reported the situation as 'very serious'.[9] By the end of September some 14,000 people on the mines had been infected and by the 3rd of October it was in Port Elizabeth, Naauwport and Pretoria. Other ports and principal towns were the first affected, reaching Uitenhage, Bloemfontein and Kroonstad by the 7th.

The onset of the influenza was often sudden, starting with a headache, dizziness, and pains in the chest, back and limbs. The suddenness of the onset was illustrated in the story of a mine cage lift operator, W.E. Hill, who having been suddenly attacked on 1st October while on duty then failed to stop an ascending lift cage of miners which crashed into the head-gear and plunged back down the mine shaft, killing 20 men and injuring eight others.[10] At the beginning of the epidemic however it was usually mild with high temperatures and a cough developing. On 1st October the Cape Times published an interview with a medical person who assured the public that there was no serious danger. But the spread of disease in Cape Town was rapid and by 2nd October hundreds were affected. At that time, after the First World War, Cape

Town was particularly overcrowded with an increase in population of 90,000, or some 50% since 1911, and many were crammed into overcrowded and insanitary houses and tenements in such areas as the Malay quarter and District Six. It was noticed that Coloureds, Indians and Malays were particularly susceptible to the disease, possibly because of worse overcrowding than the white community. By the 4th October some 5,000 in Cape Town were ill, but the Medical Officer of Health optimistically stated that he thought it was at its peak. By this time it was starting to have a visible impact on the city due to people being away from work. Milk and newspapers were not being delivered, shops were short-handed, trains were delayed and factories were closing.

Dr Ashe reported from Kimberley that, following an initial outbreak in the gaol on the 1st October, by October 4th he could not see one third of the people who sent for him in the town and from that day on it was impossible for the ten doctors to cope with the work. At every place he called the neighbours on each side almost dragged him into their houses. Assistance was given by the Defence Force Medical Department, who reorganised the doctors according to districts and shifts and supplied additional doctors, nurses and orderlies. A system of hanging out a red flag was initiated for cases where whole families were ill and unable to call for a doctor. Where they had no flag people used neckties, undergarments, a sunshade and even bathing drawers. Great assistance was given by the De Beers Diamond Company who had suffered appalling mortality amongst their mineworkers.[11] At the Zaaiplats mine however, a lower mortality amongst their 500 miners was reported, with only eight deaths out of 400 affected. This was thought to be due to the strong winds blowing through, and the fact that they had closed the African compound and made the workers sleep and live out in the open, with increased meat and soup rations. The African compound was described as a collection of rough rondavels about three metres in diameter, with no ventilation.[12]

Within just a few days, by 5th of October, 50% of the telephone department were away from work, and Johannesburg had 52,500 cases. It was noted that people involved in communications, such as post office workers, tram conductors and railway workers, were particularly affected. By 17th 17,000 cases had been treated in Rand hospitals. The Magistrate of Kimberley telegrammed Pretoria: 'Spanish influenza attacked Dutoitspan Compound population 2,000 eight days ago. Deaths from pneumonia complications began four days later, have now reached 150 and will probably be doubled'.[13]

By Monday 7th October there were 20,000 cases in Cape Town. The

Mayor called an emergency meeting of the Council and it was decided to delay the opening of schools and establish a special Executive Committee to work on the epidemic. Some 210 out of 500 members of the cleansing department were ill, and trade refuse removal was suspended. Cape Town, similarly to Kimberley, divided the city into areas with a doctor in charge of each. Standard prescriptions were agreed to, to prevent multitudes of doctors from prescribing differently which was putting undue pressure on the pharmacies, and 45 depots established where the volunteers and nurses who were undertaking house to house visits could request medical help and obtain medicines and foodstuffs. 12 marquees were erected at the city hospital and military tents. 16 Marquees were erected at the old Government house in Newlands, and various schools and other buildings were converted into temporary hospitals.[14] Wynberg and the Cape Divisional Council opened four temporary hospitals of their own and, with Simonstown, established relief organisations. Forgotten however were the Docks and Ndabeni – the location to which the poor had been removed after the plague outbreak – which fell under the South African Railways and Harbour and Native Administration Departments. Conditions were appalling in these locations and by 9th October 120 people in Ndabeni had died, with corpses being wrapped in blankets and tossed onto wagons. At this point the City of Cape Town decided to assist but by the end of the month another 134 had died. At the Docks Location the Medical Officer and Superintendant both fell ill and, after a climbing death toll reaching 74 out of the 1,400 residents, the Railways and Harbour Authorities appealed to the military for help. It was then evacuated to a tent camp and tented hospital at Green Point, in which another 22 people died.[15]

On October 8th a telegraphic circular was issued by the Union Health Department to all Magistrates to engage medical and nursing assistants, and on the 9th a circular was issued to Local Authorities urging that everything reasonable be done to combat the epidemic, and that the Government would bear half the cost. A vaccine was produced and made available for general use, with a circular going out on the 19th regarding its use. Requests from Local Authorities poured in for assistance such as hospital equipment, medical and nursing aid etc.[16] On the 14th October the disease was proclaimed a contagious or infectious disease in terms of the various Provincial Acts in force at the time which gave Local Authorities power to compulsorily remove people to places of isolation or hospital for treatment or observation. A memorandum of the Union Health Department of 22nd October was published reporting on communication with authorities on the influenza outbreak. On October

15th the Chief Medical Officer of the Local Government Boards reported that there had been a 'considerable recrudescence of influenza in England, of a type so far not very severe'. He advised that people with severe catarrh should stay at home, and to avoid unnecessary sneezing, coughing and spitting, avoidance of overcrowding and congregating in single rooms, avoidance of fatigue and alcohol. He recommended cleanliness of persons and dwellings and the use of 'anti-pneumonic vaccine'.

A Report of bacteriologists in England issued on 18th October expressed doubt as to the causative agent and thought that the existence of some virus as yet undiscovered was possible. The vaccine available was aimed at several bacteria rather than a virus. By then doctors in the Cape were reporting that, as in England, while the earlier cases were notable in their mildness there was increasing virulence as the epidemic progressed with progression to pneumonia and a higher mortality rate. They recognised three phases of the attack: firstly an initial period with fever and catarrh of upper air passages, lasting a few days; secondly a period of subsidence of fever and abatement of symptoms, then finally another period of fever and catarrh of the lower air passages, passing rapidly into influenza. Prolonged rest in bed was considered vital and inoculation was felt to lessen the severity of complications. In the same edition of the South African Medical Journal, dated 26th October, obituaries were written for 11 doctors who had died from influenza and pneumonia in the previous two weeks. This was followed by a report that the epidemic was exceptionally severe in Cape Town with many doctors affected and others having returned to clinical duties to assist.[17]

At the end of October Local Authorities were given the power to close cinemas and theatres. In Kimberley mine workers started to demand to be allowed to go home and were eventually allowed to leave in batches of 200, fanning out to various destinations across the country and taking the disease with them. Many never made it to their homes, dying on route in the packed and congested trains, and by mid-October hospital coaches were being attached to the trains to give care to the sick. Other workers dropped at the roadside and died there while walking to their kraals.[18] The epidemic spread through all the rural areas, devastating the Transvaal, Natal and the Transkei where there was little assistance available outside of the Native Commissioners, the Magistrates and a few doctors. Local relief committees were set up and supplies sought from Durban, East London and Cape Town which were largely inadequate. In some instances the medicines sent were mistrusted by the local Africans with some suspecting it was poisoned. Many refused to go to the hospitals for similar reasons. Inoculation was likewise often rejected.[19]

In Bloemfontein a 'White Flag' system was started to show those households who were unaffected by the disease, but a visitor there in October saw scarcely seven during his trip. Iron boilers were placed in the Bloemfontein Town Hall containing soup which was given to the needy and motor bicycles and sidecars were commandeered to deliver the soup night and day to families at home. Tempe and Eunice Girls School were turned into hospitals. In Theunissen 236 out of 800 people were bedridden, including the local doctor, and red flags were placed at his home, which was barricaded off to stop people going there for medical help. It was said that the spread in the Free State was aided by the weather as gales and dust blew everywhere 'carrying the dreaded microbes of influenza in all directions'.[20]

In a leading article the South African Medical Record of 9th November 1918 stated 'In face of an epidemic which stands by itself in its explosive nature, in the suddenness of its onslaught, in the rapidity of its spread, in the exceptional way in which it affects the members of the profession, and in the difficulties it presents in the way of differential diagnosis, the obstacles in the way of proper observation are altogether greater than the ordinary.' It was proving impossible to collect data 'when a third or perhaps half of the population of their neighbourhood are patients at one time'. The epidemic was thought to be affecting South Africa more severely than Britain or Spain, with much higher mortality rates and it was thought the label 'Spanish flu' was unfortunate. The greatest impact seemed to be on people aged between 25 and 45, with remarkable sparing of those over 60 years: 'young children and aged people have again and again been the only members left alive'. Various other differences were noted compared to previous epidemics, including it affecting men and women equally, whereas previously men were more affected, and the greater incidence of lobar pneumonia as a complication. Another characteristic feature was the tendency of the disease to be mild in the earlier phases which possibly aided its spread as the diagnosis was only made late into the illness. An observation was made that a dose of opium in the very early stage seemed to be helpful in warding off severe disease, although this was thought to not be of any practical use, given the difficulty of early diagnosis. Commenting on calls to clean up slums and improve sanitation the article stated:

> No amount of sanitary reform, housing or of any other kind, will prevent its recurring on some future occasion. Influenza is not a filth disease, nor a

poverty disease, nor a bad air disease, and it is, therefore, not amenable to public health control in the same way as is enteric, typhus, plague, or tuberculosis. It is, indeed, the despair of the Public Health man.[21]

Obituaries for a further 13 doctors who had died from influenza followed. Statistics record a death toll of around 4,700 in Kimberley, 7,500 in Cape Town, 1,300 in Bloemfontein and 2,000 in Johannesburg at that time. In Cape Town the entire city was in the midst of unprecedented disaster, although the Council was impressed by the way people came together to volunteer and assist, in spite of the devastation. Phillips commented that assistance across the usual barriers of race, class and religion appears to have become common, even though volunteering was not a decision to have been taken lightly given the extreme infectiousness and very real risk to life, which was all too obvious as the carts piled high with corpses passed by in the streets. Many were buried wrapped only in blankets, or even just hessian, and put into communal graves in long trenches dug by Nigerian troops who were brought in to assist the labourers and university students who were digging in the Maitland cemetery.[22]

The main symptoms reported were headache, pains in the back and limbs, high temperature, haemorrhage from the lungs during coughing and sometimes from the bowels, and delirium. Further complications other than pneumonia included gastrointestinal, meningeal and spinal symptoms, along with pericarditis and myocarditis, paraplegia, nerve paralysis, psychiatric symptoms, and nephritis. Various treatments were tried including vaccine therapy, emetics such as ipecac, potassium iodide, digitalis and mercurial and saline purges, of which only the vaccine therapy received widespread support.[23] Some doctors felt the symptoms were too severe to be influenza and motivated strongly that they were actually dealing with a form of pneumonic plague, one defending this position with such vigour that he stated in a letter 'my colleagues are trying a gigantic bluff in respect of this epidemic. I feel certain that they know they have made a wrong diagnosis at the beginning'.[24] Others suggested it was due to the gas used by the Germans during the war – that the gas had favoured the growth of a germ previously unknown.[25]

Up until 30th November a total of 104 doctors, 227 nurses and 163 medical students, hospital orderlies and vaccinators were engaged by the Union Health Department. The Doctors were sent to 81 different locations, nurses to 111 places and the remaining personnel to 56 places. Over 40,000 articles of hospital equipment were obtained from the

Defence Department and distributed, along with medical and nursing staff. All Government Departments were instructed to make available all personnel, save those necessary for emergency work, to assist in combating the disease and assistance was sent out to Local Authorities, Magistrates, Native Commissioners and others.[26] By 28th December 35 doctors had died from the disease. It was considered to be having a more drastic effect on medical staff than cholera, yellow fever or plague as they were less able to protect themselves due to extreme infectivity of the disease.

Reports came in from all over the country of the impact of the epidemic. In Ladysmith (Natal) it was claimed to have affected 85% of the population. The heaviest mortality was among Africans due mainly to pneumonia, heart failure and exhaustion. Among the White population the toll was heaviest amongst adults aged 18-32 and particularly pregnant women, with children and those over 50 being spared. The chief factors in spread of the disease were said to be the inability to procure vaccine, the overwhelming suddenness of the epidemic, incomplete clinical knowledge, lack of hospital accommodation and overcrowding in houses. Special features described included a dry, hard, leathery tongue, various rashes – blotchy patches, measly rashes, crops of spots like those in chicken pox or typhoid, an increased spleen and a heavy pungent odour, like 'the smell of a latrine left un-emptied for some days'. Various medicines were tried, including opium, aspirin, atropine and quinine, along with milk, champagne and brandy, all of which seemed to do more harm than good. Only strong black coffee with sugar was reported upon positively, along with broths, barley water and water only.[27] Ashe in Kimberley described in addition haemorrhage from the nose, mouth and throat as common, with early, heavy and persistent menstruation, severe constipation, sleeplessness and violent delirium. Deafness sometimes occurred and loss of sight, together with debility and tiredness which persisted long after recovery.[28] Cairns in Philipstown added desquamation (shedding of the skin – including sometimes almost perfect casts of the feet) and hair loss as features and also referred to the characteristic smell. He noted the loss of those in the reproductive years and commented:

> If one considered this and the whole sequence of orphanage, loss of parental control, the loss of influence of wife over husband and vice-versa, the loss of home life, the loss of infant life, the loss of the flower of the manhood and womanhood of the land, the loss of some of the best brains of the country, which follow as a natural consequence, the total appals

one.[29]

Leipoldt described its effects on the Transvaal low veld as they moved from farm to farm, establishing central farm depots for emergency treatment and transporting moribund patients to the towns in hospitals. He describes visits to outlying farms where most were dead or dying 'for the most part it was impossible to save many patients who were obviously dying when we reached them. No medicine or drug had the slightest effect on the disease ... the conditions were really appalling, for the epidemic raged with astonishing virulence, and medical and nursing assistance could only be adequately given in the larger centres'.[30]

By early November 1,147 miners on the Rand had died, and 61,000 out of the 190,000 employed on the mines had been admitted to various mine hospitals. The recruitment of replacements from Mozambique had to be stopped in order to prevent them returning to spread the disease there. This gave the Chamber of Mines serious concerns about their profits as the shortage of labour began to severely impact on production: 'The influenza has indeed played havoc with the profits and makes one very anxious about the future' and warnings of mine closures abounded.[31] Nearly 140,000 South Africans died between August 1st and 30th November 1918 as shown in the Table below: [32]

Mortality in South Africa: Influenza Pandemic of 1918

Area	European	'Other than European'	Total
Cape	5,855	81,253	87,108
Transvaal	3,267	25,397	28,664
Orange Free State	2,242	7,495	9,737
Natal	362	13,600	13,962
Total	11,726	127,745	139,471

A Commission to enquire into the Influenza Epidemic was established by Government Notice 1588 of 3rd December 1918. Their task was to enquire into and report upon:

(a) the circumstances attending the commencement of the recent epidemic of influenza in the Union of South Africa;
(b) the incidence and spread of the disease;
(c) the measures taken to combat it;
(d) the measures recommended to be taken to safeguard against or deal with any similar outbreak in future.

The Commission first met just two days later on 5th December and then almost daily, hearing evidence from private and government Medical Practitioners, Administrators, Councillors, Magistrates, representatives of Indian Relief Committees, the military, and employers such as the Chamber of Mines and the railways. They met in Pretoria, Johannesburg, Durban, Pietermaritzburg, East London, Kimberley, Bloemfontein and Cape Town, and heard altogether 192 witnesses. It confirmed that the disease had no connection with the plague, but expressed doubt as to the causative organism (postulated as Bacillus influenza). It found that 11,725 Europeans and 127,745 Africans and coloured people died, giving a mortality rate of 8.26 per 1,000 and 27.19 per 1,000 respectively.[33]

The 'Report of the Influenza Epidemic Commission', signed on 8th February 1919, highlighted the ways in which the country had been unprepared for an epidemic of this magnitude and suddenness. It particularly noted the lack of health authorities in rural areas of the Transvaal, the Orange Free State and Natal, and that no steps had been taken since the Union for the creation of an efficient central Department of Health. Up until January 1918 the Health Department had just been a branch of the Department of the Interior. It noted also that, while the Local Authorities had generally done extremely well, usually through voluntarily organised committees, the Provincial Administrations had taken no particularly noteworthy steps to combat the epidemic. It recommended that a Public Health Department should be created, filled by a body of experts of such professional standing that the general public and health officers of the country could confidently look to them for expert advice in every domain of public health. It also recommended the establishment of surgeries in rural areas, and that permanent hospitals be provided. Other points made were that travel by rail had undoubtedly facilitated the spread of the disease, particularly as workers fled the dense mining areas such as Kimberley and Pilgrims Rest, and that such travel should be limited in future outbreaks. It also was of the opinion that wider powers and great discretion should be given to local authorities to deal with all questions of sanitation and hygiene, including the power to declare a disease notifiable without reference to the Union authorities.

The Commission found that it was clear that bad housing, congestion and insanitary conditions facilitated the spread of the disease and tended to increase mortality. It strongly emphasized the need to devote immediate attention to the improvement of housing and sanitary conditions in slum areas and native locations, and that municipalities should be encouraged to install water-borne sewerage systems and public water supplies.[34] Also recommended was the training of school children over 13 years, and in particular girls, in hygiene, first aid and home nursing. In addition it laid the framework for the establishment of District Surgeons and permanent hospitals throughout rural areas and the extension of the telephone system. It suggested that schools and public buildings should be so designed as to allow them to be used as hospitals in emergencies.

It was estimated that the total amount spent on the epidemic by the Government and local authorities was £308,000. Local Authorities had found themselves without money to fight the epidemic and a compromise was proposed whereby Government would pay four-fifths of the cost.[35] This was the amount provided for in law in the Cape. The costs of the epidemic raised many questions in Parliament, with some members objecting to government bearing the cost, and others alleging that poorer authorities had been unable to provide the necessary care because of lack of funds. Some pointed out that some doctors claimed as much as £200 per day. while others had worked night and day, risking their own lives and 'passing though the most loathsome horrors they could, but tending to the dying and bringing to many the changes of salvation without charging an halfpenny'.[36] The matter of carrying the cost was highly contentious, with the debate veering between carrying all the cost in that it was a national emergency, and alternatively blaming the outbreak on local authorities 'a very large number of deaths were caused owing to overcrowding and insanitation, for which Government was not responsible at all. The responsibility of keeping a town healthy was by law placed on the municipality concerned'.[37] At the end of the debate the Assembly voted to reduce the amount of money available by £100,000, which only provided for half the costs incurred by local authorities in dealing with the epidemic.

The Public Health Bill was brought to the House of Assembly at great speed soon after the great influenza epidemic, being presented in January 1919. The terrible loss of life in the epidemic had highlighted the defects in public health legislation and had meant that many residents had discovered 'for the first time that a large number of their fellow citizens were living like animals. Coloured people and natives must live under healthy conditions if the other members of the community are to remain healthy'.[38] The bill compelled Local Authorities to appoint Medical Officers of Health, and provided that these may not be dismissed by the local authority without the approval of the Minister, in order to prevent their intimidation by Councillors into ignoring properties which posed a health hazard. The Act provided for the Minister to provide public health services where there was no local authority, or where the Local authority was failing to take effective measures.

The Government response to the epidemic was severely criticised in Parliament. The Member for Bethlehem in the Free State, J.H.B. Wessels, brought a motion condemning the conduct of the Government in connection with the epidemic, and talked of the neglect of rural districts: 'like an assassin the scourge had gone through the country and taken a terrible toll in its course'. Civil servants and railway employees had been offloaded in Bethlehem 'but the Government had done nothing, and the greatest tribute was due to the private persons who had, at the risk of their own safety, looked after the hundreds of people who had been brought in'. He talked of hundreds of cases of farmers who had died after going to deal with their cattle, and 'hundreds of cases in which women had got up from their bed of sickness to look after their children and died in doing so'. He paid tribute to the Magistrate of Bethlehem 'who may be an Englishman, but who has his heart in the right place'.[39] Much criticism was aimed at the Government for not having responded correctly to the arrival of the ship Jaroslav, and having allowed those on board to spread the disease all over the country. The government's defence was that at the time they were not aware of the severity of the disease in Sierra Leone, and that the illness on the ship appeared mild. In respect of the many children orphaned by the epidemic the Government provided for their care under an extension of the Children's Act, with 42 being provided for at Paarl, 84 at George, 70 at Dewetsdorp and 252 at Frankenwald. Grants were provided to orphanages at Kimberley.[40]

Housing had been identified by the Commission as playing a major role in the spread of the disease, and the housing shortage had been exacerbated during the War as building came to a standstill. There had been large movements of people and military men across the country, yet after the war no new houses were available to meet the demands of natural increase, migration and demobilisation of soldiers. During the War large numbers of buildings had deteriorated into slum or semi-slum conditions and overcrowding had increased. Many letters and articles were written in the Cape Town press regarding the swarming, insanitary slums, particularly by those who had had cause to see them for the first time during house-to-house visits during the epidemic. A return of the epidemic was widely anticipated and urgent action to alleviate the conditions was considered critical, as from the hovels the disease could spread back to the city.

A massive clean-up operation took place in Cape Town amid heavy public pressure for action. Following the Influenza epidemic at the Cape, Richard Stuttaford, a city councillor, was of the view that better housing might have saved many lives. He developed a scheme for a garden city, which was placed before the acting Prime Minister FS Malan in January 1919, where he proposed to donate £10,000 to a trust for a development at Uitvlugt. This was the same area which had previously been used as a location for a temporary hospital for plague patients and adjacent to Ndabeni, to which Africans had been sent to clean up the city during the outbreak of plague. The concept was to provide land where less affluent people could build their own houses, or that employers could build houses for their employees as a way to reduce the number of slums in the city. This then went on to become the garden city of Pinelands.[41] In the intervening period since the plague epidemic the location at Ndabeni had become overcrowded and the poor housing conditions had contributed to the spread of influenza in the area. Following the epidemic tents were provided as a temporary measure to ease overcrowding, and negotiations were held with the Cape Town City Council for them to take over the location.

A Government Committee, formed in 1919 to consider the housing crisis, reported on the massive shortfall in housing for Whites, Coloureds and Africans in urban areas which lead to the Housing Act of 1920.[42] Arising from the concern that the location of Ndabeni posed not just a threat to the health of the Africans, but also to the white population, a new location was built at Langa in the 1920's to replace it.

The slow response to the epidemic was not unique to South Africa and it was noted that the War had diverted the attention of governments in other countries away from public health measures. 25% of South African doctors had not been available because of the War. It was considered that the establishment of an International Bureau for the collection and dissemination of information related to the prevention and limitation of diseases and epidemics would be helpful.

On 6th March 1919 it was reported that the ship Kenilworth Castle was due to arrive in Table Bay en-route to Australia with influenza cases on board. It had been arranged since 30th November 1918 that, for vessels such as this, they would not be allowed to come to the wharf but would be kept in the Bay. Any passengers intending to land had to be examined by both the Port Health Officer but also other medical officers, and if sick they would be taken to the City Isolation Hospital. Those who were healthy could travel on to their destination, but the local authorities concerned would be notified that they were coming. There had been 29 cases on board with two deaths. Quarantining the ship was not undertaken due to it being considered both futile and a delay to shipping. This stance had been taken following events in Australia, which had imposed rigid quarantine and the wearing of masks, yet the disease had spread to Sydney and other towns. At that time there were still cases occurring in South Africa, with 80 cases in Durban at the beginning of March and two deaths, and 12 cases in Potchefstroom with one death. Members of Parliament were concerned that the measures in respect of shipping were inadequate and that the passengers should all be quarantined.[43]

By September 1919 a second wave of epidemic had come. It was more general and widespread, but while there were many severe cases the disease was less fatal. It attacked mainly those who had escaped the previous time and was particularly prevalent in Pretoria among the poorer sections of the community. However the mortality was not as high as with the previous outbreak. The public pressure to clean up the urban slums started to fade as the sense of urgency lowered, and by July 1920 the Cape Times commented:

> In spite of the tragic and appalling lessons of the Influenza visitation, the insanitary state of affairs in the slums has in no way changed for the better. If anything it has probably become worse since the housing problem has reacted more disadvantageously upon the poorer classes than upon any other section of the community.[44]

Seasonal epidemics of influenza continued to occur in the winter months, with one in 1935 following another European outbreak. Case mortality was low however, with the common complications being otitis media (ear infections), laryngitis and neuritis. Influenza was again severe in Europe in 1936 and strict precautionary measures were taken to prevent it entering by ship. 260 cases were reported on ships coming from Europe to Cape Town but did not spread inland. The ships were disinfected on arrival.

The onset of the Second World War in 1939 again gave rise to large movements of men and populations around the globe as had preceded the 1918 pandemic. In the winter of 1940 there was an outbreak of influenza at the military camp at Premier Mine, which resulted in 6,000 cases in a two month period with 650 admissions to hospital. Approximately 30% of men were affected, and it was considered that the outbreak was contributed to by a sudden onset of unusually cold weather just prior to the epidemic. It was recommended that in the winter time men should be instructed to put on greatcoats at sunset and be permitted and encouraged to have the evening meal with their coats on, where messes consisted of tents. Other factors, such as dust, sleeping conditions, and place of origin did not seem to have any significant effect –in fact the enlisted men with worse living conditions than the officers had a lower incidence of infection. It was noted that the incubation period was around two to three days, and the outbreak lasted approximately seven weeks. Around 8% developed pneumonia and relapses after several days were common, but deaths were negligible. Sulphapyridine, a sulphonamide antibiotic known as M&B 693, was used on a trial basis to half of the patients, regardless of the severity of the illness with variable dosages. It was not found to reduce the length of the high temperature and it was concluded that it made no difference in influenza.[45] A similar outbreak occurred at the Potchefstroom military camp in 1941 with 1,500 cases admitted to hospital. The hardest hit was the youth training brigade, aged from 15 to 19 years. Sulphapyridine was again used somewhat experimentally, to treat cases of high fevers and cases complicated with pneumonia with very good effects.[46]

While studies during the 1918 pandemic had identified the influenza bacillus of Pfeiffer as probably the causative organism, by the 1940's this was no longer supported as distinct influenza viruses were being isolated. Epidemics in America in 1936-37 and 1938-39 had been found to be caused by one type of virus, and in an epidemic in 1940 another type was identified. It was generally agreed that immunity after an attack of influenza lasted around twelve months, but attempts to produce a prophylactic vaccine had been disappointing.

In 1949 another epidemic started, spreading across from Sardinia, Sicily, and Italy and from there to the rest of Europe, in which 2,200 people in the Netherlands died.[47] Influenza also appeared in Liverpool of a very virulent type, which killed considerable numbers of elderly and chronically ill. Following this in 1950 there was an influenza epidemic in South Africa, but not of a catastrophic nature. In Cape Town it affected a large number of students and hospital nurses, but the disease was mild and not associated with serious pulmonary complications, with no increase in the number of pneumonia deaths during the period. The strain was similar to those isolated in Europe and America.[48] Similarly a report was made of an epidemic in Vanderbijl Park, an industrial town near Johannesburg, starting in May 1950 through until September, which affected some 20% of the population but with no deaths. Antibiotics were used frequently which reduced the duration of fever, but it was noted that those so treated took ten days on average instead of eight days to return to work.[49] The epidemic was also reported from Johannesburg, where it appeared to start, Durban, and most other towns in South Africa. However the mortality rate was very low. Influenza Type B virus was responsible for the early wave of the epidemic, and Type A for the more severe second wave.[50]

In 1952 the World Health Organisation established an Expert Committee on Influenza which reported in 1953, and which stated that it was impossible to foresee when a serious epidemic would occur, but that if it did it would spread with such rapidity that there would be very little time to institute control measures. The best approach was considered to be immunisation, and further research was needed into this.[51] A further epidemic occurred in South Africa in the winter of 1952, which was more severe in the Cape than that of 1950. Institutional outbreaks occurred in hospitals, schools and prisons. Influenza viruses were classified largely in three groups by the mid 1950's – A, B and C - with type A being the most important cause of major outbreaks. It had also become clear that the viruses were constantly changing their antigenic make-up and that once a new virus emerged it was able to spread very fast. What happened to the virus between outbreaks was less certain – whether it passed on to some other country with lower herd immunity and then on around the world, or whether it 'went underground' waiting to emerge modified or unmodified to start an epidemic some years later. As immunity after vaccination only lasted several months it was considered best to give a dose once month before an epidemic season. Effectiveness was estimated at between 25 and 40%, although it was hard to measure accurately due to the lack of accurate diagnoses.[52]

In 1956 there was an outbreak of influenza known as 'Asian 'Flu', as it started in the Far East in Hong Kong, Singapore, Manila and Taiwan, and thence to India, Thailand and Japan. This was a new variant of the type A, but found to be relatively mild. A warning however was put out in the media and local authorities urged to make plans. Preparations were made to treat large numbers of cases in existing and improvised hospitals, and clinics and at home and to feed people on a large scale, together with contingency plans to provide other essential services in the event of large numbers of workers taking ill. When the epidemic did arrive however it was neither explosive nor severe and most cases could be treated at home. The first cases were identified in gold mine compounds around Johannesburg and in African compounds in Natal late in June, where large numbers of the African labour force were taken ill. The epidemic lasted only about four weeks on the mines and, out of a total of 110,000 workers on 21 mines, over 17,000 of them were affected. Their main symptoms were cough, chest pains, headache, sore throat, loss of appetite and fever. Only three deaths were reported from pneumonia. The virus responsible was identified as the same one in the Far East - A/Singapore/1/57.[53] By the end of July there had been 60,000 cases in Africans in the Johannesburg and outlying areas. Europeans were less severely affected but there were short periods when schools, factories and business reported absenteeism rates as high as 50%.[54]

The influenza reached Cape Town around the 29th July when it was reported that pupils from Langa African Township, (as created after the 1918 epidemic) were staying away from school through illness. After a few days it spread rapidly though the location affecting all ages, sexes and groups. The Langa hospital was inundated and hospital staff started to take ill. The epidemic in Langa lasted around two weeks and was estimated to have affected 7,000 out of the 23,000 residents, although only three patients were taken seriously ill. After that reports came in from school principals from other areas of the Cape Peninsula of mounting absenteeism due to the Asian influenza, sometimes reaching as high as 80%. Health services were placed under great strain as the disease spread from the Non-European areas to the more affluent European areas of the city, although not to the same extent. However other essential services were not seriously disrupted on account of the fact that the influenza spread steadily in phases across the city, and the duration of illness was only four or five days, so that many people recovered and were back at work before the next group were affected.[55]

The disease continued across the country through 1957 but with most cases making a full recovery after a few days of fever. Samples of the influenza virus had been obtained from the World Influenza Centre in London and vaccine prepared which was first issued at the beginning of July. By September the epidemic started to wane by which time it was estimated that by then some 30-40% of the population had been affected, although there was no major disruption to essential services and relatively few deaths. The disease re-emerged in 1959, affecting those areas and people who had escaped in the first round of the epidemic, but the fact that influenza was not a notifiable disease meant that the number affected was not known. However the virus was identified as the same Asian strain of the influenza Type A2 virus, which was noted to be a virus containing human and avian influenza genes.

Influenza continued to affect the country in the winter seasons, but never again so severely as in the first 60 years of the century. While it remained a significant cause of death for the elderly and at risk, the devastation caused by the traditional strains of the influenza virus did not recur. However new viruses started to emerge around the globe posing new risks. In 2002 the first confirmed case of Severe Acute Respiratory Syndrome (SARS) occurred in November in mainland China. A second case presented in December, and a further eight people close to him developed a similar pneumonia 8-10 days after his admission. A further 1,512 people became infected in Guangdong Province of whom 58 died. From December 2003 it appeared in Hong Kong with 16 cases in the hotel where the first case, an infected physician from Guangzhou, had occurred. From here it spread to 30 countries around the world within weeks with hospitals amplifying the disease. The outbreak lasted until 5th July 2003. It re-emerged in early 2004, but never reached South Africa, possibly because of the stringent control mechanisms which had been put in place internationally.[56] These also were effective in preventing the 'Swine flu' pandemic affecting the country a few years later in 2009.

While the reason for the extreme virulence of the 1918 pandemic, and its origins, remain unclear it appears that the devastation of the earlier epidemics of influenza appears unlikely to recur. There are continued anxieties about the emergence of new strains of influenza viruses, but the surveillance systems in place are sophisticated and global in reach with international cooperation and notifications. Together with the ability to rapidly produce effective vaccines, and the existence of anti-viral medicines, it means the epidemics of the future are unlikely to repeat the massive mortality of the epidemic of 1918.

ENDNOTES

1. Orenstein A.J. 'Epidemiology' *South African Medical Journal* 11(15) 1937:529-535
2. Anderson Jasper A. 'Influenza in Cape Town' *South African Medical Record*, 17(3) January 11 1919: 36-39

3. Leading Article, 'The Influenza Epidemic' *South African Medical Record*; 16(21) 9 November 1918:317-320
4. Lagden G.Y. *Report by the Commissioner for Native Affairs, Transvaal, for the year ended 30th June 1904*, Pretoria, Government Printing and Stationery office, 1904: pA4
5. Pritchard S.M. 'Report by the Pass Commissioner, Native Affairs Department' in Lagden G.Y. *Report by the Commissioner for Native Affairs, Transvaal, for the year ended 30th June 1904*, Pretoria, Government Printing and Stationery office, 1904,:pB51
6. Lagden G.Y. *Report by the Commissioner for Native Affairs, Transvaal, for the year ended 30th June 1906*, Pretoria, Government Printing and Stationery office, 1906: pA19-A22
7. Anderson Jasper A. 'Influenza in Cape Town' *South African Medical Record*, 17(3) 11 January 1919:36-39
8. Cluver P.D. *Report of the Influenza Epidemic Commission, 1919*, Cape Times Ltd, UG 15-'19 p6-8
9. Ibid, 12,
10. Phillips H. 'Black October': the Impact of the Spanish Influenza Epidemic of 1918 on South Africa, *Archives Year Book for South African History*, vol1, Government Printer Pretoria, 1990:2
11. Ashe E. Oliver; 'Some Random Recollections of the Kimberley Influenza Epidemic' *South African Medical Record*, 17(1) January 11 1919:6-9
12. Hay-Michel A. 'Influenza on the Zaaiplaats mine' *South African Medical Record*, 17(2) 11 January 1919:24-26
13. Cluver P.D. *Report of the Influenza Epidemic Commission, 1919*, Cape Times Ltd, UG 15-'19 p12
14. Anderson Jasper A, 'Influenza in Cape Town' *South African Medical Record*, 17(3) 11 January.1919:36-39
15. Phillips H. 'Black October': the Impact of the Spanish Influenza Epidemic of 1918 on South Africa, *Archives Year Book for South African History*, Vol 1, Government Printer Pretoria, 1990:17
16. Cluver P.D. *Report of the Influenza Epidemic Commission, 1919*, Cape Times Ltd, UG 15-'19:11
17. Health Department 'Memorandum on Influenza' *South African Medical Record* 16(20) 26 October 1918:311
18. Phillips H, 'Black October': The Impact of the Spanish Influenza Epidemic of 1918 on South Africa, *Archives Year Book for South African History*, Vol 1, Government Printer Pretoria, 1990,:6
19. Ibid, 85-86
20. Report in *The Times of Natal*, 22nd October 1918: p1.
21. Leading Article, 'The Influenza Epidemic' *South African Medical Record* 16(21) 9 November 1918:317-320
22. Phillips H. 'Black October': the Impact of the Spanish Influenza Epidemic of 1918 on South Africa, *Archives Year Book for South African History*, Vol 1, Government Printer Pretoria, 1990:18
23. Marais Dr, 'Discussion on the Cape Town Influenza Epidemic' *South African Medical Record*, 16(23) 14 December 1918:353
24. Purvis Beattie W. 'Influenza and Bacteriological Facts' *South African Medical Record*, 16(23) 14 December 1918:371
25. Burman Jose, *Disaster Struck South Africa*, C Struik,1971:90-91
26. Cluver P.D. *Report of the Influenza Epidemic Commission, 1919*, Cape Times Ltd, UG 15-'19 p11,

27. Burman C.E.L. 'A Review of the Influenza Epidemic in Ladysmith and District with clinical observations' *South African Medical Record* 17(1) 11 January1919:3-6
28. Ashe E. Oliver; 'Some Random Recollections of the Kimberley Influenza Epidemic' *South African Medical Record*, 17 (1) 11 January 11 1919: 6-9
29. Cairns P.T. 'Report on an Outbreak of Epidemic Influenza, Philipstown and District, October and November 1918' *South African Medical Record*, 17(2) 11 January1919:19-24
30. Leipoldt Louis C. *Bushveld Doctor*, Jonathan Cape, London, 1937:118
31. Chamber of Mines, Cited in: Phillips H, 'Black October': the Impact of the Spanish Influenza Epidemic of 1918 on South Africa, *Archives Year Book for South African History*, Vol 1, Government Printer Pretoria, 1990:29
32. Watt Thomas, 'Question Day in the House' *Cape Times* 24January 1919
33. Cluver P.D. *Report of the Influenza Epidemic Commission, 1919*, Cape Times Ltd, UG 15-'19 p6-8,
34. 'Report of the Influenza Commission' *South African Medical Record* 17(4) 1919:51-55
35. Watt Thomas, 'Finances of the Union Reviewed' *Cape Times*, 25 January1919
36. Merriman Mr, 'Echoes of the Epidemic' Debate in the House of Assembly, *Cape Times* 28 January 1919:16
37. Ibid, 17
38. Watt Thomas, 'Public Health of Union', Speech in House of Assembly reported in the *Cape Times* 30 January1919:23
39. Wessels J.H.B. 'Aftermath of the Epidemic' *Cape Times*, 5 February1919:35
40. Watt Thomas, 'Provision for Epidemic Orphans', *Cape Times*, 12 February 1919:58
41. Cuthbertson C.C. 'A new town at Uitvlugt: the founding and development of Pinelands 1919-1948'; *Contree* vol 4, July 1978:5-9.
42. *Annual Report of the Department of Public Health, 1935*, Government Printer Pretoria, UG 43-'35, p 8
43. 'The Influenza Menace: Cases on "Kenilworth Castle"', *Cape Times* 6 March 1919:128
44. Editorial, *Cape Times*, 19 July 1920
45. Schaffer R. and Shapiro B.G. 'Studies in Influenza' *South African Medical Journal* 15(5) 1941:83-91
46. Emdin W. 'A clinical and therapeutic survey of an Influenza Epidemic at the Potchefstroom military camp' *South African Medical Journal* 16(5) 1942:101-107
47. *World Health Organisation Technical Report Series* No 64 (1953)
48. Van den Ende M. et al; 'The 1950 influenza epidemic in Cape Town' *South African Medical Journal*; 25(26) 30 June 1951:445
49. Cochrane J.C. et al, 'The Influenzal Epidemic of 1950 in Vanderbijl Park', *South African Medical Journal* 25(12) 1951:209-211
50. Westwood M.A. and Gear J. 'A laboratory study of the Influenza Epidemic which occurred in South Africa in the winter of 1950' *South African Medical Journal* 25(47) 1951:862-864
51. *World Health Organisation Technical Report Series* No 64 (1953)
52. Andrewes C.H. 'Influenza Today and Tomorrow' *South African Medical Journal* 29(1) 1955:3-7
53. Westwood M. Smit P. and Oberholzer D. 'Asian Influenza in South Africa, A laboratory and clinical study of an outbreak on the Simmer and Jack mine' *South African Medical Journal* 32(8) 1958:216-218.

54. Scott Millar J.W. *Report of the Medical Officer of Health on the Public Health and Sanitary Circumstances and Housing in Johannesburg during the period 1st July 1953 to 31st December 1957,* City of Johannesburg 1957:8
55. *Annual Report of the Medical Officer of Health, City of Cape Town, 1957,* Cape Times Ltd Parow 1958:37
56. MacLean A. et al, *SARS: a case study in emerging infections,* Oxford University Press, 2005

8 CHOLERA AND THE RURAL POOR

While the need to bring about infection control and quarantine measures at the Cape was first brought about by smallpox, it was fear of cholera, a dread disease that ravaged Europe and Asia, which finally brought about the need for strict health regulations to prevent disease entering South Africa through the Ports, and in addition started to fuel racial tensions against Indian immigrants. In February 1820 a violent epidemic raged in Mauritius, thought to be cholera, and on 1st July 1820 it was proclaimed that any vessel arriving from there was to be ordered into strict quarantine by the port captain and that the ship was to fly the flag known as the 'yellow jack'. Vessels which arrived from India, where cholera raged, were to fly a similar flag until it was ascertained that no disease had occurred on board during the voyage. The penalty for breaking quarantine was death, although this was never enforced. From 1st February 1820 1,821 vessels from the East were quarantined without exception.[1]

Dr Matthews, in Natal in the 1860's, said that Asiatic cholera had never been known in the Province.[2] However from 1860 the mass importation of Indian workers began, due to the shortage of labour on the European-owned sugar plantations. Various ships started arriving at Port Natal (Durban) from India throughout the late 1800's, as part of the indentured Indian labour scheme, and by 1875 there were some 6,500 of them, mostly initially working on the farms. However, from the late 1870's many Indians started to immigrate to South Africa unaided, and set up as traders, shop-keepers, independent farmers and business men. Cholera was a regular visitor to India, and some of these ships carried cases of cholera with them. The ship the Belvedere suffered a severe outbreak which started 10 days after leaving Calcutta, and 24 people died before the ship reached Port Natal. During 1888 the ship Quath-lamba, on its third voyage, arrived from at Durban with immigrants from India, having twenty cases of cholera with nine deaths on board, of which two were White crew members. It was quarantined at the Bluff for three weeks between December 1888 and January 1889 before being permitted to disembark its passengers, who all had their clothes burnt by the authorities.[3] Two years later the Congella arrived with 400 immigrants and nine deaths from 'acute diarrhoea'. However there was no spread.[4]

Although none of these cases resulted in outbreaks of cholera in Durban, the association of cholera with the arrivals from India added to an increasing hostility and suspicion of the White population of Durban to the growing Asian numbers in their midst. What was originally supposed to be a limited scheme to supply indentured Asian labour had since led to increasing numbers of Indians in and around the city, engaging in free farming, trade and commerce, which was seen as threatening the economic and property interests of the Europeans. Agitation against the Indian migrants had been increasing for some time, and the apparent threat of cholera made a useful lever for their arguments. The Town Council tried to end Indian immigration by steamship, urging the use of sail to lengthen the voyage so that any epidemic disease being carried would rather break out at sea before they arrived in the port. The Council also launched attacks on the government for maintaining nuisances in its immigration, harbour and railway barracks which housed large numbers of African and Indian workers. This agitation reached a head in 1897 when mobs in Durban prevented the landing of Indians from two ships suspected of harbouring cholera. The protestations against Indians over the perceived threat of cholera were a convenient outlet for rising European antagonism towards the Indian community in general, and contributed to the Immigration Restriction Act of 1897 which aimed at prohibiting their free immigration.[5]

Cholera was successfully kept away from South African shores through the early 1900's. In 1944 a cholera-infected vessel arrived in Durban from India but was contained by placing the ship in quarantine and vaccinating all contacts. In 1947 the Department of Health confirmed that there had never been a case of cholera in the country outside of those arriving on ships.

In the mid-1940's it was found that cholera responded to treatment with sulphonamides. Whereas up until then it had been found that 30-80% of all cholera victims died, treatment with sulfadiazide, along with adequate fluids, had effected a 100% cure in an outbreak in Calcutta. Sulphaguanidine had similarly been found effective. Penicillin was at first also thought to be effective, but this was later disproven. Blood plasma was also used to counteract the dehydration and shock. By 1951 the drug chloramphenicol had been found to be effective, although the disease developed so rapidly, and with such dehydration, that the use of an antibiotic was almost precluded.

The pandemics which occurred in the 19th century and first half of the 20th century were of the strain of the Vibrio cholerae organism known as Classical. Then in 1961 a new wave of pandemic started in Indonesia and spread rapidly across Asia and appeared in Africa. This was known as the El Tor strain which had some important differences from the Classical strain – firstly it was more likely to produce unapparent infection with the actually number of infections during an epidemic greatly exceeding the reported clinical cases, and secondly it was able to persist and multiply in the environment, in particular rivers, streams and food. Both of these factors increased the difficulties of control and eradication. While cholera had been made notifiable in South Africa in 1965 following the spread of the El Tor strain to Africa, there is no evidence of any known case of endogenous cholera acquired in the country until 30 September 1980. Prior to this there had been monitoring on the mines using Moore pads in the mine sewers, which commenced from November 1973 in anticipation of the disease being brought into the country by migrant workers as the El Tor strain spread down the eastern countries of Southern Africa. This had aided in the detection of people positive for Vibrio cholerae on the mines for some years, with the mine sewer pads yielding positive results. As early as 1974 migrant workers had spread cholera on a small number of gold mines on the Witwatersrand, but the outbreak was curtailed within two months. Some 20,000 miners were vaccinated and the potential epidemic prevented.[6] Altogether there were 31 cases and 32 recognised carriers, but no deaths, on the mines.

In 1979 a surveillance programme similar to that on the mines was introduced in the Northern Transvaal. The first diagnosis of cholera in the community was made in the Eastern Transvaal, at Shongwe Hospital on 2nd October 1980. During November of that year the disease spread out of the original area of the KaNgwane homeland, with cases being found in Gazankulu in the Eastern Transvaal on the 9th November and as far as Eikenhof, south of Johannesburg, on the 11th November. In December it arrived in the mid-Transvaal homeland of Lebowa, and before the end of the outbreak in winter 1,648 proven cases of cholera had been reported from the area.[7] Altogether, across the country, there were 3,950 confirmed cases and 42 deaths.

This outbreak was an extension of the seventh pandemic of cholera which was engulfing the poorer countries of the world, with the El Tor strain of the cholera organism. It had been endemic in the countries of northern Africa for the previous decade and it was considered only a matter of time before it reached South Africa. The spread was through the rural, impoverished regions through the movement of African people visiting family and friends, and drinking contaminated water. Seedat felt that the containment of the outbreak was hampered by the inadequate reticulated water system, the lack of sanitation, the overcrowding, impoverishment and very poor standard of living and the lack of full cooperation among the numerous authorities existing at that time. In Apartheid South Africa, not only were there National, Provincial and Local Authority health departments, but each so-called African Homeland was supposed to maintain separate, independent Health Departments as well. There were also three cases in Natal at Bergville, but the disease did not break out further.[8]

The second outbreak of cholera in Lebowa in 1981 began with the admission of a patient from the village of Mogoto into Groothoek hospital on 2nd November. Within a few days more were being admitted from the nearby village of Moletlane. The Gumpies River which ran past both villages, with Moletlane downstream of Mogoto, was thought to be the source of infection as Vibrio cholerae had repeatedly been isolated from it. The river was used for washing clothes, bathing, recreation and collection of drinking water. Water vendors pumped water from the river into tankers which were taken to the villages and the water sold to those unable to collect their own water, although there were also bore holes in the village, some of which had broken pumps, and rainwater tanks. Analysis found there was a close correlation between the use of river water and the risk of contracting cholera and concluded that the water vendors had a part to play in the spread of the disease. The outbreak fell off after four weeks when heavy rains replenished water tanks and reduced the villagers' dependence on the river water.[9]

In Natal the first cases were at Ingwavuma near the Mozambique border with the first bacteriologically confirmed cases in Stanger in November, in Durban in December and in the Transkei also in December 1981. The disease spread through the rural areas of the KwaZulu homeland. By mid-1982 there had been some 46,000 cases across the country of which 35,530 were from KwaZulu, and some 16,000 cases had been treated in Natal hospitals. At its height 2,000 patients were treated at rehydration centres in converted schools around Umtwalumi, south of Durban, over a two week period. Women were affected in greater numbers, thought to be due to their greater exposure to river water through their domestic chores. While the disease dropped off as the dry season approached, when rains commenced again in May there was another outbreak near Stanger.[10] 218 people were reported to have died from the 1981/82 epidemic. It was noted that the cholera infected areas all lay in regions that had an average rainfall greater than or equal to 600mm per annum.

Sitas gave an account of the disease in the rural farming area of the Umvoti Mission Reserve in the centre of KwaZulu-Natal. The disease was first recognised by the Department of Health on the 19th November 1981, although the first case had arrived on the 12th November, brought back by a family who had been visiting friends in the cholera area to the north. From there it spread to infect 148 people across the reserve, all African, most of who were living in wattle and daub or cardboard and tin shacks. Those in these poorer settlements had an incidence of 10.4 per thousand, some four times higher than those in richer, more permanent settlements, and the incidence was twice as high in those whose water source was impure compared with those using clean, treated water. Women were infected more than men, and the highest incidence was in those aged 21-40 years. This was also put down to women being more engaged in domestic chores which would bring them into contact with infected water in rivers and dams. Many cases spread within families with an intra-familial incidence rate of 34%. However many people who relied on impure water did not get sick which, combined with the high intra-familial transmission rate, suggested that the cause of the outbreak was more complex.

The results of the analysis suggested that the role of crowding, gathering and feasts which had been occurring over the December holiday period had a greater role to play in facilitating the spread of cholera in the Reserve than infected water. The spread within the home was linked to the faecal-oral route, or indirectly to the lack of water rendering households and utensils unhygienic, especially among the poor.[11] During the epidemic it was found that all 44 rivers of Natal along with their tributaries, streams and dams had become infected with the cholera bacteria. Given that 78.6% of patients stated that they used rivers as their source of water it was then no surprise that so many had been infected. In addition 74% of patients had no proper sanitation facilities beyond pits or buckets. It was noted that for this El Tor strain of epidemic there was a carrier state of between 30 and 100 for each severely ill patient. The 2% who are ill in an outbreak represent the tip of the iceberg of the pool of infected people, and the carriers are unknown. These go on shedding the bacteria into the environment. As the number of severely ill patients was reaching towards 50,000 it was estimated that there remained some two million infected people in the country.[12]

While estimates of severely ill patients went up to 50,000 for the 1981/82 outbreak, the annual numbers of bacteriologically confirmed cases were 3,786 in the 1980/81 epidemic, 11,141 for the 1981/82 season, and then in the following years 7,638 for 1982/83 and 1,977 in

1983/84.[13] The estimated, treated cases were always much higher than those which were laboratory confirmed, however, with an estimated 20,000 cases in 1982/83 and 5,434 in 1983/84. The 1983/84 outbreak gave a case-fatality rate of only 1% with 20 deaths. Natal and KwaZulu again gave the bulk of cases in 1983/4 from three main areas – Eshowe, Port Shepstone and Inanda, just north of Durban. These districts were again within the 600 mm rainfall demarcation line. The remainder of the cases came largely from the Transvaal area and homelands there, but only reported 28 cases altogether, demonstrating a shift in area from the Transvaal where the first epidemic appeared in 1980/81 to KwaZulu-Natal. The attack rate was highest at 1,226 per 100,000 in Eshowe area. The epidemic affected all ages, although worst in the elderly. The number of deaths was 42 in 1980/81, 218 in 1981/82, 62 in 1982/3 and 20 in 83/84.[14]

From 1985 onward the number of cases dropped significantly with 284 in 1986 and just 43 in 1987. Cholera took a high toll in the countries to the north of South Africa in 1991 and at the end of the year reports were made of positive sewer pads at a gold mine in the Western Transvaal. 39 positive results were received by the National Department of Health in the last month, and 10 positive rectal swabs were found during December. The Department warned that the risk of it passing into South Africa was high, given the large number of migrant workers crossing into the country to work in the mines.[15] Cholera continued to be present occasionally in neighbouring countries, being reported from Mozambique in 1992. By 10 August 1992 deaths had occurred and 11,442 cases diagnosed in eight of the country's 11 Provinces.[16]

In February 1993 a nine year old girl was admitted to Hlabisa Hospital in northern KwaZulu with cholera, although she had no history of travel or contact with cholera cases. In March there were two more cases from a different area. In April there were eight more cases, another 30 in May. and five more in June. These were all bacteriologically confirmed. However the disease did not break out further into the Province and the annual number of cases declined again so that in 1997 there were just three. In an analysis of all South African cases of cholera up to 1998 it was found that of all the cases ever diagnosed since 1980, 98% of them were in the black African population, 51.5% were female, 44.5% male and the rest unknown. The more severe disease was found in adults rather than children, with clinical disease being quite rare in children under one year of age. In newly affected areas the disease attacked adults more than children, whereas in endemic cholera children were attacked more.[17]

During 1998 and 1999 a few cases occurred in Mpumulanga Province, Johannesburg, Secunda and Durban as a result of people bringing the disease in from Mozambique, but there was no spread. However in early 2000 there were severe floods in the Mpumulanga lowveld (formerly eastern Transvaal). Cholera again came in from Mozambique with the El Tor strain occurring onto a banana plantation and Albertsnek village, but there were only 21 cases with no deaths. In August 2000 cholera returned to the country with a massive outbreak occurring, starting in the north of KwaZulu-Natal and spreading southwards predominantly, as in 1981, in the lower lying rural areas of KwaZulu. Its worst effects were felt in the areas of Empangeni, Eshowe and Ulundi, then worked down to the Port Shepstone area somewhat south of Durban. By December 2000 more than 12,000 cases had been confirmed and 52 cases.[18] The massive spread was contributed to by the late diagnosis of the initial cases, and a very slow reaction by the Provincial health authorities in implementing a comprehensive control programme, by which time the epidemic was out of control and spreading all across the province.

In that same month of the year 2000 one isolated case occurred in the township of Imbali, now within the Msunduzi Municipality (formerly Pietermaritzburg). Perhaps because the township was on mains sewerage and water supply there was no spread. In February 2001 the second case occurred in the Pietermaritzburg area, in a rural community of Maswazini, part of the Vulindlela area. The first case was reported on 1st February and large numbers of additional cases quickly followed. Upon investigation it transpired that it had started in the house of some people who had recently returned from visiting a cholera area to the north of the Province. They had then shortly after thrown a huge party, at which a great many people had contracted the disease – a scenario very reminiscent of Sitas's experience in the Umvoti outbreak 20 years earlier. Inspection revealed the most likely source to be contamination of food served at the party possibly related to the extremely poor sanitation in the area with roughly constructed, inadequate and fly-ridden pit latrines. By 9th February some 320 cases had been reported in the area. The Local Authority, Msunduzi Municipality, supported by the Province, launched an aggressive control campaign with treatment of latrines, community meetings and door-to-door inspections and education campaigns in schools, media inserts, leaflets and posters. Altogether 4,845 houses were visited and 95,000 pamphlets distributed. Some 3,500 toilets were treated – either emptied or covered with lime. An emergency rehydration centre was established in a community hall. By the end of the outbreak there had been 804 reported cases, although not all were confirmed biologically, and 13 deaths – a case-fatality rate of 1.6%. As a result of the intensive control measures the outbreak was over in five weeks. Control was aided by the fact that the population had access to clean treated water for drinking purposes, although it was a grave concern at the beginning that the water authority, Umgeni Water, was engaging in a policy of disconnection of domestic water connections for non-payment, which would have forced people back into using river water – had the municipality not been able to intervene and stop the disconnections the outbreak may have had a very different ending.[19]

The policy of payment for water and aggressive cost-recovery programmes for the rural poor was not unique to the Umgeni Water distribution authority. In rural areas of the Province the Department of Water Affairs and Forestry was also accused of forcing poor households, who were unable to pay, to resort to unsafe water sources by disconnecting piped water supplies. In the area of the Madlebe Tribal Authority near Empangeni in the north of the province, the epicentre of the epidemic, the Department had funded a water supply scheme some years before, following the cholera outbreak there in the 1980s. However the scheme was later found to have been inadequate in scope for the number of households living there, and included a R50 registration charge and flat-rate monthly R20 charge by the Uthungula District Council who administered it. By the year 2000 many had returned to using rivers and streams, exacerbated by the fact that non-payment by some households meant that the standpipe was cut off, affecting all the households in the area. The enforcement of cost recovery for water started in August, and the first cases of cholera started the same month.[20] The link between payment for water and the emergence of cholera was later acknowledged and followed by the introduction of the national government's Free Basic Water policy providing six kilolitres of water per month free to each household in the country.[21]

By May 2001 it was reported that there had been almost 95,000 cases of cholera in the Eshowe area of northern KwaZulu-Natal, although only 197 had died at that time. There had by this time been a massive control programme undertaken by the Provincial Department of Health, assisted by the local, national and international authorities including the World Health Organisation, the Ministry of Water Affairs and South African National Defence Force, yet still the disease continued to spread. The control programme included the sending in of water tankers to communities to provide safe water, the establishment of emergency rehydration centres, and community mobilisation around health messages. The South African Medical Health Services contributed to many of the rehydration centres, treating thousands of people.

A massive awareness campaign was undertaken including posters, radio broadcasts and community meetings, warning people against drinking river water and giving bleach for home treatment of water. However, problems with the education campaign included the lack of resources in poor communities to boil or clean water with bleach, and the difficulties of the hilly terrain and remoteness of many villages which made the distribution of water and supplies difficult. Hundreds of community volunteers were trained to spread the word in the villages and informal settlements. However, Taylor commented that although some adopted the advice the disease continued: 'the social context of living in poverty and patterns of rural life where drinking from streams and rivers are age-old habits, did not shift easily'. He also suggested that 'in their efforts to save precious clean water, toilet and sanitary practices may well have been lacking. Food preparation therefore became a risky business and the diseases soon spread to other family members'. This may link with observations in Umvoti in 1981 and Pietermaritzburg in February 2001, that massive spread of cholera seemed to link more with parties and social gatherings (with very large gatherings frequently occurring for funerals) than drinking contaminated river water. Taylor devised a small test tube experiment which illustrated to local people the amount of contamination on their own fingers through incubating water which they had touched in their own pockets. He commented:

> In Eshowe both the authorities and recipients of the cholera campaigns often assumed that if people stopped drinking contaminated water from the rivers and streams they would be safe from infection. Closer investigation revealed a different picture however. Once a person contracts cholera he or she may be a carrier of the disease for up to 30 days. During this time if personal hygiene is not carefully observed and hands are not washed after using the toilet, other members of the family may contract the disease from the infected person's hands. This knowledge, which only became evident through engaged experimentation and dialogue with significant others, overturned previous misconceptions and enabled a far more meaningful engagement with the issues.[22]

Taylor concluded that the learning process which had occurred during the crisis may have done a great deal to help build a new South Africa, where the knowledge of others is respected and everyone had a contribution to make despite their upbringing and rural circumstances, rather than experts perceiving Eshowe people as rural folk who needed to become the recipients of informed messages.

Other analyses after the epidemic revealed the communities' difficulties in understanding and accepting the causes of the epidemic, with some in rural areas finding it hard to distrust the river water which they had always drunk for generations. Some people believed that prayer could ensure the water was pure, and others suggested that cholera was spread intentionally by White people by aeroplane or other methods, to undermine the new post-Apartheid political dispensation. Witchcraft was also suggested as a possible cause.[23]

By the end of the epidemic in April 2002 there had been a total of 117,147 cases and 265 deaths in the country, the vast majority being in KwaZulu-Natal. The epidemic prompted the government to treat the supply of water to poor communities more seriously and urgently and, as mentioned above, introduce the policy of Free Basic Water. Greater emphasis was also placed on the provision of adequate sanitation with funds made available for the construction of Ventilated Improved Pit Latrines at various locations across the Province, including Vulindlela near Pietermaritzburg. However, Hemson found that, four years after the epidemic, the implementation of the free water policy was being implemented unevenly, that piped water services were frequently unreliable and often interrupted, that unreliable supplies led people to store quantities of water at home which posed a health risk and that those families who had previously experienced cholera still appeared to be at greater risk of related diseases such as diarrhoea. This suggested they could be vulnerable to the recurrence of cholera in the future.[24]

Cholera again appeared in Mozambique in 2008, following which some cases appeared in Mpumulanga province of South Africa. Then later in 2008 cholera broke out in Zimbabwe to the north of South Africa, across the Limpopo River. The disease broke out following years of economic collapse and subsequent breakdown of their water treatment and sewerage systems, and their health services were unable to cope due to drug shortages, insufficient medical supplies, and the general disarray of Zimbabwe's health services. This gave rise to a cholera epidemic which went rapidly out of control. By December 2008 there had been over 12,500 cases and 560 deaths since August, and the United Nations reported that the disease was present in all of Zimbabwe's 10 Provinces and in 55 of the 62 Districts. Between September and November most wards in the country's large hospitals closed and on 17 November the capital's main teaching hospital, Parirenyatwa, closed shortly after the closure of Harare Central Hospital. The closures were due largely to the failure of water supplies and sanitation systems, with toilets overflowing. Faced with the closure of their hospitals, sick Zimbabweans fled towards South Africa to try and access medical care which was unavailable in their own country. Many were admitted to the Beit Bridge Hospital in Zimbabwe, on the border with South Africa, which at its peak was trying to treat 250 new patients per day. The whole situation was then made dramatically worse by the breakdown of the town's water treatment plant and a spill of raw sewage directly into the Limpopo River, which resulted in the largest single cause of fatalities and infections. A team from South Africa went in to repair the failed and neglected sewerage system, but the disease was by then widespread in the region.[25]

Having crossed the border in November, by the 8th December 2008 there had been 633 cases of cholera in South Africa, mostly initially in Zimbabweans who had crossed the Limpopo seeking help. There were some 57 cases in the closest hospital, at the small town of Musina, where rehydration centres had to be opened to help, and eight deaths. The case-fatality rate was lower in South Africa, at 1.3%, than in Zimbabwe where it was standing at around 5% - a reflection of the poor state of the health services there. By 11th January 2009 the total cases were up to more than 1,900, from all nine Provinces of South Africa, with the vast majority in Limpopo centred around Vhembe district, followed by 144 cases in the central, urban Province of Gauteng. Musina had been declared a disaster area. The number of deaths stood at just 15 – a low fatality rate of 0.78% - but rivers were testing positive and the area of infection was spreading. A National Outbreak Committee composed of the Provincial and National Departments of Health, the WHO and other International organisations and NGOs had been established and was directing programmes of community mobilisation, health education, supply of bleach and oral rehydration fluids, and case finding. Water was being trucked in to villages without safe supplies and rehydration centres established.[26] The lessons learned from the KwaZulu-Natal outbreak were proving useful in addressing and containing the epidemic, but dealing with the source of the epidemic in Zimbabwe was an on-going challenge. A further problem was the continuing flood of refugees and economic migrants from Zimbabwe following the political instability and economic collapse of the country, many of whom were living in informal and inadequate settlements.

By March 2009 there had been 12,324 cases recorded in South Africa with 59 deaths, but the rate of new cases was finally declining. Five new water treatment plants had been rapidly commissioned for rural villages.[27] The final total by August 2009 was reported at 12,787 cases and 64 deaths, virtually all of which were either in Zimbabweans who had crossed into the country, or in poor communities with inadequate water and sanitation. Across the whole sub-continent, including as far as Angola, Zambia and Malawi, there had been over 150,000 cases, with some 12,000 in Swaziland and 14,400 in Mozambique but the vast majority of 94,000 had been in Zimbabwe. Altogether there had been 5,460 deaths from the disease. In South Africa the outbreak mainly affected Limpopo, Mpumulanga and Gauteng, with other cases, including the usually affected KwaZulu-Natal, largely spared.[28]

The number of cases in the epidemic was massive, possibly aided by an early degree of denialism within the authorities who firstly were loath to be critical of the events happening in Zimbabwe, and secondly who always seemed reticent to raise the alarm about cholera in particular, which then precluded early preventive measures which could limit a possible outbreak. This was similar to previous outbreaks where delays in response had occurred through a reluctance to admit the imminent dangers. Still it was clear that the South African Authorities had developed a rapid response capacity, with tried and tested interventions which could address cholera in the future, although the mainstay in reducing the risk of cholera remains the widespread introduction of treated, safe water and hygienic sanitation schemes. As illustrated by the explosive outbreaks which have occurred around community gatherings, as long as the rural areas remain with badly constructed, fly infested pit latrines, and while river water is cheaper than safe water, the risk of cholera returning in intermittent devastating epidemics will remain.

ENDNOTES

1   Laidler P.W. and Gelfand M. *South Africa its medical history, 1652-1898: A medical and social study* Struik, Cape Town, 1971:149
2   Matthews J.W. *Incwadi Yami or Twenty Years Personal Experience in South Africa; 1887*; Africana Book Society, Johannesburg 1976:16
3   Brain J.B. and Brain P. 'The health of indentured Indian Migrants to Natal, 1860-1911' *South African Medical Journal* 62(20) 1982:739-742
4   Laidler P.W. 'Statistics, Social Disease and Legislation' *South African Medical Journal* 14(4) 1939:71-77
5   Swanson, Maynard W. '"The Asiatic Menace":creating segregation in Durban, 1870-1900' *International Journal of African Historical Studies*, 16(3) 1983:416
6   Seedat M.A. 'Cholera in South Africa' *Modern Medicine of South Africa*, 7(9) September 1982:81

7   Sinclair G.S. et al, 'Determination of the mode of transmission of cholera in Lebowa' *South African Medical Journal* 62(21) 1982:753-755
8   Seedat M.A. 'Cholera in South Africa', *Modern Medicine of South Africa* 7(9) September 1982:88
9   Sinclair G.S. et al, 'Determination of the mode of transmission of cholera in Lebowa' *South African Medical Journal* 62(21) 1982:753-755
10 Seedat M.A. 'Cholera in South Africa' *Modern Medicine of South Africa* 7(9) September 1982:82
11 Sitas F. 'An investigation of a Cholera outbreak at the Umvoti Mission Reserve, Natal. A Non-Water Borne epidemic?' *Second Carnegie Inquiry into Poverty and Development in Southern Africa*, Carnegie Conference Paper No 151
12 Seedat M.A. 'Cholera in South Africa' *Modern Medicine of South Africa*, 7(9) September 1982:83
13 Küstner H.G.V. 'Secular trends of selected diseases' *Epidemiological Comments*, National Department of Health, 11(3) March 1984:p10.
14 Küstner H.G.V. 'Analysis of Cholera IV' *Epidemiological Comments*, National Department of Health, 11(10) October 1984:5-22.
15 Küstner H.G.V 'Cholera in South Africa' *Epidemiological Comments*, National Department of Health 18(12) December 1991:268
16 'Cholera on our Border' *Pretoria News* 10 August 1992
17 Küstner H.G.V. 'Cholera in South Africa' *Epidemiological Comments*, 24(1) January 1998:3
18 Durrheim D.N. Ogunbanjo G.A. Blumberg L. Keddy K.H. 'Cholera – The Grim Reality of Under-development' *South African Family Practice*, 23 (2) February-March 2001:5
19 Dyer J.J. 'Cholera Outbreak Control Programme' *Pietermaritzburg-Msunduzi, Umgeni, Mpofana District Health Services Annual Report 2001;* Msunduzi Municipality 2001:58-65
20 Hemson D. et al, 'Still Paying the Price: Revisiting the Cholera Epidemic of 2000-2001 in South Africa' *Municipal Services Project Occasional Paper No 10; Human Sciences Research Council*, Grocotts Publishers and Printers, Grahamstown, February 2006:13
21 Ibid, 7
22 Taylor J. 'Meaningful Learning and Social Change: the case of the Eshowe cholera crisis in South Africa' *African Wildlife* 59 (2) 2005:12-14.
23 Hemson D. et al, 'Still Paying the Price: Revisiting the Cholera Epidemic of 2000-2001 in South Africa' *Municipal Services Project Occasional Paper No 10; Human Sciences Research Council*, Printed by Grocotts Publishers and Printers, Grahamstown; February 2006:22-23
24 Ibid, 37
25 Bateman C. 'Cholera: getting the basics right' *South African Medical Journal [online];* 99(3) Cape Town March 2009:132-136
26 Mugero C. 'Cholera Outbreak in South Africa' *National Outbreak Committee Situational Report* (Sitrep 29); Pretoria, 11 January 2009.
27 Page L. and Khumalo T. *Report of the Department of Water Affairs and Forestry*, South African Government Information Service, 12 March 2009
28 Ramatuba R. 'Cholera Response and Mitigation' *Report of the Directorate of Environmental Health*, National Department of Health, Pretoria, 27 August 2009.

9   THE CURSE OF THE BUSHVELD: MALARIA

Mentzel, in his description of 1787 of the Cape, states that 'the cold quotidian, tertian and quartan fever is, however, quite unknown here'.[1] However malaria is mentioned as being in existence around Delagoa Bay from 1822, where a description of 'Hottentot' treatment is given:

> On the first appearance of symptoms the patient retired to his hut and kept warm. Water was boiled in a pot and placed between his legs while he sat on a stool enveloped in mats and leant over the steam inhaling it. Suddenly the whole was thrown off and a shower of cold water poured over him, and he was hurried to the side of a large fire, placed in a recumbent position, bled by light incisions of the shoulders, breast and backs of hands.[2]

There is also mention of it being present in Cape Town in the summer, when mosquitoes flourished in the canals, or 'grachts' which ran through the city carrying water from Table Mountain. Most of these were filthy, smelly and filled with refuse at this time. The city generally had become insanitary, with many streets still lacking sewers and with rudimentary sanitation. Water was available from 60 or so fountains or pumps in the city.[3] The cold winters, however, prevented malaria establishing itself as a year-round disease.

As the Voortrekkers migrated out from the Cape in the 1830's to escape British rule malaria was mentioned as experienced by them when they reached the north-eastern low-lying regions of the Transvaal, where it wiped out whole families. One of the early pioneering parties lead by Louis Trichardt was devastated by malaria once they descended onto the low veld, below the high plateaus, and he and practically all his party fell ill with the disease and eventually died. The later arrivals chose to make their settlements close to rivers and streams, but within a generation had been forced to abandon their early sites due to the malaria problem. The few settlers who escaped moved to found a new town in 1849 which they named Lydenburg, or Town of Suffering, in memory of the high mortality in their earlier location. However they were just as exposed in their new settlement and also died, although in lesser numbers.[4] In the dry season of the winter malaria usually subsided, but in the summer when the rains came it started again every year. After a while the pioneer families began to realise that it meant death to camp near water, and that it was safer to pitch camp or build their homes on a barren, stony hill. In particular they learned to rest above the line of white mist that lay above river beds, as they believed the poisonous air was heavier and settled in low lying areas.[5] However malaria continued to take its toll and these early migrants to the Eastern Transvaal had a difficult time with little available by way of treatment for the disease.

Quinine Sulphate had been discovered in 1820, and in 1847 Hare published a pamphlet on the treatment of malaria with quinine which, following an investigation by the Calcutta Medical Board, resulted in the routine use of quinine to treat malaria. This was before the transmission by mosquitoes had been proved. Prior to the introduction of quinine, from 1804 to 1847 cinchona treatment had been used along with violent purging using calomel. This was later replaced by Magnesium sulphate which was thought to enhance the absorption of quinine.[6]

Following the discovery of gold in 1872 miners rushed to the Eastern Transvaal, as had the Voortrekkers before them, into the area of Pilgrims Rest where malaria was known to be endemic. Many of them suffered from it and so devastating was the disease that new arrivals on the diggings were regarded as another pilgrim coming to his rest. In 1878 the seasonal outbreak of malaria was so severe that emergency hospitals and to be erected. Malaria stalked many of the mining areas, including those at Barberton, and a temporary hospital was started there in two corrugated iron shacks.[7] Malaria was also known to be prevalent around the coastal and northern areas of Natal and during 1866-68 malaria spread out of Zululand and the coastal areas as far west and north as the Orange Free State and Transvaal, and as far south as Port Elizabeth in the eastern Cape.[8] Dr Matthews reported an outbreak in 1869 where he had had 120 cases among whites and Indians on a sugar estate near the mouth of the Umgeni river, now close to the centre of the city of Durban. Malaria was also reported from around Verulam, further north.[9] In 1880 Laveran discovered the malaria parasite, and Ross proposed the malaria-mosquito theory in 1897.

During the Anglo-Boer War malaria also took its toll, particularly in the Concentration Camps which were established for Boer women and children across the Transvaal. Devitt reported malaria in camps in the towns of Volksrust, Middleburg, Standerton, Irene and Belfast, possibly brought to the camps by families who were already carrying it from the low veld. The disease killed many, exacerbated by the dire shortage of nurses and particularly those familiar with the condition.¹⁰ The Ladies Commission, established by the War Office in Britain in July 1901 to investigate conditions in the Camps, reported of the Pietersburg camp:

> A large number of refugees arrived from the Lowveld absolutely saturated with malaria. One party of 21 persons had trekked north with the Boers all the way from Johannesburg and had finally surrendered at Pietersburg; eight of these people had died on the trek, one was lying dead in the wagon when they arrived, six died soon after and the remaining six are now slowly recovering thanks to better climate, medical care and good food.¹¹

While malaria as an overall cause of death in the camps was largely overshadowed by measles, pneumonia and typhoid, it still caused significant morbidity and morbidity in the Eastern and Northern Transvaal camps.

Cape Town still suffered from malaria up to the end of the nineteenth century with 40 cases being treated in the Somerset Hospital in 1900 with two deaths.¹² However by the early 1900s anopheline mosquitoes were no longer being found in the Cape Peninsula, although a case of malaria was reported in Cape Town in 1918 which appeared to be locally contracted.¹³

Haydon and Hill described an outbreak of malaria in Durban in 1905 due to A. coastalis, later known as A. Gambiae, in which 4,177 cases occurred, with 42 deaths, during the first six months of the year.¹⁴ Park Ross reported on another outbreak in Northern Zululand known by the locals as Isigwebedhla Umkhuhlane. He advocated the use of quinine, screening of dwellings and bed-nets plus protective clothing.¹⁵

Up in the Transvaal malaria continued to feature in reports of that era with it being referred to repeatedly in the reports of the Transvaal Administration, Department of Native Affairs. 1906 appears to have been a particularly bad year with many District Commissioners referring to it. Wheelwright, Commissioner of the Northern Division based in Pietersburg stated that the district was notoriously bad for it in many parts and the disease was that year worse than for many years, having been intensified by heavy rains. He refers to its interference with the collection of revenue such as rentals on Crown lands 'a great portion of which lie in malarious areas; the people are very scattered and the collectors suffered much from fever'. It also affected the collection of Native Tax:

> In the more unhealthy parts of the district it is found necessary to exempt

many more natives from taxation than in the healthier parts. In the former, probably as the result of fever, many men grow prematurely old and are practically unable to leave their own locations and proceed to higher and cooler altitudes, as the fever lies latent in their systems and readily appears on changing from their warmer homes to the high veld.[16]

The Native Tax had been in place for many years, standing at that time £2 for every adult male, and was aimed at forcing the men into waged labour on the mines and other places where they were needed. The rental for Crown lands was imposed from 1904 on Africans residing or cultivating such lands.

Dr Spencer, District Surgeon in Middleburg, investigated a serious epidemic at Pokwani from where he reported that the disease was Intermittent Malarial Fever, attacking mainly those working on the land growing mealies and corn, usually women. He described the illness as lasting a week or two, after which the sufferers often returned to work only to be attacked again after three or four days with the process repeating for a period of some three months. He estimated the number affected to be around 600-700. Spencer commented 'the rainfall has steadily increased in this district for the past three years and this year has in this respect been similar to the year before the war when the sickness was as rife as now'. He continued 'Those carried off by the fever were mostly aged, or young children, a small number occurring amongst young men or women whose resistance to disease was probably lowered by some physical condition – perhaps by syphilis contracted or inherited. Pneumonia and high temperature was responsible for most of the deaths'. Spencer said that the deaths were contributed to by 'the absence of the antidote to all malarial fevers – quinine', and an absence of milk due to the steady loss of cattle to disease over the previous two years.[17] Quinine was then distributed free of charge to all the sick through their chiefs, but still some 400 deaths were reported.

Malaria spread all across the Transvaal that year – the Commissioner from Rustenburg commented that fever in this Division was at times very bad and whole families had been carried off by it; reports were also made of severe illness in the Barberton and Piet Retief areas. From Sekukuniland in the central Transvaal L.C.R. Harries, the Sub-Native Commissioner, reported that the state of health was very bad, 'Malarial fever, consumption and syphilis having been very prevalent. With regard to the first it is stated by old residents in the District that it was exceptionally severe'.[18] Malaria was also reported by District Health Officers in certain parts of the Cape, being reported upon in Barkly West where the first serious outbreak had occurred in 1900 with many children and old people dying. In the early years of the century it reappeared seasonally according to the rainfall.

Through the early 1900's the Resident Magistrates and Native Commissioners continued to report the toll of malaria in their areas, across mainly Zululand, Natal, and the Transvaal but extending to parts of the Orange Free State, the Cape and the Transkei. In the Transvaal in the reports of 1910 and 1911 extensive mention is made of the presence of malaria.

Despite the regular reports of the Native Commissioners, amongst others, in 1922 Spencer wrote that the ravages of malaria upon the Transvaal were being generally ignored, save for the distribution of quinine tablets, and that they were being given less attention than cattle diseases. He stated that there was progressive retrogression and retardation of the country owing to the prolonged disability, physical apathy, anaemia and mental impairment produced by acute and chronic malaria affecting all those in habiting the low veld and many on the middle veld. In the low veld (low lying eastern areas) he reported that the disease killed 15 out of 1,000 people in the healthiest seasons, and more than double that in epidemic seasons. It also caused invalidism and disability for long periods. The farmers almost all succumbed and after repeated attacks were too weak to work, and 'as for the women and children and the natives on the low veld, they simply die and are buried without record, like so much flotsam and jetsam'.[19]

On the higher middle veld, where it was less severe, malaria was largely ignored by the authorities yet large numbers were disabled by the disease with chronic rheumatism, bronchial catarrhs, weak hearts, physical apathy, anaemia, chronic headaches and mental debility. Often these symptoms were misdiagnosed and not attributed to malaria. The mosquitoes were thought to be breeding in the streams, marshes and ponds of the area, but most importantly in the small dams for irrigation purposes to be found close to almost every house and farm. Occasionally epidemics occurred, during which the Africans suffered the most and men worse than women and children, although deaths occurred mainly in children. During the malarial season, the hottest time, the men would sleep outside the huts while women and children slept inside the smoky huts. With 20 years experience in the area Spencer thought that the deaths from malaria were often misdiagnosed as croup, bronchitis, and convulsions, and that many would have responded to quinine treatment. He estimated that half of the deaths of Europeans on the middle veld were due to malaria.

Malaria was acknowledged to be responsible for the non-development of the low veld, delaying European settlement and being responsible for most of the sickness and death of the African population. It was considered an economic loss to the state whose control was greatly hindered by the cost of interventions. Malaria was also endemic through the north eastern areas of Natal around Kosi Bay, St Lucia and Pongola throughout the year, with the heaviest epidemics occurring in summer when there was both excessive heat and heavy rains. It was noted by Dr Park Ross to affect the wealthy less than the poor – 'dump a colony of poor whites or persons on relief works down amid an infected native population, and one heads for a certain epidemic'. Non-immune immigration was also a factor: 'malaria breaks out when non-immune Cape labour is sent to a sugar estate in a malarious area in Natal in spite of good housing and food conditions, whereas local natives are not so much affected'. The situation was much worse when they were lodged under poor economic conditions in an even mildly malarious area. Park Ross prepared a map in 1921 showing the relative intensity of malaria across the country, which showed a large swathe of country where malaria was continuously present in severe form throughout the year, stretching from the north, through Mozambique to east of the Ubombo mountains. A survey undertaken by him in that area found that 53% of children under 10 had parasites, and 70% had enlarged spleens. The Africans in this area showed a fair degree of immunity. However in the surrounding areas, where there were summer epidemics, 96% of children had parasites and there was a high proportion of malignant cases.

The recommended preventive measure was the distribution of quinine to reduce both the amount of fever and the number of carriers, and to distribute it liberally via Magistrates' offices, police posts and selected stores. Anti-malarial measures of drainage, filling in borrow-pits, and removal of undergrowth from streams to reduce mosquito breeding sites were considered effective if planned and carried out with meticulous attention to detail. The protection of African houses was described by Park Ross thus: 'a native wants to sit round a fire at sundown, and he does not mind smoke. In fact he seems to like it. I give him a house where he can have his fire in the open, and sit sheltered from rain near that fire. I make the only entrance to a set of rooms a single door and I place it so that even if it is left open, the adventurous mosquito has to face a smoke smudge before it can possibly get a human meal'. The settlement of poor Whites on the low veld was seen as a particular problem, as the development of the land required that they keep free of fever, and 'a great number of poor whites and nomads who haunt the low veld can never be depended upon to use means to keep themselves free of it without constant and unending supervision'. It would require that the Government netted their houses, undertook drainage and supervised the quinine distribution, and it was thought this would be an expensive undertaking. With the better-off settler antimalarial measures for both himself and his labour could be insisted upon. However, some had a tendency to reject preventive measures, which would make then themselves carriers and a risk to the community.[20]

In 1923 Spencer again lamented the lack of government action in respect of malaria in the Transvaal. He reported how the lack of action had resulted in potentially prosperous farming area being decimated over the previous 10 years, with most of the settlers having died of the disease or its consequences. The effect of epidemics on the local population was described as unchanged over the past 50 years, and many had suffered and died from malaria during the construction of the Delagoa railway line, which opened in 1895. The symptoms on the low veld were more severe than the middle veld, and the impact on the heart and nervous system persisted long after the initial attacks. Enormously enlarged spleens were also common, with anaemia and weakness. Some suffered from loss of speech and memory, and inability to walk. Those with chronic malaria often became dull, slow and irritable.[21] Spencer noted that dry summers favoured general or epidemic malaria, while wet summers, with regular and frequent rains, produced sporadic disease. Some of the blame for infection he laid with the settlers who thought that they would acquire immunity if they didn't take preventative measures. Indeed it was true that some people were never affected by the diseases, and he queried whether it was some condition of their cutaneous secretions which protected them. However in the main he did not observe much in the way of immunity either acquired or inherited. He recommended a great extension of screening measures, to include schools, houses, hostels, hotels, boarding houses, and public servants quarters. [22]

Malaria continued to be prevalent in the Transvaal throughout the 1920's with Tzaneen described in one report as being severely affected. It was concluded that a proposed colony of non-immune White people in the area would suffer greatly from malaria and that the death rate would be high – an estimated 80% would go down with the disease. 'It is only people of high stamina and good spirit who are prepared to fight through such conditions, and I understand that these are not the distinguishing characteristics of the colonists whom it is proposed to put there'.[23] Malaria was also prevalent in the Zoutpansberg, Potgietersrust, and

Waterberg areas.

In 1930 sporadic cases had started appearing in areas of Natal previously thought to be malaria-free. The incidence had been increasing since 1929, with a severe outbreak in the coastal districts of Zululand and northern Natal in 1928 and then becoming more widespread in the 1929/30 season, reaching as far as Umzinto in the south and as far west as Weenen and Ladysmith. Isolated outbreaks even occurred in places such as Harding and the Transkei at altitudes of over 3,000 feet due to the infection being carried by labourers. The total mortality was 1,653 compared with 2,758 in the previous season, and the epidemic caused widespread disruption to the sugar mills and plantations because of the large number of labourers affected. In addition work on the railway line around Stanger was virtually halted. The wider spread was thought to be due to favourable rains and climatic conditions promoting the rapid multiplication of mosquitoes and the movement of people. A malaria team including a Doctor, inspectors and African assistants were organised to carry out surveys, education and advisory work. The Assistants were trained to measure spleens, take temperatures, identify mosquitoes and larvae, hunt for breeding sites and apply anti-larval measures. Quinine distribution depots were formed at police posts, missions, stores and animal dipping tanks.[24] However, there was widespread resistance to the tablets largely due to the intervention of Traditional Healers who cautioned that it may result in death or sterility. The attitude of non-compliance of the Healers has been attributed to the recently passed law which restricted their activities (Act 13 of 1928). The information pamphlets were also written in English which was not widely understood. In addition the government continued to understate the epidemic and the quinine supplies were inadequate. The outbreak continued even into the winter months of June and July due to unusually mild weather.[25] In the southern parts of Natal, such as the coastal resort area of Umzinto, people were unprepared and mosquito netting, Paris green (recently introduced as a larvicide) and repellent had to be brought in. In 1931 it extended even further south to Port St Johns. The exceptionally dry summer had caused many of the rivers to dry up leaving small pools where mosquitoes could breed.

Epidemics of varying intensity continued to occur in Natal, with the highest number of deaths, an estimated 10,000, in 1931/32 when all but four of the 45 magisterial districts were affected.[26] 2,252 cases were admitted to two hospitals in Durban alone. Various factors were noticed to predispose to increased malaria, including an exceptionally wet spell of weather followed by humid warm weather; a tendency of the public to try and treat themselves, and those who ignored advice regarding prevention. The malaria season of 1932 was the worst in the history of the Natal coast up until then, due to the favourable meteorological conditions. The epidemic of 1932 was associated with prolific breeding and infestation of dwellings of A gambiae throughout the province of Natal at altitudes up to 3,000 feet (914 metres) above sea level. The incidence was particularly severe in the African areas, and an attempt was made in the Tugela Valley to control the disease by weekly fumigation of huts with sulphur dioxide. However this failed due to its rapid diffusion out of the grass huts, although popular with the African population as it killed cockroaches. In the remote rural area of Msinga pyrethrum and paraffin insecticide was introduced with such striking results that it was then extended to other areas of the province, including farms and sugar estates. The serious impact of the epidemic on the sugar industry resulted in the organisation of the sugar belt into local control areas, and in 1932 a Natal Provincial Ordinance was promulgated to establish rural malarial committees with power to levy rates for malaria control. 17 coastal and two inland committees were set up, and employed malaria inspectors. Anti-larval work continued, but was found less effective than anti-adult measures in controlling the disease.[27] Overall the mortality was estimated by Magistrates to be 22,132, although this proved very contentious with the Department of Health putting the figure at more like 10,000. The lack of consensus was partly due to there being no registration system of African deaths.

In the period from 1929 to the early 1930's malaria hit the city of Pietermaritzburg in Natal severely. Prior to that there had been no cases except for a few in 1906, probably due to the city's position 80 kilometres inland from Durban at an altitude of some 700 metres. No further cases occurred until 1929 when a handful were reported, and again in 1930 and 1931. However between January and May 1932 1,500 cases occurred with 105 deaths, followed by 239 in the same period of 1933 with 25 deaths. Due to the absence of cases no anti-larval measures had been taken until 1931, but during the 1933 season extensive drainage, anti-larval and anti-mosquito measures were taken to which was ascribed the reduction in cases. In an area outside the boundaries, Bishopstowe, where no measures were taken, 48 out of 52 residents were affected with five deaths. Extensive analysis was undertaken with 1,500 anopheline larvae studied in 1933. Each of the three peaks of infection recorded during the 1933 outbreak was found to occur three weeks after a sharp rise of mean daily temperature, usually accompanied by a fall in relative humidity. It was therefore proposed that anti-mosquito measures should be intensified after a rise in mean daily temperature. Spraying of houses was undertaken which seemed very effective. The spread of malaria from the coast to the midlands of Natal was postulated to be due to an unusually high rainfall, although some suggested it was due to the increase in the number of cars with closed windows travelling from Durban. 14 out of 52 male Europeans infected were railway employees, most of which were infected while on night shift on railway property where trains from endemic areas arrived.[28]

While there were localized outbreaks in other parts of Natal, including Port Shepstone to the south, Camperdown to the east and Weenen and Greytown to the northwest, many rural parts of Natal however had considerably less malaria in 1933 than the year before. According to the Department of Health Reports appreciation was expressed at the annual Hindu celebration in Isipingo, south of Durban, with thanks given in the form of offerings and prayers for the reduction in malaria. This was put down to more vigorous preventive measures being taken by the rural malaria committees and local authorities from Richmond to Ladysmith. The area under anti-malarial measures now extended 250 miles in length. The Transvaal was threatened in the 1933 season due to torrential rains in January. Fortunately, however, the rains dropped off in the following months, so the mosquito breeding was limited.[29]

Preventive measures for malaria in the 1930's were grouped into various categories: measures against the larvae and adult mosquitoes; protective measures such as screening, bed nets and repellents, and actions directed at human hosts. One measure suggested against the latter, related to the carrier status of African children, in which Booker and Annecke proposed 'the only immediate measure at our disposal to mitigate this danger is to compel natives to live a safe distance from European habitations and from dangerous breeding grounds'.[30] They also however recommended the thorough treatment of cases to prevent them becoming carriers using quinine and magnesium sulphate as a purgative. In 1931 atebrin, a synthetic derivative of quinolin, was also introduced along with plasmoquine and neosalvarsan, more commonly used for the treatment of syphilis, was also recommended by some as an adjunct to quinine and plasmoquine, particularly in benign tertian cases. Malaria was at this point endemic in the Transvaal, Natal and the Transkei.

In 1933 the Malaria Commission of the League of Nations produced its Third General Report. This detailed the reaction to treatment of the different strains of malaria. It proposed that treatment with quinine should aim at assisting malaria patients to acquire as much immunity as possible by assessing the stage of the patients disease, and prescribing a dose of quinine just sufficient to be effective at that stage without interfering with patients defensive mechanisms. Treatment after the patient had had several paroxysms of fever was considered preferable to early treatment. Patients were recommended to go to bed early in the disease to promote perspiration, and take a purgative and a drug to induce a good flow of bile before quinine. Caffeine given intravenously or hypodermically before quinine was also recommended.[31]

Leipoldt, who was Medical Inspector of Schools in the Transvaal from around 1911, described malaria as 'the Curse of the Bushveld' and felt it was given inadequate attention in that Province. 'It rarely kills. If it did the bushveld folk would be much more interested in it and would combine in a mass attack against it. But what it does is more insidious, more nationally detrimental. It weakens, it saps the energy and the spirit of its victims, it stunts their growth, it changes their outlook on life itself, it causes widespread physical and mental deterioration. Therein lies its greatest danger'. Writing in 1937 he said that the position was not much better than on his first arrival. 'In times of epidemic, when the mortality from it is slightly greater than in ordinary seasons, a mild flutter of apprehension runs through the Bushveld, but it is never sufficient to stir folk into active, organised attack upon a scourge that is endemic'.[32] He maintained that all Bushveld dwellers suffered from malaria to some degree, and that both whites and Africans were infected, but that the government had shown no interest until under D. Malan as Minister of Health, when he had commissioned a Report from Professor Swellengrebel.

Leipoldt had instituted the distribution of quinine to schools and urged that it be taken regularly in summer. However such an initiative had not been without problems, in that teachers did not comply with the instructions in the early years – one had used their administration as a punishment. Part of this he put down to the poor quality of the teachers: 'the small climatic allowance made to teachers in malarious districts attracted the inferior type rather than the superior'. Leipoldt suggested rather replacing this with extra service bonuses, with an annual bonus to teachers who kept their schools free from malaria. He also recommended that no schools be built on the small malarious farm areas, but rather that larger ones be built in safer areas with hostel accommodation. However his recommendations were not accepted, which he ascribed to the indifference of the highveld decision makers, and ignorance of what the disease was doing on the lowveld – the stunted physique and widespread malnutrition. Following the report to the Government of Professor

Swellengrebel in 1931 malaria control in the Transvaal was improved, although Leipoldt felt that it had still not attained the importance it required:

> With the change in government malaria has again become a minor consideration, and while the legislature has trifled with dozens of subjects of ephemeral importance it has done nothing, during the past five years, to cope effectively with the scourge of the Bushveld. Preventive measures, so far, have been confined to regulations, and to research work.[33]

Arising out of Swellengrebel's report a Research Station had been established at Tzaneen in the low veld, where the disease was hyper-endemic, under the South African Institute for Medical Research (SAIMR). The Department of Health had a Control Unit which visited each farm to give advice. The main mosquito vectors had been identified by Ingram and De Meillon as Anopheles gambiae and Anopheles funestus, the former of which bred in shallow depressions, such as pools or puddles, with full such exposure. Anopheles funestus preferred streams of water at the edges with rank vegetation and slow current. The spread and distribution of these mosquitoes depended upon the weather, with A. gambiae spreading only with rainfall and being able to survive through winter. A. funestus required a mean monthly temperature of 15°c, and was less dependent on rainfall as it bred in perennial streams, and was the dominant type in the low veld. Both mosquito types were dormant during the day and chose to lurk in secluded, quiet and confined spaces inside the house, usually behind or under furniture or amongst hanging clothes in a bedroom. The habits of the mosquitoes were of importance in determining the best control measures for the larvae, with oiling or removing puddles being important for A. gambiae, and removal of vegetation along streams, together with oiling, being needed to control A. funestus. The difficulty of the latter meant that personal protection from mosquitoes by nets and insecticides etc was important in the A. funestus areas. The Department of Health also recommended repellent smears and wiping of furniture with paraffin rags. The extent of area to be covered around an individual's house was up to a kilometre.

Progress in controlling malaria in the Transvaal was said to be hampered due to the vastness of the areas, apathy, and the cost of the preventive measures to farmers. Lack of knowledge about malaria in the days of the early settlers had resulted in farmers always building their houses on the bank of a river or stream, which complicated prevention. In addition farmers were said to be in very poor circumstances in the

1930's, with poor nutrition and reduced resistance to disease: 'in many homes there is not the wherewithal to buy the daily mealie meal, let alone think about prevention of malaria'. The African population were considered a 'menace' from the perspective of malaria: 'the unscreened native hut is ... a very great danger to the farmer', and 'these squatter native families on Transvaal farms are a malarial menace on account of their being the reservoir of infection for the newly born mosquito vector seeking its first blood meal'. Farmers were advised to keep the huts at least a mile from their houses, and practice daily mosquito spraying in them.[34] The Department of Health continued to urge farmers to pay more attention to the state of their employees' houses, and to realise that better housing made economic sense as it would be easier to protect their staff from infection. In some areas the farmers themselves were poor, such as around Piet Retief near the Swaziland border, but those who took preventive measures soon realised the benefits. Education outreach work was done from the centre in Tzaneen, with school headmasters, the Railways and Harbour Administration, local authority Health inspectors and the anti-malaria staff from the Pongola Irrigation Scheme being trained. The latter was particularly at risk and it was found in a survey in 1932 that 50% of both European and African staff were infected.[35]

Further research into the local mosquitoes revealed that A. funestus bred in the permanent streams originating in the Drakensberg mountains and was independent of local rainfall. Its seasonal fluctuation was dependant on temperature, needing a mean temperature over 61°F (16°C), giving it a fairly stable population and levels of malaria in warm areas. It could cover distances up to two miles, but 80% of adults were found within a half-mile (800 metres) from their point of origin. Its habits changed at around 2,500 feet, (762 metres) below which it frequented houses and gave rise to intense malaria. However, above this level up to 3,500 feet, (1,067metres), while larvae were still numerous, the adults no longer entered houses and malaria was absent, as it preferred to bite hosts when in confined spaces. In contrast A. gambiae preferred small temporary pools hence showing seasonal fluctuations related to the distribution of rain. In winter it was limited to altitudes below 2,000 feet and a mean temperature of over 61°C but covered a much wider area in summer. With summer rains it could spread much further into normally dry countryside, such as Rustenburg in 1928. Because of its wide fluctuations in coverage it was A. gambiae which gave rise to epidemics, as it spread to areas where there were people without immunity and no knowledge of prevention and treatment. In Rustenburg many were suspicious of quinine, and deaths were a feature of such epidemics. A. gambiae was not generally a house dweller but often found roosting in crevices and hollows.[36] However by monitoring the rainfall in the Transvaal area and subsequent A gambiae breeding it was possible to predict with some accuracy when an epidemic was due.

Anti-larval work included drainage and tree planting of marshland and fencing to exclude cattle from marshes and limit water-filled hoof prints. Problems were experienced with this approach in some African reserve areas of Zululand due to suspicion of these activities, with the local population fearing Government interference with water supplies and movements of cattle. Fumigation of huts with sulphur was allowed, but proved a failure. However the acceptance of the process by the Africans meant that control by spraying with a reliable insecticide could prove tolerable and effective. Weekly spraying with pyrethrum was then systematised in the reserves. After a two year trial hut spraying was then undertaken on a very large scale in Natal and Zululand, with focussed attacks added for a mile around any outbreak. The success of these measures encouraged the local population to engage in further anti-malarial measures, including draining of water and planting of gum trees, with the Department of Native Affairs establishing plantations at strategic locations to drain the swamps.[37] In addition the drainage and plantation measures resulted in financial saving of some 60% on oil and wages in the forthcoming years as breeding spots were brought under control

In the coastal city of Durban one of the focus areas for malaria control was the elimination of major breeding sites in marshes and river banks. The Eastern Vlei (wetland) was reclaimed with major engineering works, raising its level to eliminate breeding places. The Umbilo River was trained and reclaimed with a concrete canalisation at Congella. Land reclamation at the Bay was undertaken as part of the harbour extension. Still larvae and malaria were found extensively around Mayville, Stamford Hill, Durban North, the Umlaas River, Wentworth and all the peripheral parts of the city. Only the Berea and Congella suburbs were considered safe. The Railways and Harbours had their own programmes covering 30 stations, 564 miles of railway in the Transvaal and 418 miles of line and 62 stations in Natal. In addition they had to look after some 7,000 employees. Part of their measures included netting and improving African housing, but also keeping it far from European housing to reduce the risk to Europeans. Trains and buses were sprayed and inspected at various points and mosquitoes captured and analysed, although only two female anopheles were found in 1933, leading to the conclusion that public fears of the risk posed by trains was probably exaggerated.[38]

In major urban areas and European towns generally larval control took precedence over adult spraying, with measures such as tree planting and draining employed to eradicate breeding areas and provide a permanent solution. This was also used in rural areas, with approximately 750 hectares of Eucalyptus saligna ('gum trees') being planted in African coastal reserves to drain low-lying, water-logged areas. In the African urban areas spraying for control of adults was more important, and in rural farming areas both measures were employed. At that time some 932 people were employed in the local authorities and other organisations to control malaria. Weekly insecticidal spraying of houses using pyrethrum was based on the principle that the female anopheline mosquito became a transmitter of malaria parasites approximately 12 days after injecting infected blood, therefore spraying weekly meant the vector didn't live long enough to transmit infection. Insecticide spraying took place from Pongola in the north to the Umkomaas valley in the south, and up the river valleys as far as Pietermaritzburg and Paulpietersburg, representing an area of 9,000 square miles (more than 2.3 million hectares) or half the Province.[39]

The organisation of the anti-malaria strategy became more and more successful with Malaria Committees, farms and estates, local authorities and an extensive network of European Inspectors, African sprayers and malaria assistants, all playing a coordinated role. The anti-malarial measures had succeeded in dramatically reducing the incidence of malaria in Natal during the 1930's, with a reduction in rural malaria deaths from 3,677 in 1932 to 36 in 1939, despite unfavourable weather conditions in 1939. However the Minister of Posts and Telegraphs, speaking on behalf of the Minister of Public Health in Parliament, commented in 1939 that in the epidemic areas of the Transvaal malaria had never been known to occur on such a scale before. Heavy rains in December, January, February and March had provided ideal breeding conditions for A. gambiae. Malaria inspectors and health visitors were placed in the Province to advise farmers and local authorities with preventive measures. Treatment and quinine depots were started, and gangs of African sprayers engaged. Quinine was distributed to scattered African populations through 'quinine runners', and pumps and insecticides made available.[40] On the Witwatersrand occasional cases of malaria were reported even around Johannesburg, at an altitude of 1,750 metres. While A. funestus remained to the east of the Drakensberg mountains, A. gambiae had a wider distribution in the western and central Transvaal, and would occasionally under abnormal conditions approach the Witwatersrand. In years of little frost and heavy rainfall the mosquito could spread as far as Pretoria, Germiston, Springs and Johannesburg. Such exceptional conditions occurred in the 1938/39 season. Evidence suggested that breeding had spread along the courses of rivers and streams, aided by motor transport and trains.[41] The epidemic raged across the Transvaal including Pietersburg, Middleburg, Barberton and Rustenburg and dragged on as long as June in some areas. Altogether there were 9,311 deaths – almost 1% of the population in the rural areas, and as high as 2.7% of the entire population in Potgietersrus district.[42]

In order to reduce the morbidity and mortality amongst African labour the Department of Public Health discouraged the recruiting of southern non-resistant Africans for work in the Zululand malaria-endemic sugar belt. It was recommended rather that Portuguese (Mozambican) labour be brought in as they were malaria-tolerant. It was also proposed, in order to conserve these resistant labour forces for the sugar plantations, mills and malaria gangs, that recruitment by other industries and areas be prohibited.[43] However, movement of labour from farms in malaria-free zones to malarious northern and eastern areas continued, and placed their lives at risk. The control measures put into place certainly started bearing fruit in the Natal and Zululand areas, with the incidence in 1940 being the lowest recorded. The number of positive blood slides detected in the Government Laboratory at Durban dropped from a high of 4,605 in 1933 to 135 in 1940, the number of cases in the African reserves fell from 31,270 in 1934 to 428 in 1940, and the number of deaths from 1,000 to 13 in the same period. The amount of quinine issued fell from 3,000,000 tablets in 1932 to 300,000 in 1940 – a 90% drop. Malaria in the Province was controlled by 40 local authorities, 20 statutory Malaria Committees, four voluntary groups and the South African Railways, as well as the Department of Public Health. Thousands of gallons of anti-malaria oil and insecticide were used, and over 600 acres of gum trees (Eucalyptus saligna) had been planted to dry out swampy areas which proved very effective in removing prolific vector breeding sites.[44] In the Transvaal also the incidence came down from the terrible levels of the previous year, with only a few cases occurring on the Witwatersrand which appeared to have been brought in by motor car. People were advised to spray their cars when returning from malarious areas as mosquitoes were found to hide behind the dashboard and under the bonnet. However in 1944 a further severe epidemic broke out in the same region as that affected in 1939, in the Olifants river valley.

The early work on the insecticide DDT was done during the war by the British and American Military, and remained classified during that period. It was found to be a stable, soluble compound which was insecticidal by contact. It was used by the British Army against lice in the form of impregnated clothing, for dusting of the clothing of labourers in the Middle East, against mosquitoes in the Middle East and Italy, by aeroplane spraying against mosquitoes in Burma and the Far East, and against mosquitoes, flies, sandflies, fleas, cockroaches and bugs in the form of residual spraying on walls and ceilings. It had been found to be quite safe and considered the most generally effective insecticide for dealing with insects of medical importance that had ever been produced. It was described as one of the few momentous medical discoveries of the Second World War, and the greatest single weapon yet developed in the fight against insect carriers of disease. In respect of malaria it was used against both larvae and adults. With larvae it was applied as a 5% spray in oil on water, while for adults a spray was used both as a knock-down spray and as a residual spray, which was round to be remarkably effective. It dramatically transformed the war effort in the Pacific by rendering formerly untenable areas safe for the Allied fighting troops. A 5% kerosene solution was sprayed, sufficient to apply 100mg per square foot, onto walls, ceilings, etc and was similarly effective against flies, bugs and fleas.

By 1945 trials were underway in South Africa for a variety of uses, including the removal of the Aedes mosquitoes which could carry both yellow fever and dengue. While it was not yet available for use it was predicted to be an effective agent in the control of malaria, typhus, plague, relapsing fever and fly-borne disease.[45] Aerial spray by aeroplanes was also being investigated and tried in Zululand on the waters of the Umfolozi River. Further trials were undertaken in 1946 in Zululand spraying a 5% solution on the inside of the traditional beehive-shaped thatched hut. As the entrance doors were only up to 2ft by 4ft (just over one metre) in size, the carrier and his spray knapsack had difficulty entering – he had to enter on all-fours, and bring a length of hose inside. DDT was found to be highly effective (99.2%) in eradicating adult mosquitoes, even 14 weeks later - far more so than the previous spraying with pyrethrum, and at a lower cost. It also reduced the flies and cockroaches.[46] Some people had started to buy their own DDT privately, often using it incorrectly. But while DDT was highly effective it was also known to be toxic, although the kerosene it was diluted in was more toxic and the early cases of accidental poisoning were rather due to the ingestion of kerosene than DDT.

Also in 1945 the drug Paludrine was discovered, which found to be useful as a preventive drug, which was used along with Atebrin during the second world war as prophylactic for troops in the 2nd World War, and in 1946 the first results were published on trials of a new antimalarial drug, chloroquine, known initially as SN 7618, which was found to be both effective and well tolerated. In that year some 1,600,000 tablets of quinine had to be issued in the Transvaal alone.

In 1949 some 92,476 huts were sprayed were sprayed with DDT in Natal and Zululand, which gave a considerable cost reduction over the methods previously employed. Some areas were so remote and inaccessible that the DDT had to be carried in on pack donkeys, but as the hut spraying remained effective in killing mosquitoes for up to three months the process was much more efficient and many more huts could be covered. This, along with the drainage of areas where heavy mosquito breeding occurred through the planting of eucalyptus trees and a range of other measures, considerably reduced the incidence of malaria in the Province.[47] The spraying of DDT on the railways also had dramatic effects when it was applied to the rolling stock and living quarters of their staff such that only eight A. gambiae mosquitoes were found in over 13,000 huts checked in the Eastern Transvaal in 1947.

By the mid 1950's the use of DDT in pest control was seen globally as a dramatic success, with its use reducing cases of malaria in Italy from 500,000 in 1945 to 400 just six years later. Within ten years the number of cases in Ceylon (Sri Lanka) had fallen from around three million cases to 7,300. However resistance was starting to appear, which spread to other insecticides. This partial failure of control with insecticides revived interest in the older public health measures such as draining stagnant water and eliminating breeding places. It also stimulated research into biological methods of control, such as the use of naturally occurring enemies of the mosquitoes, and larvae-eating fish. Awareness was also increasing of the toxicity of insecticides with greater caution urged in their use, such as protective clothing and respirators. Poisoning from insecticides was declared notifiable in South Africa from 1951.[48]

It was calculated by the World Health Organisation that, if transmission could be interrupted for a period of three years, there would no longer remain a source of infection in the population for anopheline mosquitoes to feed on and malaria could be eradicated. This then called for intensified action by national governments so that it could be achieved as quickly as possible before resistance appeared in the mosquitoes. The impact on South Africa of bringing malaria under control was dramatic. The Minister of Health broadcast a statement in 1952 that, with the almost complete disappearance of malaria in the northern Transvaal, the town of Groblersdal had grown from only a handful to over 300 families. In Pongola there was a chance that within five years the area would be producing 20% of the country's sugar, and in the area around the Limpopo 15,000 to 20,000 acres were now producing tobacco and groundnuts. In Letaba the irrigated land had grown from 700 acres in 1940 to 12,000 acres in 1952.[49] This wasn't to say that epidemics no longer occurred – in 1953 1,610 cases were notified following particularly favourable weather conditions – but they were rapidly brought under control by tried and tested routines using DDT spraying and larvicides, and deaths were much rarer due to the greatly improved medical treatment. Even in areas which were no longer malarious, such as Cape Town, DDT was added to larvicidal oil and applied to standing water to prevent mosquito breeding for the nuisance value of the insects.

The World Health Assembly adopted the Global Malaria Eradication Campaign in May 1955 focussing largely on vector control with rapid and intensive DDT spraying programmes before resistance, which had appeared in Greece, the Middle East and northern Nigeria, became a problem. The control of the disease made such progress that by 1958 malaria was considered eradicated from large parts of the Transvaal and well over 80% of the population at risk in the Northern Transvaal, who had been at risk of malaria just 10 years previously, were protected and free of risk. Concern about resistance to both insecticides and anti-malarial drugs was growing however, and control measures had to intensify, with the objective being to totally eradicate the disease before resistance became a problem. Resistance was already appearing to the drug daraprim (pyrimethamine), but fortunately had not yet been seen to DDT.

One of the problems for South Africa in achieving total eradication was the fact that it bordered onto four other countries – Botswana, Zimbabwe (then Rhodesia), Mozambique and Swaziland – where malaria was still endemic. This was a particularly difficult problem in view of the large amounts of migrant labour that passed through the Transvaal on the way to work in both farms and the gold mines and reported cases remained clustered close to the borders, particularly adjacent to Swaziland and the then Rhodesia. The Kruger Park game reserve formed a kind of buffer between South Africa and Mozambique in that there was not much human traffic across it, although it was also a risk zone in that not much vector control could take place there. The Anopheles gambiae mosquitoes and their larvae were still found mainly along the Limpopo and rivers draining into it, including the Oliphants,

Sabie, Crocodile and Komati rivers, and intensive anti-larval work was undertaken there, although 'the only drawback with Native labour is their fear of snakes, crocodiles, hippopotami and buffalo near the larger rivers' and protection and compensation was required.[50] The handling of DDT posed risks to workers in particular from absorption from the skin, which was greater than that of inhalation, and protective clothing was required. Acute DDT poisoning could lead to convulsions and death from respiratory or heart failure, although actually in many cases it was the solvent used in the solution that was responsible for the poisoning. However chronic low level exposure to the insecticide was thought quite safe - experiments were cited of giving oral doses up to 200 times the daily rate of normal exposure to volunteers over an 18 month period which did not produce any symptoms or signs of illness.[51]

The disease was declared notifiable in 1956. By the 1960's total notifications were hovering around the 200-300 level. These cases mostly occurred in the north and east of the Transvaal and Northern Natal, although an outbreak did occur in the Northern Cape in 1961. In that year a National Malaria Organising Committee was appointed to coordinate all anti-malaria activities in the country. Survey and prevention activities were still intense with regular house spraying and routine blood smears to detect and treat carriers – some 113,000 being tested in 1964.[52] By 1965 only relatively small malarious areas remained, at low altitudes along the north-eastern coastal strip. It was considered possible that eradication could be achieved, but for the continuous flow of migrants moving between South African mines and surrounding countries. This was at a time when most African states had gained independence from their colonial masters and were hardening attitudes to the increasingly hard-line and racist South African government. As Mansell Prothero observed:

> From the point of view of malaria eradication any reduction in labour migration will be desirable. But if large scale schemes for eradication are to be planned in East and South-central Africa inter-territorial cooperation will be as necessary for achieving success here as elsewhere on the continent; this may be difficult to obtain if relations continue to deteriorate between independent African states and those which remain controlled by European minorities.[53]

Around 230,000 African huts in South Africa were being sprayed annually. While ever present in the background the systems in place were proving so effective that the numbers of cases were down to a few hundred, although occasionally there were outbreaks with 1,790 cases in the Northern Transvaal in 1972. One of the problems of the success of the malaria control programme was that people there were no longer exposed hence did not acquire immunity, and non-immune people were at greater risk from the disease should it re-emerge. Following this outbreak the control programme was further enhanced with additional, better trained field teams, large scale active surveillance and the upgrading of hospitals, clinics and laboratories. Increased surveillance and improved detection meant that more cases were notified following these measures. The number of cases again rose sharply in 1978 to 7,103. Following this numbers of notified cases hovered at just over 2,000 cases per year until the late 1980's. During this period it was noted that the White population appeared to have been at greater risk than the African. However from 1983 Africans were at greater risk, which in 1987 stood at about three times the risk of Whites in the non-endemic areas and four and a half times the risk in the endemic areas, the peak being in the 15-19 year age group.

Although the comprehensive control programmes were being implemented on a routine basis, in 1984 there was a four-fold increase in the number of notified cases of malaria, which coincided with the arrival of a tropical cyclone. The research centre at Tzaneen reported that there had been a 'mosquito explosion' mainly of the A. gambiae complex following good rains in the Eastern Transvaal in November and December 1983. Soon after cases began increasing and presumptive treatment with chloroquine was given to those judged to be at greatest risk. Some 20,000 people were involved, mainly along the Mkomati and Mlomati rivers. Then, on 28 January cyclone Demoina struck the eastern side of South Africa, which brought further rain to the Eastern Transvaal along with torrential rains in northern Natal. While the Transvaal rains were not as severe as Natal, the Mkomati and Mlomati Rivers came down in flood in the Transvaal and created large areas ideal for mosquito breeding. In northern Natal the areas of Ingwavuma, Ubombo, Hlabisa and southwards to the Tugela River were badly affected by the cyclone and an increase in cases of malaria prompted by increased mosquito breeding lead to the start of presumptive treatment regimes on a large scale. In the week of 12 March almost the entire population of Ingwavuma were given treatment. The cyclone also damaged roads and infrastructure, disrupting the routine anti-malaria programmes.[54]

In 1985 numbers of notified cases continued to rise sharply with 11,358 cases reported in that year. The disease maintained a seasonal pattern with the peak time of year being February to May. There were variations however between regions with the homelands of KaNgwane and Gazankulu in the Eastern Transvaal having an earlier start to their malaria seasons, commencing from October each year.[55] Cases numbered 9,081 in 1987, 8,651 in 1988 and 5,798 in 1989, although the case-fatality rate was low at less than 1% due to many of the cases being detected due to active case finding rather than people reporting ill. The areas of highest prevalence were still the Transvaal and its internal homelands and northern KwaZulu-Natal. In the Transvaal the highest rate was in the Barberton district where intense irrigation was practiced and a considerable proportion of farm workers migrated in from Mozambique. It was estimated that some 20% were infected with malaria on arrival in contrast with local inhabitants where surveys had shown a prevalence of between 0.3 – 0.7%. Other cases arose from the numerous game reserves in the Eastern Transvaal. Northern Natal also had large irrigation schemes established in the Makhatini Flats area which had increased potential breeding sites. In addition 1987 in particular had suffered particularly heavy rainfall and severe flooding had affected parts of Natal, with heavy rains falling in the malaria areas of Ingwavuma and Ubombo in the far north of the Province. This combination of factors was leading to increasing levels of malaria and complicating control.

It was noted that, amongst the African population, rates were similar among both males and females, thought to be due to the fact that both men and women were equally active outdoors – men working in the fields, and women also fetching water and washing by the rivers. Among the White population however, men were affected far more than women, probably due to White women being less active outdoors. The border with Mozambique continued to pose challenges in respect of malaria control and some 40% of cases were imported.[56] Case fatality rates were low at around 0.86% in the Transvaal and Venda for 1990. This was higher, at 2.26%, if the actively detected cases were excluded and was thought to be mostly due to delay in seeking and receiving treatment. 93% of deaths were in Africans.[57] A further challenge was a growing resistance since 1982 to the preferred treatment chloroquine, and sulfadoxine-pyrimethamine was being recommended instead in Natal and KwaZulu. In addition changes in the mosquito vector were also being noted. After decades of systematic residual insecticide spraying in the endemic areas Anopheles gambiae had been almost eradicated, but its place was being taken by Anopheles arabiensis as the main vector which bit both indoors and outdoors. Epidemics of malaria were preceded by sudden, explosive increases in the A. arabiensis vector population despite the on-going spraying and larvicidal activity. It had also been noted that cessation of spraying lead to re-emergence of the vector within four years of spraying having stopped, and numbers of mosquitoes, including A. gambiae, growing quickly to their previous levels.

By this time around one million structures were being sprayed annually in endemic areas and 400,000 blood slides were being examined. These revealed that over 98% of South African malaria infections were due to Plasmodium falciparum, P. vivax, P. ovale and P. malariae being rarely seen.[58] The endemic areas remained in the northern and eastern Transvaal (including its Homelands) and northern KwaZulu. Occasionally a few cases also occurred in the northern Cape in the Upington-Kakamas districts and in the vicinity of the Kuruman and Molopo rivers, with a handful of cases notified each year, although many of these were infected outside the region and were simply notified there. Still there was a malaria control programme in place, and in 1988 the mosquito vector Anopheles gambiae was first sighted in the Kalahari Gemsbok National Park in the northern area bordering Botswana and Namibia. A small outbreak of 37 cases ensued shortly after a period of exceptionally heavy rainfall, which led to massive flooding in what was usually an arid part of the country.[59] The extensive flooding led to standing pools of water and increased mosquito breeding. It was a reminder of how susceptible people remained to an increase in malaria brought about by sudden changes in environmental conditions.

From 1994 the relaxation of border controls with the new political dispensation resulted in increasing numbers of migrants crossing from Mozambique, still a malarious country, into South Africa. Asymptomatic carriers of the disease brought drug-resistant strains into KwaZulu-Natal in particular, and by 2000 it was estimated that 56% were resistant to the preferred drug, sulfadoxine-pyrimethamine. However the new political dispensation in South Africa meant that international co-operation on malaria between it and Mozambique became easier and more productive.

From the early 1960's concerns had been started to be raised by environmentalists about the effect of DDT on the environment, precipitated in 1962 by Rachel Carson's book *'Silent Spring'*. Following much debate and controversy DDT was banned by the United States Environmental Protection Agency in 1972, and by many other countries soon after. South African banned its use for agricultural purposes in 1974, but retained its use for malaria control. Internationally support moved towards programmes which avoided pesticide spraying, rather focusing on such interventions as the distribution of impregnated bed nets. While the banning of DDT and other insecticides was comparatively simple for developed northern nations without malaria and other insect-borne diseases, it was noted by developing countries that these countries had benefited extensively from them in their development, and their prohibition would significantly inhibit poorer nations from achieving the same. It was also noted that the scientific evidence for harmful environmental health effects of DDT was equivocal at best, and considered by many to be unsubstantiated and unscientific, while the life-saving impacts through malaria control were demonstrably enormous. It was estimated by the World Health Organisation to have saved some 25 million lives during the period of its use. In addition the indoor house-spraying programmes used in malaria control had been shown to have very little dissemination of DDT into the wider environment. Still the global campaign by international environmental groups gained momentum.[60]

Bowing to international pressure, amongst other largely environmental reasons, and also due to complaints from communities that bed bugs were becoming resistant, South Africa Malaria Advisory Group took a decision in 1995 to phase out the use of DDT in its malaria control programme. It was phased out of KwaZulu-Natal and Mpumulanga in 1996, and out of the Northern Province in 1999. Synthetic pyrethroids such as deltamethrin and cyfluthrin were used in place of the DDT, which were initially effective and more tolerated by the population – being less irritant to other nuisance insects such as bed bugs and being less visible and unsightly when sprayed onto house walls. However the cost of the newer insecticides was far greater than DDT and more complicated to administer, with cyfluthrin costing some four times that of DDT per structure sprayed. In addition there was increased resistance by the mosquitoes to the new insecticides, and by the late 1990's A. funestus, which had disappeared from South Africa some 25 years earlier, started to reappear. More disturbing still was that within three years the cases of malaria had risen astronomically, and deaths had risen from 32 in 1996 to 214 in 1999. The return of A. funestus had contributed to an increase in incidence in northern KwaZulu Natal from 9.5% to 40%. Cases increased from 8,693 in 1996, which would have been mostly from active case finding, to 27,238 in 1999 with many pouring into local hospitals seriously ill from the disease.

It was clear that A. funestus was resistant to the synthetic pyrethroid insecticides which had been used to spray houses instead of the tried and tested DDT. In addition parasite resistance had appeared to the first line drug treatment, sulphadoxine/pyrimethamine, used in KwaZulu-Natal. The outbreak culminated in a massive outbreak in the summer months at the end of that year, with a total of 61,935 infections being reported nationally for the year 2000, which prompted the Department of Health in March 2000 to take the decision to revert to using DDT for malaria control.[61] Although this decision was taken in face of continuing international opposition to the use of DDT, it was confirmed by the Southern Africa Development Community (SADC) Health Ministers in May 2000 who agreed to its continued use. The impact on the epidemic was dramatic and the disease was once again brought back under control, with the case load dropping 75% from the previous year. In neighbouring Mozambique, where they still did not use DDT, there were over 67,000 deaths from malaria in 2001, and 13,672 in Zimbabwe.

The SADC meeting followed Malaria Consultation Meetings attended by Ministers of Health from Botswana, Mozambique, Swaziland, South Africa and Zimbabwe, which had started in response to the increased risk of malaria epidemics in the flood-affected areas after Cyclone Elaine. One of the outcomes was the endorsement of a regional framework for malaria control, and a Task Force was established to draw up an effective SADC malaria control plan. This was adopted in April 2001 and included policies on house spraying as a major strategy, surveillance, epidemic preparedness, case management, procurement of insecticides and drugs, research, community mobilisation and capacity building. In addition the WHO has had the Southern African Malarial Control Programme in place since 1997, and the Lubombo Spatial Development Initiative: Malaria Control Programme (LSDI) has been in place since October 1999, covering Eastern Swaziland, southern Mozambique and north-eastern KwaZulu-Natal.[62]

These regional initiatives reflected the changed political dispensation in South Africa in particular, which recognised the regional nature of the malaria problem and resolved to work with neighbouring countries with which there had existed poor relations pre-1994. Since the initiatives began, by 2007 they had markedly reduced the numbers of cases of malaria in areas of South Africa – KwaZulu-Natal and Mpumulanga – bordering Mozambique. From the 1999/2000 season, when the cases in KwaZulu Natal were 41,077 and in Mpumulanga 13,856, to the 2006/2007 season the caseload fell by 99% and 84% respectively. The decrease was attributed to the LSDI, the re-introduction of DDT spraying, and the change of first-line treatment to the drug co-artemether following increasing resistance to Sulphadoxine-pyrimethamine. In addition to these two Provinces malaria was still reported from Gauteng and occasionally the Orange Free State, where the cases were all in people who had travelled to malarious areas. There remains also still significant malaria in the Limpopo Province with the highest number of cases, both imported and through endogenous spread, with 2,898 cases in 2007 and 34 deaths. Overall the case-fatality rate for malaria in 2007 was only 0.9% of a total national caseload of 6,615, and the national target is reduction to 0.5%.[63]

Malaria remains a risk in these low-lying areas of South Africa bordering other Southern African countries, and is likely to remain so for the foreseeable future. The peak districts are the Vhembe district of Limpopo bordering Zimbabwe and the uMkhanyakude district of KwaZulu-Natal, bordering Mozambique. The other challenges posed by the borders are that those crossing in from outside are often silent carriers who do not visit health facilities and are fearful of detection and deportation. In addition the continuous movements of population across the porous boundaries can bring in drug-resistant strains of the disease. The age group most at risk is the 20-24 year group, males more than females, although 37% of the 2007 cases were in children under 18 years and 9% in children under five years. The incidence of malaria peaks in the hot, rainy, summer months of January, February and March, and preventive measures are still required by those travelling to these north-eastern areas in summer. However the control programme remains active and intense and, with inter-country collaboration through the Southern African Malaria Control Commission, is proving effective. South Africa is a key participant on many expert regional and multi-national committees due to the experience and expertise gained over the last two centuries. The lessons learnt from the changes introduced in the late 1990s were a sharp reminder that a change or reduction in effort could once again lead, within a very short space of time, to devastating outbreaks.

ENDNOTES

1. Mentzel O.F. *A Geographical and Topographical description of the Cape of Good Hope; 1787;* Translated by Marais G.V. and Hoge J. Edited by Mandelbrote H.J. The Van Riebeeck Society, Cape Town, 1944.
2. Cluver E.H. *Public Health in South Africa*; Central News Agency Limited, Fifth Edition (undated):163
3. Phillips H. 'Cape Town in 1829' *Contree,* 8, July 1980:5.
4. Leipoldt Louis C. *Bushveld Doctor*, Jonathan Cape Ltd, London, 193: 95
5. Searle C. *The history of the development of nursing in South Africa 1652-1960*; The South African Nursing Association; 1980:79

6   Booker C.G and Annecke S. 'The General Practitioner in the Prevention of Malaria' *South African Medical Journal* 7 (3) 1933:80
7   Searle C. *The history of the development of nursing in South Africa 1652-1960*; The South African Nursing Association; 1980:82
8   Laidler P.W. 'Medical Establishments and Institutions at the Cape: Through Epidemics to reform' South African Medical Journal 13(7) 1939:223-229
9   Matthews J.W. *Incwadi Yami or Twenty Years Personal Experience in South Africa; 1887*; Africana Book Society, Johannesburg 1976:16
10 Devitt Napier, *The Concentration Camps in South Africa during the Anglo-Boer War of 1899 – 1902*; Shuter and Shooter, Pietermaritzburg 1941:31-33
11 'The Report of the Ladies Commission' cited in Martin A.C. *The Concentration Camps 1900-1902: Facts, Figures and Fables*; Howard Timmins Cape Town 1957:16
12 Collins V.E. *Report of the Resident Surgeon Somerset Hospital, in reports on the Government and Aided Hospitals and Asylums, 1900*, WA Richards, Cape Town, 1901, G41-'1901 p 3
13 Dunley Owen A. 'Notes on Malaria', *South African Medical Record* 16(9) 1918:136-8
14 Hill E. And Haydon L.G. 'The epidemic of malaria fever in Natal' Journal of Hygiene, 5, 1905:467-484.
15 Le Sueur D. Sharp B.L. Appleton C. 'Historical Perspective of the malaria problem in Natal with emphasis on the period 1928-1932', *South African Journal of Science*, 89, May 1993:232-239
16 Wheelwright C.A. 'Report of the Native Commissioner, Northern Division, Zoutpansberg Province', in: Lagden G.Y. *Report by the Commissioner for Native Affairs, Transvaal, for the year ended 30th June 1906*, Government Printing and Stationery office, Pretoria,1906 pB45.
17 Spencer H.A.cited in Lagden GY, *Report by the Commissioner for Native Affairs, Transvaal, for the year ended 30th June 1906*, Pretoria, Government Printing and Stationery office, 1906 pA14-15.
18 Harries L.C.R. 'Report of the Sub-Native Commissioner, Sekukuniland' in Lagden G.Y. *Report by the Commissioner for Native Affairs, Transvaal, for the year ended 30th June 1906*, Pretoria, Government Printing and Stationery office, 1906 pB59.
19 Spencer H.A. 'Malaria as it Occurs upon the Middelveld of the Transvaal' *South African Medical Record* 20(18) 1922:342-249.
20 Park Ross G.A. 'Control of malaria in the Union', *South African Medical Record* 20(23) 1922:450-459.
21 Spencer H.A. 'Malaria on the Lowveld', *South African Medical Record* 21(1) 1923:3-7
22 Spencer H.A. 'The Treatment and Prevention of Malaria' *South African Medical Record* 21(4) 1923:84-87
23 Watson M. in: *Annual Report of the Department of Public Health, Union of South Africa, 1930*, Government Printer Pretoria, UG 40-'30, p66-73
24 *Annual Report of the Department of Public Health, Union of South Africa, 1930*, Government Printer Pretoria, UG 40-'30, p37
25 Le Sueur D. Sharp B.L. Appleton C. 'Historical Perspective of the malaria problem in Natal with emphasis on the period 1928-1932', *South African Journal of Science*, 89 May 1993:232-239
26 Truter P. 'Malaria, an increasing threat' Letter to the Editor; *South African Medical Journal*, 73, 16 April 1988:501.
27 Cluver F.W.P. 'Malaria Control in Natal and Zululand' *South African Medical Journal* 14(6) 1940:113-17

28 Anning C.C.P. 'Meteorological factors in the incidence of malaria in Pietermaritzburg' *South African Medical Journal* 8(23) 1934:875-878
29 *Annual Report of the Department of Public Health, Union of South Africa, 1933*, Government Printer Pretoria, UG 30-'33, p27
30 Booker C.G. and Annecke S. 'The General Practitioner in the Prevention of Malaria' *South African Medical Journal* 17 (3) 1933:79
31 'The Treatment of Malaria, Report of the Malaria Commission of the League of Nations', *South African Medical Journal* 7(16) 1933:540-544
32 Leipoldt Louis C. *Bushveld Doctor*, Jonathan Cape, London, 1937:93
33 Ibid, 98
34 Annecke S. 'Malaria Control in The Transvaal' *South African Medical Journal* 9(1) 1935:3-7
35 *Annual Report of the Department of Public Health, Union of South Africa, 1933*, The Government Printer Pretoria, UG 30-'33, 29
36 De Meillon B. 'Distribution of A Gambiae and A Funestus, Report of the Malaria Research Station of the South Afrian Institute for Medical Research', in: *Annual Report of the Department of Public Health, Union of South Africa, 1933*, Government Printer Pretoria, UG 30-'33, p61-64.
37 *Annual Report of the Department of Public Health, Union of South Africa, 1935*, The Government Printer Pretoria, UG 43-'35, p29-31
38 *Annual Report of the Department of Public Health, Union of South Africa, 1933*, The Government Printer Pretoria, UG 30-'33, p31
39 Cluver F.W.P. 'Malaria Control in Natal and Zululand' *South African Medical Journal* 14(6) 1940:113-117
40 Clarkson C.F. Minister of Posts and Telegraphs, *Debates of the Senate of South Africa*, 23 March 1939:251
41 De Meillon B. and Gear J. 'Malaria contracted on the Witwatersrand' *South African Medical Journal* 13(9) 1939:309-312
42 *Annual Report of the Department of Public Health, Union of South Africa, 1939*, Government Printer Pretoria, UG 52-'39, p 41
43 Ibid, 46
44 *Annual Report of the Department of Public Health, Union of South Africa, 1941*, Government Printer Pretoria, UG 46-'41, p 25
45 Gear H.S. 'A Note on the Use of DDT in Medical and Health Problems', *South African Medical Journal* 19(16) 1945:290-292
46 Cluver F.W.P., 'Report on Malaria Control in rural Native Areas by using DDT insecticide', *South African Medical Journal* 20(13) 1946:368-370
47 Cluver F.W.P. 'Modern methods of malaria control' *South African Medical Journal* 24(18) 1950:327-328
48 'Editorial: Acquired resistance to insecticides', *South African Medical Journal* 28(19) 1954:390
49 *Annual Report of the Department of Health, Union of South Africa, 1952*, Government Printer Pretoria, UG 40-'1954, p8
50 Brink C.J.H. 'Malaria Control in the Northern Transvaal', *South African Medical Journal* 32(32) 9 August 1958:805
51 Sapieka N. ' Modern insecticides: their toxicity and control', *South African Medical Journal* 33(50) 12 December 1959:163-'166
52 *Annual Report of the Department of Health for the Five Years ended 31st December 1964*, Republic of South Africa, 1966, Government Printer Pretoria, RP11/1966, p8
53 Mansell Prothero R. *Migrants and Malaria*; Longmans Green and Co Ltd, London, 1965:97

54 Hansford F. and Theron D. 'Malaria Update' *Epidemiological Comments* 11(4) 4 April 1984:18
55 Küstner H.G.V. 'Malaria: Problems Old and New', *Epidemiological Comments*, 15(1) 1988:2-55
56 Hansford C.F. and Muller H. 'Malaria in South Africa 1987-1989', *Epidemiological Comments*, 17(12) October 1990:2-9.
57 Muller H. 'Deaths due to Malaria during 1990' *Epidemiological Comments*, 18(4) April 1991:86-90.
58 Küstner H.G.V. 'Malaria: Problems Old and New' *Epidemiological Comments*, 15(1), 1988:p2-55
59 Küstner H.G.V. 'Malaria in the Northern Cape' *Epidemiological Comments* 15(5) 1988:19-25
60 Tren R. and Bate R. 'Malaria and the DDT story' *Institute for Economic Affairs*, London, 2001:45-54
61 Ibid, 68-72
62 Balfour T. 'TB and Malaria in SADC countries' in: *South African Health Review 2002*, Health Systems Trust ,Durban, 2002:315-320.
63 Makubalo L.E. et al, *Annual Report 2007: Prevalence and Distribution of Malaria in South Africa,* Report by the National Department of Health, Directorate of Epidemiology and Surveillance, Pretoria, March 2008

MEASLES: A HARROWING TOLL

The name measles may have been derived from the term 'mezils' which was used first by John of Gaddesden in England, 1280-1361, who applied it to both measles and certain leprosy lesions. Measles and smallpox were often mixed in both Arabic writings and in Tudor times, with measles being thought to be a milder form of smallpox. The distinction was only really accepted in the 1600's when measles appears as a separate item in Parish returns in London. The epidemic in England of 1670 was when the features were first described clearly by T. Sydenham.[1] Measles is mentioned as far back as the 18th century as being present on ships arriving in South Africa. As with most other infectious diseases it appears to have been introduced through ships arriving at the Cape, the authorities in St Helena declaring on 9th March 1807 that ships leaving the Cape had introduced it to the island, and produced a devastating outbreak. However there is no record of a severe outbreak in Cape Town until June of that year, where the outbreak was also described as giving rise to horrible devastation.[2] Following this the Supreme Medical Committee of the Cape instituted an enquiry into the 'present state of the Medical Art' where, amongst other problems, the Committee found ignorance of the medical practitioners and a prevailing custom of preparing medicines themselves, to the 'manifest injury of the patient'.[3] Burchell refers to measles having spread inland to Klaarwater in 1809, which was thought to be the first time it had spread so far into the interior of the country.[4] The first medical society in the country was later established in the Cape in 1827, known as the South African Medical Society, following which a marked improvement in the standard of medicine and surgery was noted.[5]

Several ships bringing the 1820 settlers also carried measles, and were forbidden to land in Simon's Town on their way to Algoa Bay.[6] The first mention of a serious threat was from the ships Balcaras and the William Fairlie, in March 1822. Troops were sent to Robben Island to be quarantined for up to 40 days.[7] The next severe epidemic to be mentioned is that of February 1839 which also started in the Cape, and was thought to have come from Mauritius. Many of Cape Town's residents refused to be moved to the temporary hospital, which was established at the former Slave Lodge, as it was originally in a mild form, although it was believed the overcrowded housing conditions were aggravating the disease. By March it was still spreading and becoming more virulent, with several deaths occurring in children under eight years. It moved rapidly across the country through to the frontier settlers and communities, spreading from the European communities to the Coloured and African communities. By 22nd April there had been 9,467 cases with 123 deaths, and by May it was thought that 15,000 out of 25,000 had been affected.[8] By the middle of 1839 the epidemic had spread throughout the Eastern Cape and affected most of the 1820 settler families.[9] From there it moved through the Afrikaaner communities on the Great Trek where, in a laager of 1,000 wagons, hundreds of people lost their lives.[10] It reached as far as the newly established settlement of Andries Pretorius at Pieter Mauritsburg (Pietermaritzburg) in Natal where it also had a disastrous impact.

In London in 1849, the first year after the first Public Health Act, measles was the sixth leading epidemic cause of death with 1,154 deaths out of 26,243 recorded. It was massively overshadowed by cholera in that year with 14,215 deaths, and significantly behind diarrhoea, typhus, whooping cough and scarlatina. However its incidence and mortality were noted to have increased over the previous decade, alongside the increasing urbanisation and urban poverty. Epidemics came in waves across the country during the 19th century, every two or three years, growing in severity up to the end of the century and the early twentieth century. There was significant evidence that mortality from the disease was related to social class and economic conditions. Studies showed that mortality in families confined to living in one room was six times greater (9%) than in those wealthy enough to afford four rooms or more (1.5%). Measles was also found to affect particularly badly those living in institutions, and numerous studies had shown the rapid spread that occurred through schools.[11] Significant epidemics also took place in South America in 1865, in North America during the American Civil War, and in Paris in 1871. When the disease was introduced into populations who had no previous exposure its attack rate was up to 99%, and mortality was devastating. When it attacked the Pacific island of Fiji in 1875 it wiped out 25% of the population.[12]

Measles was also brought out to Natal not just from Europe and the Cape, but on the ships bringing migrant Indian indentured labourers to the Colony. Passengers on the ship Malabar were ravaged by a particularly severe form of measles which resulted in a number of deaths.[13] Measles was said to be prevalent in the Transkei in the 1880's, in particular 1882, when it was said to be proving very fatal to children. Six to eight deaths per day were reported from some districts.[14] Passing reference is made to measles by District Surgeons in Natal in the 1890's, but it seems generally to have been described as a lesser infection, not associated with fatal epidemics and not featuring as a significant cause of admission to hospital. That may have been because of a practice of treating sufferers at home in order to prevent the spread to other hospital patients which may also have been why numbers reported were quite low.

However, during the Anglo-Boer War of 1899–1902, measles arose with devastating impact, particularly in the camps which the British had established to accommodate thousands of women and children removed or fleeing from the farms. The camps commenced from July 1900 when the first one was established at Mafeking to accommodate refugees from the western areas. From then throughout 1900 and 1901 further camps were established across the country - from Port Elizabeth up to Pietersburg, as far east as Pietermaritzburg and west through to Klerksdorp. During the 1901 winter the camps started to grow faster than the authorities could cope with them, with women and children arriving by the thousand before the tents and supplies were ready. Many of those arriving were in poor condition with Dr Van der Waal commenting

> These people came into camp ladened with disease ... they brought in whooping cough and diphtheria, diseases of which the camp was clear when they came in. They also brought a malignant type of measles which was spread like wild-fire. This form of measles closely resembles typhus fever and is very deadly.[15]

By 24th July 1901 there were 82,408 people in 25 European camps and 23,489 Africans, rising to 38,547 by September with some 22,795 Coloureds. The death rates in the camps at this time were between 1,000 and 1,500 a month for Europeans, rising up to 2,411 in September 1901 – 2.2% of the inmates - and between 500 and 1,000 Coloured deaths. The highest monthly mortality was estimated to be in October 1901 at the Brandfort Camp where there were 345 deaths in a child population of 2,122.[16] However many of the inmates of Brandfort had been in terrible condition before they arrived with the Superintendent commenting:

> Most of them had been taken from a Boer laager in the District of Hoopstad and had been with the commando for several months. The

privations and hardships this had induced had told with great effect on the health of the women and children, many of whom were most scantily clad.[17]

Many arrivals at camps were reported to be half-starved and riddled with diseases, hence re-introducing infectious disease to the camps and preventing their eradication. Of these deaths in the second half of 1901 some 80% were due to measles which struck in the greatest epidemic seen in the country. The community had very little immunity hence when a particularly virulent strain of measles, often appearing as haemorrhagic or black measles, struck it killed thousands of infants. The complications of bronchitis and pneumonia were particularly fatal due to the cold winters, inadequate and overcrowded shelter in tents, change in diet and the shortage of medical and nursing care. It has also been noted that the last great epidemic of measles had been suffered by the Boers during the Great Trek of the 1830's which possibly had led them to a psychological fear of the disease.[18]

Other contributions to deaths were reported as being strange and dangerous home remedies applied by the Boer women to their children, including one woman who painted her sick children with green paint, following which they died of arsenical poisoning. Still these were minor in the context of the epidemic, and Emily Hobhouse calculated the total deaths in the camps as 20,177 while others reported it as high as 27,800. Following the attention drawn to the conditions in the camps by Emily Hobhouse in Britain in 1901, and with the end of the measles epidemic, conditions in the camps started to improve. In 1902 more camps were opened in East London and throughout Natal as far as Wentworth in Durban, but the mortality was lower than the terrible period of July to December 1901.[19]

During the aftermath of the war measles continued to be mentioned by Resident Magistrates and Medical Officers in the Reports of the Department of Native Affairs, and by District Surgeons across the country, with outbreaks being reported in rural towns such as Cradock in 1902, which killed 28, Adelaide in 1907 with 200 cases and six deaths, and townships such as New Brighton (outside Port Elizabeth) in 1910, but they do not usually seem to have been associated with very high mortality. In Bloemfontein it was reported as causing only five deaths out of 346 in the city that year, compared to 21 for whooping cough. There seems to have been a general air of fatalism about the disease, there being no vaccine or specific treatment, and measles is remarkably absent from South African medical literature in the early 1900's after the

Anglo-Boer War. Perhaps it was because there were so many more dangerous diseases to contend with at the time – typhoid and other hygiene-related diseases, smallpox, plague, syphilis and diphtheria were causing much more concern, perhaps also due to there being measures would could be taken regarding these infections.

Yet measles remained a prevalent disease and occasionally, such as in Cape Town in 1916-17 where there were 167 deaths, caused significant fatalities. Perhaps this was a more virulent strain as it coincided with a time of high prevalence in Britain and the movement of people associated with the First World War. Similar high mortality rates from measles had been noted in Australia related to their large troop movements, exacerbated by the long period spent travelling at sea – up to eight weeks. Australian troops returning from the Anglo-Boer War in 1902 had likewise suffered high losses from measles. On the returning troopship Drayton Grange there had been six deaths from measles and 154 hospitalised with the disease. In America also measles was closely linked to mobilisation for the war effort, with a high incidence from April 1917 to December 1918. What was noted was that it was essentially a disease of rural recruits coming for the first time into a densely crowded environment in the military Camps, and starting with the congestion in the trains bringing them in.[20] However, generally in Cape Town there were only a handful of deaths reported annually. In England around this time after the First World War the number of deaths from measles started to fall dramatically, and it was becoming a far less significant disease.

1,056 cases were reported in Europeans in Pretoria in the period from 1931-1934, and 14 deaths. In Non-Europeans there were 76 cases and 17 deaths, illustrating its more fatal character. In 1935 there was an epidemic in the city with 665 cases of which 43 were aged over 16 years. Pietermaritzburg reported an outbreak of 50 cases. This followed outbreaks internationally, such as that in 1934 in the United States with over 600,000 cases in the first six months. The use of convalescent serum was recommended to mitigate outbreaks in schools or elsewhere, for example to contacts in a hospital ward. It could also be given between four and six days from the onset of the rash to attenuate an attack.[21]

In Cape Town measles again was found to be more severe in Non-Europeans and the poorer classes, although the number of fatal cases during the 1920's and 30's was not great. While in 1924 there had been a total of 136 fatalities, that dropped significantly the next year and from 1925 until 1939 there were between 3 and 86 fatal cases per year. Some of these arrived by ship, particularly from Japan in 1936. In 1940 there were no reported fatalities at all. The mortality was said to be greatest during the first two years of life and very rare after the age of five. Convalescent serum was found to be of great value as a post-exposure prophylaxis, if injected within five days of exposure to infection, and which lasted for around 14 days. If the child was injected between the 6th and 9th days after exposure they suffered a modified attack of the disease which then conferred immunity, and it was used for healthy children over two years of age.[22]

The discovery of the sulphonamide series of antibiotic drugs was hailed as a great breakthrough in the treatment of various infections, following the publication of test results in 1935. While unable to specifically treat measles, in the late 1930's it was found to cause a reduction in ear and lung complications. It also was found generally to shorten the period of pyrexia by two days on average, and to reduce the time spent in hospital.[23] There was still a dearth of information and statistics around measles nationally however, although the Medical Officer of Health for Pietermaritzburg reported that outbreaks were common in schools and their boarding establishments. Yet during the Second World War, as with the First, measles increased, at least during the first few years. Measles peaked in both the British Royal Navy and the United States Army in 1941, coinciding with major measles years in the civilian population. However its importance had declined since the First World War, possibly due to improved general health and nutrition, along with specific prophylaxis and antibiotic treatment.[24]

There was no further mention of measles in the 1940s in any of the Annual Reports of the Department of Public Health, even in sections dealing with health services in poor rural areas and infant mortality. However the City of Cape Town Annual Reports of the Medical Officer of Health do report measles deaths from 1914 and show that, since the last epidemic in 1924, deaths averaged around 30 per year, mostly non-European. The 29 deaths in non-Europeans in 1950 were all in children under five.[25] An analysis of 557 deaths of Non-European children in the Coronation Hospital, Johannesburg that same year did not make reference to a single death from measles. The commonest causes of death were pneumonia and gastroenteritis, neither of which were linked to measles.[26] Similarly an analysis in Pretoria of causes of death of children aged under five years gave the commonest causes as neglect and malnutrition with pneumonia or enteritis. Again there is no mention of measles.[27] In the Annual Reports of the Native Commissioners for that period, even though infant mortality is reported as being high, still measles is not mentioned as a cause – the major causes being pneumonia and diarrhoea.

Measles in the 1950s was considered rarely fatal, except from the complications. In the United States 90% of deaths from measles were due to bacterial pneumonia. In Pietermaritzburg and other South African cities it was noted to affect African patients more severely. The introduction of antibiotics had helped in the treatment of these complications except for measles encephalitis, which fortunately occurred only rarely. In the Western world, and indeed in South Africa, the mortality had declined significantly, which commenced before the introduction of sulphonamides and antibiotics. Factors influencing the spread and severity of measles included the host's immunity and the physical, social and biological environment, and schools were noted to play a great role in the spread of the disease, spreading it between pupils and thence to their siblings at home. It was the pre-school children that suffered the most complications. There was little specific in the way of prevention or treatment - no satisfactory vaccine had been developed, and isolation and quarantine proven of little use. Perhaps because of this feeling of inevitability of measles there was little mention of it in South African medical literature.[28] In fact some advocated 'measles tea-parties' for children under five years, so that the disease would be contracted young, and in a household it was thought advantageous for all the children to have it together if possible. Measles infection was thought to give life-long immunity. Passive immunisation with gamma globulin could be used for protection up to five days after exposure, but if given up to the tenth day it could accentuate the disease.[29]

Spencer wrote of epidemics of measles being frequent in South Africa but that the mortality statistics failed to reflect morbidity and also frequently the mortality resulting from complications. His statistics from Johannesburg for the period 1957 to 1961 show between 17 and 56 deaths annually in the city, slightly above diphtheria, and he commented that although measles was a greater problem in the African than in the European, he thought it less of a hazard than in other African countries such as Nigeria or Upper Volta [Burkina Faso]. He estimated that by the age of five years most African children in Soweto had contracted measles.[30] In the City of Cape Town's Annual Report of 1957 it talks of an increase in measles with 30 deaths, followed by 20 in 1958 with 116 cases admitted to the city hospital, 52 of which came from outside the city. In 1960, after several years of increasing numbers of cases and 223 admissions that year, the Medical Officer of Health Professor Cooper sounded what seems to have been a lone voice of warning – bearing in mind that as measles was not a notifiable disease it was only the hospital admissions that were coming to their attention. He commented that these admissions were exacerbated through bad home environment, poor nutrition and lack of proper nursing and observed 'this is however an impression, contrary to what is at present occurring in the London County Council area, that measles is today more virulent than it was ten years ago and more children develop complications such as bronchopneumonia than was the case previously'. The conditions of the Non-Europeans in the city at that time were described for the Cape Coloured population thus: 'there is much under nourishment and housing accommodation is expensive and bad'. A majority were described as living in slum conditions. Of the Africans it was said that they were mostly slum dwellers or living in unsanitary shacks on the Cape Flats. Their social and economic conditions were even worse than those of the Coloured people.[31]

Cape Town again reported increasing problems with measles in 1961 with 282 cases admitted to the City Infectious Diseases Hospital and 34 deaths - the highest number of deaths recorded since 1944 – most of which were in children under two years. The Medical Superintendent remarked on the very serious condition of the cases admitted to hospital. The Medical Officer of Health commented that 'it is quite obvious that measles cannot be regarded as one of the minor ailments of childhood'.[32] The steady rise in measles cases continued to be remarked upon by the Medical Officer of Health of Cape Town, Professor Cooper. He commented again in 1963 on the increasing morbidity and mortality with 523 hospital admissions and 87 deaths, 85 of which were in children under five years. Practically all the cases were in Non-Europeans and associated with gross malnutrition. All those admitted were gravely ill and frequently required tracheotomies. Measles started to appear as a cause of infant mortality (deaths of children under 12 months) from around this time, at 2.1 per 1,000 live births. In 1965 again Professor Cooper reported that measles had become established in a bi-annual cycle with the average deaths in the last five years far exceeding any previous period. Special arrangements had had to be made at the City Hospital for Infectious Diseases to cope with the admission and treatment of the disease.

The disease remained non-notifiable however and remained absent from the National Department of Health's reports throughout the 1960's - yet in the homeland of Gazankulu in the Eastern Transvaal it was found that measles in conjunction with malnutrition accounted for 41% of child blindness between 1967 and 1972. In Port Elizabeth first mention was made of it in 1968 when the Medical Officer of Health, J N Sher, commented 'measles in the malnourished infant with concomitant pneumonia and gastro-enteritis continues to take its harrowing toll'. In that year there had been 62 deaths from measles, 50 of which were in Africans, and 184 admissions for complicated measles to the Elizabeth Donkin and Empilweni Hospitals in the area, but as a cause of children's death it was far behind gastro-enteritis and pneumonia.[33] However by 1975 it had increased in incidence and was second only to tuberculosis as a cause of admission to the Port Elizabeth infectious diseases hospital with 269 admissions, although it was still not a major cause of death. Coovadia noted that measles often pre-disposed children to tuberculosis, his impression being that, at least in Black children, a severe attack of measles not infrequently led to pulmonary tuberculosis.[34]

Measles vaccination was added to the national schedule of immunisations in mid-1975 and was offered as a free service with other routine childhood vaccinations, a first dose being given at nine months and a second at 15 months. Following this Cape Town noted a reduction in notifications from around 800 in 1974 down to around 200 in 1979. Between 1983 and 1985 the strain of vaccine used was the Schwarz vaccine and the age of first dose was reduced to six months, although in 1986 it was put back up to nine months as it was not as effective when given at the younger age.

The disease was still not made notifiable until 1980, which contributed to the dearth of statistical information before that time. In addition, during the 1970's most areas where Africans were forced to live – the homelands and townships – were removed from provincial health and local authority governance and reporting systems. The African Townships had been removed from White local authorities around 1970 and placed under separate Boards administered centrally, and the nominally independent 'Bantustans' had their own separate Departments of Health. This meant that there were few reports coming from the poorer areas worst affected by measles, and with the worst side-effects from the disease, as the health statistics were no longer included with either the City Medical Officer of Health Reports or the National Department of Health Reports. The Health Department Reports from these homelands were mostly comprised of administrative details – budgets, staffing complements etc - with little in the way of informative health statistics. Hence South Africa had achieved almost a complete reporting silence on the health events taking place in these impoverished African areas. In particular this included the growing deadly menace from measles – a disease which seems to have developed from being a relatively mild childhood infection to being an infectious disease causing significant morbidity and mortality amongst infants, perhaps due to increasing poverty and malnutrition in the rural areas in particular.

It appears to be only when the disease finally spilled over into the City of Port Elizabeth, in the Eastern Cape, that the White-led health departments were finally forced to take notice of the rising problem of measles. Port Elizabeth was hit by a major measles epidemic between December 1982 and July 1983 which claimed the lives of nearly 300 children and affected some 2,000, a case fatality rate of 15.3%. 88% of notifications and 91% of deaths were in Africans with most of the remainder being in Coloureds. The infection incidence per 100,000 people was 448 amongst Africans, with 250 deaths, compared with only 11.8 in the White population, with only one death. The vast majority of African cases and deaths were in children aged between seven months and two years of age. It led to the appointment of a special committee by the City to investigate conditions and it was noticed that the measles attack rate correlated with the areas with the lowest standard of hygiene, housing and sanitation. The African population lived in several low-cost housing areas and squatter areas where it was calculated that the average occupancy was around eight people per house and 10.8 people to a shack in the sprawling squatter area known as 'Little Soweto'. There was an estimated shortage of 17,000 housing units for the black population. In Little Soweto a survey found that over 42% of black pre-school children were malnourished, being below the 3rd percentile for weight, and the average household income was below the level estimated necessary for African subsistence. Appalling sanitary and sewerage conditions were found with overflowing pit latrines, and in addition there was only one inadequate clinic serving a population of somewhere between 100,000 and 170,000 people. The relationship between overcrowding, poverty, malnutrition and measles had already been established and the Port Elizabeth outbreak of 1982/83 confirmed that the conditions in South Africa's African townships were ripe for such epidemics, particularly where inadequate health services resulted in inadequate immunisation levels.[35]

The Port Elizabeth epidemic was reported at the Second Carnegie Enquiry into Poverty in South Africa, and was a wake-up call that the time had finally come to take measles in South Africa more seriously. In June 1984 the National Department of Health and Welfare published an analysis of the first four years of notifications which showed it to be predominantly a winter disease (April to October) with an incidence of around 60/100,000 population and a mortality rate of about 1.25/100,000. The highest rates were reported from the Eastern Cape, which in 1983 stood at 190/100,000 However absent from their figures were the large, impoverished 'independent' homelands of Transkei, Ciskei, Bophuthatswana and Venda which would certainly have resulted in an under-estimation of the severity of the disease in the country as a whole. Indeed the total number of cases notified from the 'white' Provinces was probably a massive undercount of the total cases occurring.[36]

In 1978 an international conference had been held on Primary Health Care at Alma Ata in the then Soviet Union, following which a Declaration was made on a world-wide goal of attaining Health for All by the Year 2000. Following this commitment the World Health Organisation (WHO) launched a programme on immunisation known as the Expanded Programme on Immunisation, or EPI. While measles was made notifiable in 1979, with effect from 1980, (19,193 cases were reported) this policy was still not adopted in South Africa until February 1989 when it was endorsed by its Health Policy Council and a 'Measles Strategy' was decided upon as part of the overall plan. By the late 1980's measles had become by far the commonest notifiable disease aside from tuberculosis, with a peak of 22,559 cases reported to the National Department of Health in 1987 and 18,268 cases in 1989. However these figures still excluded the so-called independent states of Transkei, Bophuthatswana, Venda and Ciskei which were the poorest parts of the country where the impact of disease would have been worse.

Annual peaks occurred around September of every year. The incidence rate was recorded as 32 per 100,000, with the highest rate being in the desperately poor and barren homeland of Lebowa in the north, (not a fully 'Independent State') at 94, although other African homelands such as KwaZulu were also badly affected. Amongst the poor, measles had come to be considered the most serious and severe disease encountered by children, frequently complicated by pneumonia, gastroenteritis, encephalitis and blindness, with a case fatality rate in African children of 1.8%. Prior to the implementation of the Measles Strategy there was an initial assessment of the situation across the country, with a national survey being undertaken to measure existing vaccination coverage rates amongst children. The coverage rate was estimated at only 63% overall across the country before the implementation of the measles strategy.[37] The organisers of the campaign, launched officially on the 1st of January 1990, decided to try to make it integral to existing primary health care services rather than running a parallel campaign with special 'vaccination days' or services. It was thought that in this way it would strengthen and re-enforce existing services and promote their continued use as part of the Primary Health Care service. Special outreach teams and door-to-door campaigns were aimed only at those communities remote from existing services or in high risk areas such as informal 'squatter' camps. Publicity was high with use made of the media, schools, health facilities, and community structures and the plan was to improve access to vaccination, making it available at all health facilities, on every day that they were open. The vaccine used was the new Edmonston-Zagreb (EZ) strain which could be administered at a younger age than the previous vaccine – at 6 months of age.[38] Later, in 1991, this policy was modified to separate children into 'high risk' and 'low risk' categories using different titres of vaccine (High Titre or Normal Titre) accordingly. This was further amended to give high titre EZ vaccine to so-called high-risk children at six months and the Schwarz vaccine to the low-risk children at nine months due to shortages of the EZ vaccine.

The vaccination campaign brought about a decrease in measles cases in 1990 to 10,623, and further down to 4,763 in 1991. While the overall vaccination coverage rate only rose to 71%, the drop in cases and mortality was dramatic. By the end of 1991 the deaths had fallen by 90%. The Department estimated that notifications under-stated the true number of cases by a factor of nine, so that the true average figure for the period 1980–1989 was not 16,832 but 151,488. It estimated that the number of cases prevented in 1991 was as high as 109,000. Following statistical corrections the Department estimated that there were probably an average of 2,865 deaths per year between 1980 and 1989. In 1991 just 261 deaths were reported and it was estimated that over 2,600 lives had been saved by the Measles Strategy. Küstner, Editor of the Department of National Health's periodical *Epidemiological Comments*, noted the political context in which this strategy had played out, where dramatic changes had been taking place in the closing years of Apartheid:

> Perceived adversaries became partners and old friendships were dashed on the rocks of political perceptions and preferences. There was violence to such an extent that the post-implementation coverage evaluations could not be performed the way they were before implementation, because entry into certain afflicted areas was too dangerous. Yet those who agreed on the basic correctness of the new policy ... forged ahead. It was accomplished together: across political divides, across geographic divisions, and across the often artificial divisions between the various authorities in the public sector.[39] [there were then 14 separate Departments of Health in South Africa, separated by homeland and 'race']

However the gains of the vaccination campaign were short-lived. From a low of just under 4,800 cases in the 1991/1992 season, there was a massive epidemic of 22,745 cases - starting in July and running through into the following year – known as a 'post-honeymoon epidemic'. The epidemic largely affected older children, possibly explaining why reported mortality was only 53. The percentage of cases aged under five years had dropped from 69% to 39% from 1990 to 1992.[40] Coetzee reported on the 1992 epidemic as it affected Cape Town. It started at a private primary school in August then spread to other school-going children. Notifications in the City rose to 755 cases between September and December. The outbreak mainly affected older White and Coloured children in the higher socio-economic groups – presumably because these had not been considered a priority group in the vaccination campaigns, being seen as 'low risk'. Certainly they were at lower risk of getting serious complications and dying from the disease as hospital admissions remained low. This group was also more likely to have had the Measles/Mumps/Rubella (MMR) vaccine, often by a private General Practitioner, than the monovalent measles vaccine given at government clinics, and this was found to be less effective – only 74% in general and just 53% if given by a private doctor. The outbreak was probably brought to an end by the onset of school holidays in December.[41] The City of Johannesburg reported on their similar epidemic over the same period when they had 596 notified cases, of whom 48% and possibly an additional 28% (76% in total) had previously been immunised, in this case mostly at local authority clinics, and the outbreak was ascribed to a combination of non-vaccination and primary vaccine failure creating a pool of older susceptible children. They recommended introducing compulsory vaccination on school entry.[42]

The vaccination policy changed again in January 1993 to give three doses in high risk areas, at 6, 9 and 18 months, and two doses in low risk areas – 9 and 18 months, and vaccination coverage was up to 85%. By 1994 the number of notified cases had dropped back to just 3,390 cases and 12 deaths, although reporting still excluded the homeland of Bophuthatswana and some of the Transkei data where there was an epidemic occurring. It was estimated that vaccination coverage needed to be maintained at 92% to prevent future epidemics.[43]

By the end of the decade, and after intensive action around the Expanded Programme on Immunisation, measles was rapidly disappearing as a significant infectious disease, having become massively overtaken by HIV/AIDS and the accompanying infections of diarrhoea and pneumonia as a cause of child deaths. In 1998 the incidence was 1.9 per 100,000 population dropping to 0.02 per 100,000 in 2001, and with a case fatality rate of zero.[44] Hospital wards which had once been solely for measles cases had long-since been changed to accommodate infants with the complications of HIV infection and, provided that the immunisation levels can remain high, the toll taken by measles on children's health in South Africa appears to be over.

ENDNOTES

1. Gale A.H. *Epidemic Diseases* Penguin Books London 1959:99
2. Laidler P.W. and Gelfand M. *South Africa its medical history, 1652-1898: A medical and social study*; C Struik, Cape Town, 1971:151
3. Botha Graham C. *History of Law, Medicine and Place Names in the Cape of Good Hope*, C Struik Cape Town, 1962:191
4. McKay Helen M. 'William John Burchell: His Experiences as a Consulting Physician while in the Interior of Southern Africa 1810-181' *South African Medical Journal* 14(4) 1940:78-80
5. Blumberg C. *The provision of Medical Literature and Information in the Cape 1827-1973*, M Bibl Thesis Unisa, 1974:5
6. Bryer L. and Hunt K.S. *The 1820 Settlers*; Don Nelson; Cape Town, 1984:26
7. Laidler P.W.and Gelfand M. *South Africa its medical history, 1652-1898: A medical and social study*; C Struik, Cape Town, 1971:270
8. Ibid, 270 ;
9. Jeal M.E. *The Dell Chronicles 1750-1979*, Parkhurst, 1979
10. Devitt Napier, *The Concentration Camps in South Africa during the Anglo-Boer War of 1899-1902*, Shuter and Shooter Pietermaritzburg, 1941:29
11. Cliff A. Haggett P. Smallman-Raynor M. *Measles: An historical geography of a major human viral disease; from global expansion to local retreat, 1840-1990*, Blackwell, Oxford, 1993:81-83
12. Brincker J.A.H. 'A historical, epidemiological and aetiological study of measles' *Proc. Roy Soc. Med.* 31 1938:807
13. Brain J.B. and Brain P. 'The Health of Indentured Indian Migrants to Natal, 1860-1911' *South African Medical Journal* 62(20) 1982:739-742
14. Nankivell J.H. 'Report of the District Surgeon, Transkei' *Blue Book of Native Affairs 1882*, Cape of Good Hope, Volume 1 part 1,WA Richards and sons, Cape Town, p20
15. Dr van der Waal, cited in Martin A.C. *The Concentration Camps 1900-1902: Facts, Figures and Fables*; Howard Timmins Cape Town 1957:15
16. Devitt Napier, *The Concentration Camps in South Africa during the Anglo-Boer War of 1899-1902*, Shuter and Shooter Pietermaritzburg, 1941:20-21
17. Martin A.C. *The Concentration Camps 1900-1902: Facts, Figures and Fables*; Howard Timmins Cape Town 1957:17
18. Devitt Napier, *The Concentration Camps in South Africa during the Anglo-Boer War of 1899-1902*, Shuter and Shooter Pietermaritzburg, 1941:59
19. Ibid, 37-38
20. Cliff A. Haggett P. Smallman-Raynor M. *Measles: An historical geography of a major human viral disease; from global expansion to local retreat, 1840-1990*, Blackwell, Oxford, 1993:147

21 Donnolly F.A. and Nelson H. 'Some Observations on the Control of Infectious Disease', *South African Medical Journal*, 9(18) 1935:629-641
22 Cluver E.H. *Public Health in South Africa*; Central News Agency Limited, South Africa, Fifth Edition (undated) p257
23 Humphries S.V. 'Sulphapyridine as a specific for measles in Adult Natives', *South African Medical Journal* 17(5) 1943:72
24 Cliff A, Haggett P, Smallman-Raynor M, *Measles: An historical geography of a major human viral disease; from global expansion to local retreat, 1840-1990*, Blackwell, Oxford, 1993:157-159
25 *Annual Report of the Medical Officer of Health, City of Cape Town, 1950*, Cape Times Ltd Parow 1950:38
26 Levin S. 'Hospital deaths in non-European children' *South African Medical Journal* 24(48) 1950:993-997
27 Buhrmann M.V. 'Investigation of stillbirths and deaths of children under 5 years of age', *South African Medical Journal* 26(42) 1952:835-839
28 Editorial, Measles, *South African Medical Journal* 29(12) 1955:271-272
29 Slome R. 'Immunisation' *South African Medical Journal* 31(18) 1957:422
30 Spencer I.W.F. *Various Studies in the Prevention of Disease*, Thesis for Doctor of Medicine, University of Witwatersrand, Johannesburg 1969:10-11
31 Cooper E.D. *Annual Report of the Medical Officer of Health 1960*, City of Cape Town, 1960:4
32 Cooper E.D. *Annual Report of the Medical Officer of Health 1961*, City of Cape Town, 1961,:5
33 Sher J.N. *Annual Report of the Medical Officer of Health for Port Elizabeth, 1975*, Longs, Port Elizabeth 1975: p(i)
34 Coovadia H.M. *Host Allergic Response Variation in children with measles infection;* Thesis for Doctor of Medicine, University of KwaZulu-Natal, Durban 1977:17.
35 Fisher S. 'Measles and Poverty in Port Elizabeth, Carnegie Conference Paper No 172', *Second Carnegie Inquiry into Poverty and Development in Southern Africa*, Cape Town, 13-19 April 1984: 3-11.
36 Küstner H.G.V. 'Measles Update', *Epidemiological Comments*, Department of Health and Welfare, 11(6) June 1984:24-31
37 Küstner H.G.V. 'The six vaccine-preventable diseases' *Epidemiological Comments*, 17(10) October 1990:3-18.
38 Küstner H.G.V. 'The measles strategy, South Africa 1991 – an evaluation of its effect' *Epidemiological Comments*, 19(7) July 1992:112-127
39 Ibid, 117.
40 Küstner H.G.V. 'Downward trend in measles', *Epidemiological Comments*, 22 (4) April 1995:76-81
41 Coetzee N. Hussey G.D. Visser G. Barron P. Keen A. 'The 1992 Measles Epidemic in Cape Town – a changing epidemiological pattern' *South African Medical Journal*, 84(3) March 1994:145-139
42 Naidoo S. and Meyers K. 'The Measles Epidemic', *South African Medical Journal* 84(3) March 1994:125.
43 Küstner H.G.V. 'Downward trend in measles', *Epidemiological Comments*, 22 (4) April 1995:76-81
44 Day C. and Gray A. 'Health and Related Indicators', in *South African Health Review 2002*; Health Systems Trust, Durban, South Africa 2003:444.

11 A CENTURY OF POLIOMYELITIS

Epidemics of poliomyelitis (polio) were probably unknown in South Africa prior to the First World War. While polio is a very old disease, described first by Underwood in 1784, it had been a relatively rare condition which only become an epidemic disease since the mid 1800s, with an outbreak affecting the island of St Helena in 1836, and it was really only since the start of the 20th century that extensive epidemics occurred. The transition from an endemic to an epidemic disease began in Scandinavia then moved to North America. Initially small primary outbreaks occurred. Then gradually increasing attack rates were observed for a few years, followed by severe epidemics. In the early periods children under four years of age were mainly affected, hence the disease was also known as 'Infantile paralysis'. New York had an epidemic of some 2,000 cases in 1907-08 with a mortality rate of 6-7%. The contagious nature of the disease was established early in that century, particularly in the Swedish epidemic of 1911-1913, when there were 10,000 cases. Because of the horrors of the paralysis caused by the disease, and the lifelong disabilities resulting from it, it started to become a disease to be greatly feared. The First World War was responsible for the spread of many diseases world-wide, including polio, due to the massive movements of troops occurring from one country to another. New York suffered a terrible second epidemic in 1916, the worst ever recorded, with a 27% mortality. Altogether there were 8,500 cases notified with some 2,100 deaths in New York alone.

The first polio epidemic in South Africa occurred at the end of 1917, continuing into early 1918, and prior to this outbreak cases had been sporadic and isolated. The epidemic of 1917-18 occurred on the towns around Johannesburg, and mostly affected children under five years.[1] The disease started with features unlike those usually seen in the sporadic cases of previous years. The mortality was high from the beginning, and with symptoms resembling cerebrospinal meningitis. Between February and August 1918 there were 181 cases with 20 deaths in Johannesburg, and several hundred cases occurred altogether. Baumann, in giving a detailed account of the clinical features of the disease at the start of the 1918 outbreak, stated that he learnt from the epidemic that:

> Poliomyelitis must no longer be regarded as an occasional disease of childhood in which individuals suffer from a flaccid paralysis in the distribution of the lower motor neurone. We have learnt that it is a disease of communities and not of individuals.[2]

It was also a disease affecting adults, no longer just 'infantile paralysis' and with a high mortality. The only treatment described at that time was 'that of any acute infection, namely rest in bed, liquid diet, attention to the bowels, relief of pain by the exhibition of analgesics and the treatment of symptoms as they arise'. Applying ice bags to the spine or doing 'counter-irritation' with mustard leaves was also suggested, but the major emphasis was on absolute rest. 'The child with an over-fond mother who insists upon dandling the patient in her arms, jarring the irritable brain and cord and straining the weakened muscles is much more likely to be permanently crippled than one who is rationally treated'.[3] There was little cause for optimism once a limb was afflicted and paralysed. The mode of spread of the disease caused much debate, with some maintaining that it was not transferred from sick to healthy, others proposing flies as a vector, but some maintaining that all evidence pointed to spread by a micro-organism through the naso-pharynx. The disease was not notifiable in the Transvaal at that time as, prior to the Public Health Act of 1919, it was notifiable only in the Cape Province and the Orange Free State. It was reported that there were 48 cases in the Cape and 11 in the Free State in 1918.[4]

An outbreak of 40 cases occurred in Bloemfontein in December 1933 and January 1934, of whom 17 were admitted to hospital and eight died within a month. Only nine made a complete recovery and 17 were left with a residual defect. The organism had been found to be resistant to both high and low temperatures, and spread in the nasal and pharyngeal secretions of health carriers. Spread was then by droplet infections. These healthy carriers were considered the cause of isolated cases which occurred in sparsely populated areas with no obvious source of transmission. Most outbreaks occurred in the hottest part of the year, summer and autumn, which had led to the idea that the disease was carried by flies and insects. It was also noted that cases were greater in children under five years in towns, and the incidence at this age diminished with the density of the population. The incidence in adults and children over six years was greater in rural areas, which related to the acquisition of immunity at a young age being less in sparsely populated areas.

In the Bloemfontein epidemic 50% of cases were aged between five and eight years, with all cases being under twenty years. Of the seven cases aged up to four years all survived, and increasing mortality was related to increasing age, with all five of those aged over 13 years dying. The onset in the Bloemfontein cases had been sudden with pains in the neck and back muscles and a high temperature. Pain on slightest touch (hyperaesthesia) and sweating were also frequent. Paralysis often started in the legs, then the arms, inability to pass urine and faeces, followed by paralysis of the respiratory muscles of the chest and diaphragm. 'The patients remained conscious to the end, straining themselves at each inspiration, which ended with a long sighing expiration until death supervened'.[5] Very little treatment was available except for the administration of 'convalescent serum, or Pettit's serum' given intramuscularly, but trials had shown little effect. Intramuscular injection of parents' blood was recommended by some along with repeated therapeutic lumbar puncture. Artificial respiration only appeared to prolong the agony of the conscious patient. The most effective method of prevention seemed to be keeping children away from school or crowds during an epidemic.

The use of convalescent serum continued to be evaluated internationally and many concluded that it was effective in minimizing the severity of the attack if given at the pre-paralytic stage. Others however thought it of little or no value although it at least appeared to do no harm. Experiments continued internationally to find a vaccine. Passive immunisation with an injection of adult blood or serum to uninfected individuals appeared to confer some protection.[6]

Outbreaks continued worldwide through the late 1930's with children largely affected. Males were generally affected more than females. The age incidence seamed to vary with the density of the population, with the more densely populated areas having younger age groups involved, probably due to the variation in acquisition of herd immunity. Epidemics occurred more in the late summer and autumn months, with a tendency to revisit the same areas the following summer. They extensively involved schools and institutions, and were noted to follow along lines of communication such as roads and railways. There were two main types of the disease – the classical paralytic type and another described as the abortive type. The latter, perhaps 80-90% of cases, were mild illnesses with no neurological involvement and often undiagnosed, which hence contributed both to the spread of the disease and the acquisition of immunity in adults. The route of spread was still uncertain, but thought to be by inhalation and ingestion as the virus had been isolated both from the nose and faeces. It had been particularly noted to be present in sewage during an epidemic, and spread by flies was a possibility. The virus had been found to be able to survive in chlorinated water, and had been isolated from food, milk, books and drawings. There was also a possibility that it could enter though a skin wound, and recent tonsillectomy and tooth extraction were linked to cases.[7] The number of cases nationally was 26 in 1936, rising to 82 in 1937, but the National Department of Public Health was on the alert due to its previous serious outbreaks and the tragically crippling sequelae of the illness. It was undertaking investigations as to the best method of treatment practised in Australia.[8]

Notifications rose again in 1938 to 92, and in 1944 it was noted that cases were increasing again. As outbreaks occurred across the country with Natal, Cradock in the Cape and Johannesburg being most affected, plans were started to deal with a possible outbreak, it being noted that the movement of troops could facilitate an epidemic. There was still no preventive vaccine in use, and activities focused on the establishment of treatment centres, with the Cape opening a special hospital, Montebello, to which all cases were admitted. A special 'War car' was obtained from the railways to transport cases from Cradock to Cape Town. In the Transvaal special units were opened in Pretoria and Johannesburg. The South African Red Cross had twenty 'iron lungs', or mechanical ventilators, manufactured.[9] Other preventive measures included quarantine of cases and close contacts for six weeks; strict sanitary measures and disinfection of faeces; anti-fly campaigns and general hygiene measures; wearing of masks and gloves; disinfection of hands and utensils – although few disinfectants were effective against the virus; boiling of water of milk; cancellation of non-urgent tonsillectomies and dental extractions; burning of contaminated articles where possible and closing of schools, swimming baths or places where children gathered. The few effective disinfectants included copper sulphate and mercuric chloride. Gargling with 1% hydrogen peroxide or potassium permanganate was suggested, along with the painting of wounds with mercurochrome or methylene blue. Fruit and vegetables could be disinfected with potassium permanganate or copper sulphate which, being rather bright in colour, could be washed off before use. Vigorous campaigns against rats and mice were to be considered. There was no known drug treatment. However Turner, in proposing such precautionary measures in the face of an impending epidemic, concluded that as there was good reason to believe that poliomyelitis was so widespread that practically all individuals were infected before reaching adult life, it appeared that 'elaborate precautions to control epidemics are really futile, and at best all that such measures can do is temporarily postpone an inevitable infection'. The future lay in the development of an effective vaccine, not yet available.[10]

In the Transvaal the incidence stood at 41 per100,000 population in Europeans and 3.65 per 100,000 in Africans. Sure enough, as with the outbreak in 1917, this rising incidence was associated with the vast movements of people during the Second World War, and was worldwide. Serious epidemics occurred successively in many countries – the New Zealand and Australian Expeditionary Forces in Egypt were affected in 1941. In 1942 it affected American soldiers in the Middle East, and Malta suffered its first recorded epidemic in 1942 with 483 cases following its relief from prolonged siege. In all these outbreaks the adult indigenous population largely escaped, suggesting an immunity acquired from previous exposure to infection not enjoyed to the same extent by the immigrant soldiers from Northern Europe and America. In North America there was an epidemic of over 13,000 cases in 1943-44. South Africa was affected in 1944 and it had assumed epidemic proportions by October, probably due to the arrival of soldiers returning from the Middle East, who disembarked at Durban. From there it spread widely and was seen in most districts, except for the rural Transkei, where only seven cases were reported. This was presumed to be due to their having been exposed early and repeatedly to endemic strains of the virus, which then conferred immunity.[11]

Kaplan reported on the epidemic as it hit Durban, starting in September 1944. Up until January 1945 he had seen 63 cases in the Durban Children's Hospital, 50% of which were under nine years of age. Cases came from both poor and better-off homes and districts, causing great alarm amongst the public who blamed various causes such as whale meat, increased pork and bacon consumption, vaccination and malnutrition, Durban at that time suffering from food shortages. Troops disembarking from the United States of America were thought to have brought it to the port, from whence it spread inland. The public were encouraged to swat flies, to protect their food, keep children away from crowds and from persons with colds and coughs. Most cases presented with a rapid heart rate, which lasted several weeks; muscle pains, irritability, constipation, and variable degrees of paralysis. The paralysis could affect various parts of the body, including limbs, facial muscles, shoulders and hands, although the legs were the commonest affected. Treatment was largely symptomatic and supportive, with no specific drugs available.[12] The disease spread inland from Durban affecting 37 out of the 45 districts in Natal with 294 cases, but the worst hit were mainly the Durban, Pietermaritzburg, and Inanda and Verulam areas to the northwest of Durban.

It was said that polio increased as the distance from the equator increased, and in epidemic times it attacked at the rate of one per thousand, or up to between three and five per thousand in severe epidemics. In America it had been noted that the smaller the town, the higher the case-rate and death-rate. Case-fatalities were greatest in years of low prevalence, and low in years of high prevalence. In rural areas there was a tendency for older the older age-groups to be attacked. Before an epidemic hit a locality it was common to misdiagnose the earliest cases. They presented with fever, headache, vomiting, pain in the back, muscle spasm, tremor, and increased reflexes, which could be confused with other meningeal or encephalitic infections until diagnosed with a lumbar puncture. In Cradock, a small town in the Eastern Cape, 27 cases occurred in October 1944, with similar outbreaks occurring in other inland, small Cape towns including Graaff-Reinet and Paarl and also in small Free State towns such as Bethlehem and Harrismith.

Dr Hanson in Springs, a mining town near Johannesburg, reported that the first case of the disease in the town was on 28 October 1944, with 23 paralytic cases then reported over the next five months. The epidemic peaked during the hot and humid summer months, and affected Europeans more severely with 94% of cases being under 10 years of age. The seasonality was noted to be similar to that of typhoid fever and summer diarrhoea, suggesting it was similarly related to insanitary conditions and flies. An analysis of the epidemic suggested that flies were the main vector, and this was thought to be linked to the spreading of human excreta from the trains which crossed the area from all directions along with cattle grazing. Droplet infection appeared unlikely. The fact that there had not been a case in the town for 20 years, and the young age of those affected, suggested that there was a new and relatively non-immune generation who succumbed.[13] It was also discovered that silent infections were common in households in which a case of polio had occurred, and that such infections could persist for at least a month. It therefore indicated that the entire family and household contacts should perhaps be isolated for at least six weeks after contact with a case. A study in a small children's home in Johannesburg where a case occurred found that two out of seven healthy contacts were excreting the virus in their faeces, one continuing for a month.[14] In Johannesburg altogether nearly 200 cases were reported with some 542 cases overall in the Transvaal. Fear and confusion spread as the disease spread across the city, Wade, in her thesis on the Johannesburg epidemic, noted that the general public became distraught as friends, family members and neighbours were struck down. She commented that:

> For many in Johannesburg the reality of the 1944-45 epidemic was completely novel, while it reminded an older generation of their first experience of polio and their fear of the unknown, which was so much a part of the 1918 epidemic.[15]

The lowest incidence was reported from the deeply rural area of Transkei, and the incidence in Africans over the whole country was only 5.5 per 100,000 population compared with 35 in Europeans and 18 in Asians. 49% of cases were in the under 5s, but the highest mortality rate was in the age group 5-10 years.[16]

The treatment of patients after an attack focussed on bed rest and the splinting of affected limbs for several weeks, with splints being used on those muscles which remained weak or were likely to produce contractions and deformity. Circulation was maintained with massage, heat and passive movement, and as muscles regained slight movement exercises were commenced gently, sometimes under water. Bad immobilisation could give rise to deformities and joint stiffness. The greater part of muscle recovery took place within the first year, and if no improvement was seen in the first four months then the paralysis was permanent. If no muscles were found completely paralysed immediately after the acute phase then the prognosis was good. If the spinal or abdominal muscles were involved recovery took from 6 months to 24 months in bed.[17]

The disease fell off a little in 1946 and 1947 but in 1948 the South African Medical Journal warned again of an 'incoming tide of Poliomyelitis'. The rate appeared, somewhat paradoxically, to be increasing in proportion to the level of sanitation – as water and sanitation improved in North America and Europe, so the rate of polio increased. It was noted that the number of cases in America had been increasing over the previous five years, with a total of 80,000 cases reported. The United Kingdom had just suffered an epidemic five times greater than any previous outbreak, and throughout Europe the tread was upwards. There were concurrently record-breaking epidemics in Austria and Berlin.[18] In line with the warning in 1948 another considerable epidemic occurred, with 1,925 cases notified, of which 1,366 were European and 423 were African, giving rates of 57.6 per 100,000 for

Europeans and 5.4 per 100,000 for Africans. This was similar to the 1945 epidemic when the incidence in the Transvaal was 41 per 100,000 Europeans and 3.6 per 100,000 in Africans. In Africans the highest incidence was in the 0-5 year age group, whereas in Europeans there were as many in the 5-10 year age group.[19] It was suggested that the relatively low incidence in Africans was due to an immunity of the older age groups acquired as a result of previous infection as infants. This was supported by serological surveys which showed that in all age groups a greater proportion of Africans had neutralizing antibodies, probably as a result of previously silent infection. Studies done on African township populations had found that, under slum conditions, the majority of infants were infected with three types of polio virus before they were five years old and developed antibodies to each type.[20] It had become apparent that the more deprived the hygiene of the community, the earlier the immunity was acquired, and conversely the higher the standard of living, the later immunity was acquired. As Wade noted, 'a terrifying aspect of polio is that it operated within the sanitised environment of the home, away from the familiar sources of disease such as squalor and filth.[21] The epidemic began in January, peaked in March and gradually subsided in May. Johannesburg was the most affected, with over 800 cases notified. Durban was also severely affected later in the season, with the maximum incidence being in May.[22]

Following the epidemic of 1948, the then Lady Mayoress of Johannesburg, Mrs E. Gordon, called a public meeting and established a Poliomyelitis Research Foundation, which commenced with a national committee chaired by Mrs Gordon and followed by the establishment of local committees, with an appeal for funds to all the towns and villages in the country. The concerns of the Foundation were to pursue research into a disease about which there was dispute about how it spread, there was no specific remedy, no effective method of prevention and of which there were likely to be more epidemics. More than £250,000 was raised and it was hoped to build a virus research institution.[23] This would eventually be officially opened by the Minister of Health in 1953 and included the study of many other viral diseases such as coxsackie virus, rabies and Rift Valley fever.

Heymann, speaking of his experiences during the 1945 and 1948 epidemics in Johannesburg, commented that cases could appear with dramatic onset of paralysis, but also with a gradual onset of symptoms such as headache, fever, and vomiting. Often during an epidemic panic lead to over-reporting of suspected cases with these general symptoms by parents, which later turned out to be negative These could either resolve after 48 hours as an abortive case, or else continue into development of muscle pains in limbs or the back, diarrhoea followed by constipation, rapid pulse, loss of balance, neck rigidity and spinal rigidity. Paralysis usually began suddenly with loss of reflexes and low muscle tone. Legs and arms were both affected, but not usually symmetrically. Intestinal paralysis could occur, causing constipation and abdominal swelling, together with respiratory failure due to involvement of the muscles of respiration in the chest and diaphragm. Bulbar involvement affected the cranial nerves causing difficulty in swallowing, change in speech, inability to cough and pooling of secretions in the pharynx. There was no specific treatment, convalescent serum having proved disappointing and been generally discarded, hence treatment was aimed at the symptoms and making the patient as comfortable as possible in the face of a severe illness and paralysis of different muscles.[24] The worst cases required being placed on a respirator for artificial ventilation, sometimes for long periods of time, as in the case of one anonymous victim who wrote of having been dependant on an Iron Lung for seven years, and lamented their lack of maintenance.[25]

It was observed in 1951 during the recent polio epidemics that relatively more paralytic infections occurred in Europeans than Africans. The rate of paralysis also seemed to be increasing with 40% left with residual weakness or paralysis in 1948 compared with 28% in the epidemic of 1944-45.[26] It had also been noted that the spread of disease sometimes occurred after diphtheria and whooping cough inoculations, which raised the possibility of it being spread through repeated use of unsterilized needles. As one doctor put it:

> During my 33 years of private practice I invariably carried a hypodermic syringe in a spirit container – and most GPs do – and felt quite justified using it repeatedly without boiling. We now know that viruses are most resistant to spirit.[27]

He presumed that the same pertained in clinics and other mass inoculation sites.

Rising numbers of cases were reported in 1954 with the first appearance being in Durban in September and 870 cases by the end of the year. The city of Cape Town reported its highest number of cases on record at 66 residents and 55 cases in hospital from outside the City. The manufacture of formalinised polio virus vaccine was started on a large scale. The epidemic continued in 1955 when a change in pattern was noted. Both in Johannesburg and East London, the worst affected cities, there were as many cases among African as amongst Europeans, although with Africans it was still worse in the 0-5 year age group, compared with older children and adults for Europeans. In adults the disease tended to be more severe, with a large number ending in death.[28] There were 184 cases notified in the first two weeks of January 1955 and the Ministry of Health ordered seven new iron lungs for distribution to rural areas. A particularly distressing outbreak occurred at the nursing home at Addington Hospital in Durban, with 104 cases among the nurses, mainly aged between 18-25 years, in the early months of 1955, although the features were not completely typical of the disease and it was later given the name 'Icelandic disease', and thought that it may have been encephalitis. It had been noted by the World Health Organisation that epidemics had tended to affect older age groups as the century progressed. This shift in age groups was explained by improvements in hygiene and in living standards which resulted in children becoming infected increasingly late in life in the more developed countries and towns.

Recommended precautionary measures during epidemics included frequent washing of hands, protection of food from flies, washing of fruit and vegetables, avoidance of over-exertion, closing down of all un-chlorinated swimming pools, avoidance of operations for the removal of tonsils and adenoids and suspension of vaccination campaigns and intramuscular injections of an irritant nature. Injections were found to predispose the inoculated limb to paralysis when the patients became infected, particularly in respect of the diphtheria-pertussis vaccine and heavy metals. It was not recommended to close schools, although their opening could be delayed if the epidemic occurred during summer holidays, but pre-schools and crèches should be closed.[29] In South Africa researchers at the Poliomyelitis Research Foundation Laboratory were experimenting on the formula used in producing the Salk vaccine in the United States. The period of immunity induced by this vaccine was as then unknown and results of American field trials were awaited. Experts met in Cape Town on 10th March 1955 to consider the question of mass immunisation following which it would be distributed to local authorities.[30]

Maister, at a symposium in Pietermaritzburg, described the epidemiology of polio, noting that the portal of entry was decidedly the mouth, oro-pharynx and alimentary tract with the virus being found there 3-5 days before and 3-7 days after the onset of illness. Almost every patient excreted the virus in their stools for between 3 and 12 weeks. There was thought to be between 10-100 infected-but-asymptomatic, individuals for every person with symptoms. Flies and cockroaches could carry the virus, but the use of DDT in epidemics had not been helpful. Factors influencing paralysis included exercise prior to the onset of illness, local trauma, operations and in particular tonsillectomy, which predisposed to the more severe bulbar form of the disease. One doctor at the symposium described in poignant detail his treatment of his own five year old son, recently stricken by a paralysing form of the disease three weeks after a tonsillectomy, and how the paralysis had spread rapidly over two hours after the giving of an injection.[31]

The American field trials of the Salk polio vaccine covered 211 study areas in 44 states. In one study population of some 750,000 the vaccine was given to 'volunteers' in the second grade of school [if young children can truly volunteer for medical research], with 200,745 children receiving three doses of the vaccine, and another 201,229 receiving three doses of a placebo vaccine. In another study area 221,000 children out of a population of 1,080,680 received the vaccine. Out of the total study population of 1,829,916 there were 863 cases of polio reported over the next six months of which 79% were paralytic. These numbers were much higher in the unvaccinated or placebo groups, and the effectiveness of the vaccine against paralytic polio was estimated at between 80 and 90%.[32] Under pressure to initiate vaccination in view of the polio outbreak at the beginning of the year, with some 50 cases a week being reported, the Minister of Health J.F. Naudé, stated that it would be tested 'doubly and doubly and yet again doubly' before the vaccine would be used in South Africa and a full analysis of its use in America was still awaited. The initial supply of vaccine would be sufficient for 25,000 people, and it was thought that the South African vaccine would be more effective than the Salk vaccine, although a shortage of monkeys and baboons to test it on was reported. There were concerns about the safety of the vaccine, M.P. Mr C. de Wet being concerned that children might be sterile when they grew up, and he did not think there was any hurry – while it was a dramatic illness it was not as common as diphtheria. However he cited only deaths, and not the tragedy of the paralysis which damaged so many of the victims.[33]

Minister Naudé appointed a special committee to advise him on the use of the vaccine in April 1955, which met on several occasions and reviewed the developments which followed the mass immunisation campaign in America. Six manufacturing companies had participated in the production of the vaccine, one of which, the Cutter Laboratories vaccine, was found to be responsible for subsequent cases of polio through the presence of live virus in the vaccine. 69 cases occurred amongst the 409,000 recipients of the Cutter vaccine. Following an investigation in America the manufacturing process was modified with additional safety measures put in place. At its final meeting the South African Ministerial Advisory Committee of Experts advised the Minister that the Poliomyelitis Research Foundation's laboratory, which used a different strain of the polio virus, was safe, efficacious and cheaper than the American vaccine, which was not yet available in South Africa.[34] The Cutter incident raised much concern however amongst the medical profession, such that Dr L.L. Alexander, Chairman of the Division of the Medical Association of South Africa in East London, released a public statement accusing the Department of Health of 'almost stampeding the public into having their children vaccinated with a vaccine the effects of which – and this is admitted - may even be harmful and dangerous'. Minister Naudé then issued a press statement, following a speech on 27 July 1955, on the findings of the Committee. He stated that the vaccine would not be made compulsory, but that it would be made available for all children up to the age of five years and up to 15 if necessary. Parents of pre-school children who wanted to have their children vaccinated had to register with their local authorities so that adequate quantities of vaccine could be made available. The Minister refuted the East London claims and stated that their statements were incorrect and irresponsible, and that the members of the Expert Committee had decided to have their own children inoculated.[35] Altogether that year some 16,000 children were vaccinated and no cases of paralytic polio attributed to the vaccine were notified with only a handful of minor side effects.

In April, May and June of 1956 another epidemic occurred particularly in East London and the Transvaal, but none were confirmed in children who had been vaccinated. The location in East London raises the question as to whether the negative views of the local medical establishment had influenced the uptake of the vaccine amongst parents. The stocks of vaccine had run out in the early part of 1956, and the issue was only resumed in July, which was used to give second doses to those who had already been vaccinated. From August the next batch was available to start immunizing more children with priority given to those aged between six months and six years. The delay was partly due to the rigorous testing introduced after the Cutter affair, which took four to six months to complete. During the epidemic the Boksburg-Benoni Isolation Hospital received 370 cases, of which 55 needed artificial respiration in the tank respirators ('iron lung') in which the patient was immersed up to the upper chest or neck. The stress of the procedure often necessitated sedation, not just for the patient but often also for the parents. Some parents tragically had more than one child affected. Two thirds of the cases were European, and of the non-European cases it was noted that the age incidence was lowering, affecting largely the under-tens. 27 of the patients on respirators, or 49%, died. All the rest were left with severe disabilities.[36] Several of the female cases were pregnant when they contracted polio but fortunately most went on to have normal deliveries and babies after they recovered. One needed to be placed on a respirator, and went into labour shortly after. The baby was found to be normal but the mother, when she recovered, had a residual paralysis of her right leg and partial paralysis of the other three limbs.[37]

In all there were 3,349 cases reported in 1956, of which around half were in Europeans and half in Non-Europeans. The disease was very widespread and the various Provinces ended up more or less equally affected. In Cape Town there were 127 cases, the highest number ever recorded in the City, and it was noted that for the first time the number of cases in Non-Europeans was more than double that in Europeans – a reversal of the usual racial distribution. It was also noted in Cape Town that the disease was more prevalent in areas where living conditions were bad and overcrowding rife, and which had been described as 'a septic focus' for many years. Mainly the under-fives were affected, possibly due to the older age group having already been exposed in the 1954 epidemic.[38] In the following year the epidemic continued with another 271 cases and 18 deaths in Cape Town. The supply of South African vaccine was running short and more had to be imported from America while 600,000 doses were under manufacture. The epidemic finally came to an end in May 1957 after two waves of infection had occurred: the first due to Type 1 and the second due to Type 3 poliovirus. Some 2,442 cases were notified in 1957.

The Minister of Health, Mr de Wet Nel, put out another appeal to the public to utilise the immunisation services in the middle of 1958 before the on-coming summer months. He warned that another increase in incidence could easily occur and that the only means of prevention was immunisation on as wide a scale as possible. While the immunisation was not giving full protection is was protective to a large extent against the paralysis, and he pleaded with the public to ensure that, in particular, children, youth and young women who may get pregnant complete a course of three inoculations:

> We in the Union should take full advantage of the fact that, as one of the few countries in the world which produces its own vaccine, we have plentiful supplies and we should ensure that all those who need to be

protected against this disease are immunised.[39]

The high prevalence continued in the late 1950's to 1960 with Cape Town reporting 76 cases of whom five had apparently been previously immunised with the Salk vaccine. A further 101 cases were admitted to the City's infectious diseases hospital from outside the city area and two from ships in the harbour. The new Sabin oral poliomyelitis live vaccine had been eagerly awaited, and was described by Wannenburg as:

> the brightest beacon that has yet shone for suffering humanity ... much is expected from this vaccine and the expectation is proportional to the alarm and anxiety with which the community has come to regard poliomyelitis and its complications.[40]

Successful tests in Russia in 1957 and 1958 had resulted in it being rapidly extended to a national campaign with several million children vaccinated across the USSR by May 1959, with a total target of 75 million people by the end of 1960. It was introduced in South Africa in November 1960, after the International Conference held in Copenhagen during July at which it was found to be safe and effective. A pilot vaccination campaign was conducted in larger towns and cities during which 2,200,000 doses of Type 1 vaccine were administered. It immediately led to a reduction in cases. In Johannesburg alone 275,000 people were immunised in the first campaign and only 18 cases were notified – the lowest for many years.[41] The number of polio cases in Cape Town also plummeted, with only eight cases the following year compared with an average of over a hundred per year for the previous five years. The recommended method of administering the vaccine then was by a syringe which squirted the dose to the back of the throat. However Cape Town decided against this and worked with a local sweet manufacturer to devise an absorbent sweet onto which the vaccine was dropped, carefully from a height of some two centimetres, and the success of their campaign was attributed to some extent to this method of administration.[42]

The pilot campaign was followed by a country-wide campaign for all three types of virus during the cold months of 1961 for which 18,000,000 doses were prepared. South Africa was stated to be the first country after Russia to embark on such a vast campaign, which was launched by the then Minister of Health Albert Hertzog and widely publicised, and it was estimated that 80% of susceptible people were reached through it. Across the country the notifications fell from 1,054 in 1960 to 107 in 1964, and the success of the Sabin vaccine meant that there was now the exciting possibility being raised of being able to completely eradicate polio from South Africa, if not the entire world. However the vaccination programme still was not reaching everyone across the country so in 1963 it was decided to make it compulsory, with local authorities compelled to establish and maintain a free immunisation service. Parents or guardians were compelled to start immunising their children within three months of the child turning three months of age. Each immigrant under the age of forty was similarly obliged to be immunised within three months of arrival in the country.[43] This compulsion was on occasion enforced, as with a case in Cape Town where legal proceedings were instituted in 1964 against a father for not immunising his child. A suspended sentence was given pending immunisation within 12 months, after which the father was imprisoned. Similarly the following year a father of five children, whom he had refused to immunise, was also imprisoned.

The annual number of cases fell for a while, but started to climb in the late 1960's again, with over 700 cases in 1969 and in 1972 they were back up at 1,000 predominantly in Natal, the Orange Free State and the Southern Transvaal. Spikes occurred every three years, again in 1975. It was clear that the vaccine was still not being 100% effective, probably due to failure to maintain the cold chain of the very temperature-sensitive vaccine. In 1975 21 cases were notified in Port Elizabeth with the Medical Officer of Health noting that eight of these had been fully vaccinated, commenting 'this aspect is mystifying'.[44] The three year cycles were thought to be due to the build-up of a critical mass of non-immune children every three years or so. As soon as an outbreak got underway, and ill children started excreting the virus, it started to spread and involve other children and cause the epidemic. Gradually the time interval between outbreaks increased with the next outbreak in 1981/82 in the then homeland of KwaZulu. KwaZulu reported 63 of the 127 national cases in 1981, Lebowa (Northern Transvaal) 72 cases in 1982 and Gazankulu (in the eastern Transvaal) had 481 cases in 1982.

Having managed to bring the numbers down in KwaZulu-Natal, with only four cases reported in both 1985 and 1986, the next outbreak occurred between December 1987 and April 1988 when 275 patients were admitted to hospitals across the province. All but one was African, living mainly in the coastal regions stretching from Hlabisa in the north down to Port Shepstone in the south. 76.4% were in children under five years, giving an incidence of 24.2 per 100,000 in that group. The case-fatality rate was 10.2% and 94% were of the Type 1 strain. The response of the National Health Department to the epidemic was to launch a vaccination campaign using monovalent Type 1 vaccine, as it was noted that the normal trivalent vaccine usually failed to protect against the type 1 virus after a single dose and 200,000 doses were given. Attention was paid to what could have caused the outbreak. While it could have been contributed to by low levels of vaccination amongst children, it was recorded that a significant percentage of those affected (16.7%) had in fact received three doses of polio vaccine, and a further 17.8% had had one or two doses, which suggested problems with the potency of the vaccine. It was also noted that the epidemic had occurred shortly after the severe floods which had occurred in the Province in September/October 1987. This could have significantly increased the faecal contamination of the environment which, combined with low herd [population at risk] immunity, could have precipitated the epidemic.[45] While controlling outbreaks remained a problem the number of deaths decreased significantly from the early 1960's with the case-fatality rate falling from 7.7% in 1965 down to 0% in 1983. The incidence rate had fallen from a high of 22 in 1956 down to 0.3 in 1983.[46]

In May 1988 the World Health Organisation had announced a plan to try and eradicate polio by the year 2000. The Global Poliomyelitis Eradication Initiative included the achievement of at least 80% vaccination coverage among children between age one and four years. In addition it had to be ensured that the vaccine was still potent when administered, which meant the maintenance of the cold chain, the vaccine becoming inactive if not kept cool. This goal would entail the involvement of all sectors of society globally, from the community to global leaders. The vaccination levels in South Africa at the time were 81% in the urban areas and 61% in the rural – clearly not yet high enough to eradicate the disease, or even prevent the next anticipated outbreak in 1992.[47] The overall vaccination levels in 1991 were estimated at 73%, varying from a low of 51% in the Orange Free State to 100% in Natal – although this was presumably an over-estimate. Due to intensified vaccination efforts the anticipated epidemic didn't arrive, with only two cases being reported in 1991 and none in 1992. Further mass campaigns were held in 1995, 1996, 1997 and 2000, and continue on a regular bases thereafter.

Immunisation programmes and surveillance systems intensified both nationally and internationally with a Polio Expert Committee established in 1996 and by 2002 the transmission of polio was down to seven countries in the world, with 80% of cases occurring in India, Pakistan and Nigeria. Three regions of the world had been certified free of wild polio virus – the Americas, the Western Pacific and the European region. The last case of wild poliovirus in South Africa was in 1989 and South Africa appears now to be rid of one of the most terrifying and upsetting diseases of childhood. However there remain these few countries where a comprehensive vaccination programme has not been successful and cases still arise. The target date for eradication was revised to 2018, although by 2011 global cases had reduced from 350,000 cases in 1988 to less than 1000. In 2013 Pakistan, Nigeria and Afghanistan remained the only countries with endemic polio, although Somalia also has had a case, prompted by the breakdown in vaccination campaigns due to the on-going instability. Monitoring remains based on the detection of all cases of acute flaccid paralysis (AFP) which is a condition which could be caused by several neurological and infectious diseases. However each case needs careful surveillance and analysis to exclude polio as a cause. In South Africa the National Institute for Communicable Diseases has hosted a WHO-supported AFP surveillance network serving seven southern African countries.[48] With increasing immigration into South Africa from some of those countries where wild polio virus is still being found – in particular Pakistan, Congo, Somalia and Nigeria – vigilance cannot be dropped, and continuous effort to maintain immunisation coverage levels is required to prevent the re-emergence of this disease.

ENDNOTES

1 Gear James; 'Epidemiological Patterns of Poliomyelitis in Southern Africa' *Medicine in South Africa* Supplement to the South African Medical Journal 1957:19
2 Baumann E.P.' Poliomyelitis', *Medical Journal of South Africa*, XIII (6), January 1918:87
3 Ibid, 92
4 Allen Peter, 'Some general aspects of Poliomyelitis', *South African Medical Journal* 19(1) 1945:2.
5 Brink C.D. 'An Outbreak of Acute Anterior Poliomyelitis,' *South African Medical Journal* 8(15) 1934:560-563
6 Brink V. 'Poliomyelitis: Experimental and Therapeutic aspects', *South African Medical Journal*; 11(15) 1937:536-538
7 Turner R. 'Some Epidemiological and Public Health Aspects of Poliomyelitis', *South African Medical Journal* 19(1) 1945:2-7
8 *Annual Report of the Department of Public Health, Union of South Africa, 1937*, Government Printer Pretoria, UG 52-'37 p63
9 *Annual Report for the year ended 30 June 1945*; Union of South Africa Department of Public Health, Pretoria, 1946

10   Turner R. 'Some Epidemiological and Public Health Aspects of Poliomyelitis', *South African Medical Journal* 19(1) 1945: 2-7
11   Gear James; 'Epidemiological Patterns of Poliomyelitis in Southern Africa' *Medicine in South Africa*, Supplement to the South African Medical Journal, 1957:19-25
12   Kaplan M.W. 'Epidemic Poliomyelitis in Durban' *South African Medical Journal* 19(4) 1945:55-57
13   Hanson J. 'An Epidemiological study of the poliomyelitis outbreak in Springs, 1944-45', *South African Medical Journal* 19(22) 1945:422-426
14   Gear J. and Mundel B. 'Studies in Poliomyelitis' *South African Medical Journal* 19(15) 1945:262-264
15   Wade M.M. *Straws in the Wind: early epidemics of poliomyelitis in Johannesburg 1918-1945*, Thesis for Degree of M.A. UNISA, December 2006:242
16   *Annual Report of the Department of Public Health, 1945*, Government Printer Pretoria, UG No 6-'46, p12-18.
17   Du Toit, G.T. 'The After-care of Convalescent Poliomyelitis cases', *South African Medical Journal* 19(11) 1945:193-195
18   'Incoming Tide of Poliomyelitis', *Chronicle of the World Health Organisation*, 11(25) 1948.
19   Scott Millar, J.W. Poliomyelitis in Johannesburg, Public Health, 13, May1949: 143
20   Gear J. Measroch V. Bradley J.and Faerber G.I. 'Poliomyelitis in South Africa: studies in an urban native township during a non-epidemic year'; *South African Medical Journal*; 25(18), 5 May 1951:297.
21   Wade M.M. *Straws in the Wind: early epidemics of poliomyelitis in Johannesburg 1918-1945*, Thesis for Degree of M.A. UNISA, December 2006:243
22   Gear James; 'Epidemiological Patterns of Poliomyelitis in Southern Africa' *Medicine in South Africa* Supplement to the South African Medical Journal 1957:19-25
23   Editorial: 'The Poliomyelitis Research Foundation', *South African Medical Journal* 23(45) 1949:906-907
24   Heymann Seymour, 'Diagnosis and Treatment of Poliomyelitis in the Acute Stage', *South African Medical Journal* 24(20) 1950:373-379
25   'Polio, Maintenance and Care of the Iron Lung', *South African Medical Journal* 26(11) 1952 228
26   *Annual Report of the Department of Health, Union of South Africa, 1952*, Government Printer Pretoria, UG 40-'1954, p9
27   Coetzee C.H.H. 'Inoculation and Poliomyelitis', Letter to the Editor, *South African Medical Journal* 24(22) 1950:432
28   Gear James; 'Epidemiological Patterns of Poliomyelitis in Southern Africa'; *Medicine in South Africa* Supplement to the South African Medical Journal 1957:19-25
29   *Poliomyelitis 1955*, World Health Organisation Monograph series No 26, 1955.
30   'Statement in Parliament by Minister of Health on Union Supplies of Vaccine, J.F. Naude', *South African Medical Journal* 29(18) 1955:411
31   Maister M. 'Epidemiological and Public Health Aspects of the disease: Proceedings of a Symposium on Poliomyelitis, Pietermaritzburg' *South African Medical Journal* 29(18) 1955:416-417
32   Korns R.F. Abstract of Summary Report, Francis T and Korns RF et al, 'Evaluation of 1954 Field Trial of Poliomyelitis Vaccine', *South African Medical Journal* 29(19) 1955: 447-452

33 Naudé J.F.T. 'Statement on Poliomyelitis', *Debates of the House of Assembly, Union of South Africa,* Third session 21st January to 23rd June 1955, Vol 87, p2485-2487

34 Turner R. 'Active Immunisation against Poliomyelitis: A review' *South African Medical Journal* 29(36) 1955:833-844

35 Naudé J.F.T. 'East London Complaint: Further Statement by the Minister', *South African Medical Journal* 29(36) 1955: 848-849

36 Kaplan L. 'A Discussion on 55 respirator cases in the recent poliomyelitis epidemic of 1956', *South African Medical Journal* 30(45) 1956:1073-1083.

37 Kaplan L, 'Poliomyelitis and Pregnancy: case report of a birth in a respirator during the acute phase of poliomyelitis', *South African Medical Journal* 31(12) 1957:278-279

38 *Annual Report of the Medical Officer of Health*, The City of Cape Town, 1956:35

39 De Wet Nel M.D.C. 'Poliomyelitis: Statement by Minister of Health' *South African Medical Journal* 32(23) 7 June 1958:600.

40 Wannenburg H.R.J. 'Administrative Aspects of poliomyelitis in isolation hospitals' *South African Medical Journal* 33(4) 24 January 1959:76

41 Scott Millar J.W. *Report on the Health of Johannesburg in 1961*, City of Johannesburg, 1961:9

42 Cooper E.D. and Robertson W.I. 'Problems resulting from the use of live attenuated poliomyelitis virus type 1 in a mass campaign in a large urban area' *South African Medical Journal* 35(11) 18 March 1961:233

43 *Annual Report of the Department of Health for the Five Years ended 31st December 1964*, Government Printer Pretoria, 1966, RP 11/1966, p6

44 Sher J.N. *Annual Report of the Medical Officer of Health for Port Elizabeth,* 1975, p(ii).

45 Küstner H.G.V. 'Poliomyelitis Epidemic in Natal and KwaZulu', *Epidemiological Comments*, Department of National Health and Population Development, 15(3) 1988:2-30

46 Küstner H.G.V. 'Secular trends of selected diseases' *Epidemiological Comments*, 11(3) March 1984:10

47 Küstner H.G.V. 'The eradication of Poliomyelitis from South Africa', *Epidemiological Comments*, Department of National Health and Population Development, 17 (8) August 1990:3-9

48 Gumede-Moeletsi N, Suchard M. Schoub B. 'Update on Polio Eradication in Africa' *Communicable Diseases Surveillance Bulletin*, 11(2) 2013:42-47

12   DIPHTHERIA: IMMUNISATION AND INDIFFERENCE

The earliest reference to diphtheria in South Africa occurs in the 18th century, when it is referred to as the 'white sore throat', and considered the most common dangerous disease of the Cape.[1] Children usually succumbed to the disease after three or four days. Matthews refers to an outbreak in Natal in the 1850's which he states to have been the first time that the disease had been known in that region.[2] Diphtheria also occurred in the early days of diamond mining in Kimberley. At that time the precise cause was unknown and a Dr J. Mathias in 1887 postulated to the Griqualand West Medical Association: 'I am inclined to believe that it is due in a more limited extent to the inhalation of germs being taken in with the fluids and solids which are swallowed. In this respect diphtheria seems very like typhoid fever'.[3] The causative organism had actually been isolated by Loeffler in 1884, which then made it possible to start to fight the disease. Prior to this period, between 1855 and 1893, the rate in England of the disease had fluctuated between 2 and 51.7 per 100,000. The case-fatality rate also varied, but declined steadily after the use of antitoxin therapy. Antitoxin was first prepared in small animals by von Behring and Kitasato in 1890, and in horses by Roux and Martin in 1894, and the use of horse serum in the preparation of antitoxin continued from thereon. In New Jersey the case-fatality rates had shown a decrease from around 20% without treatment down to 4.4% in 1915 when Antitoxin was used.[4] It had been introduced in an immunisation programme in 1914 by Park and Zingher in New York City.

Diphtheria also featured as a significant cause of illness in children in the Concentration camps established during the Anglo-Boer War of 1899-1902, but as a cause of death was not significant and hugely overshadowed by measles in the high mortality there. It was reported across the country in the early 1900's, with small outbreaks and a handful of deaths before they were contained using isolation procedures and doses of antitoxin. Presumably this disease was spread around the country by the troop movements, as with many other infectious diseases at the time, and exacerbated by the overcrowded conditions and military enclosures, as with an outbreak in De Aar and Fraserburg, amongst other

Cape towns, in 1902. In Fraserburg it was reported to be the largest single cause of death for that year with 20 out of 141 deaths reported. It was also commented that the disease was under-notified to the authorities. The District Surgeon of Richmond reported 41 cases, all aged over two years, with 14 deaths which he studied intensely, concluding that they were due to the flow of polluted air down from a large dumping site for refuse. He also experimented giving the new antitoxin in different ways – subcutaneously, orally and rectally – of which the first seemed to give satisfactory results.[5] In 1907 Diphtheria was added to the list of diseases which fell under the provisions of the Public Health Acts of 1883 and 1897, and which was then notifiable. During that year 654 cases were notified in the Cape, the fourth highest after typhoid, tuberculosis and scarlet fever. These came in handfuls of cases from many towns in the Cape, but not in epidemic form.[6]

In the 1920s there were approximately 1,200 to 1,300 cases of diphtheria per year in South Africa, with a case-fatality rate of about 14%, or around 180 deaths per year. One particular outbreak occurred in the Observatory area of Cape Town in 1925, which affected some 30 people and spread to Worcester, causing schools to be closed. By 1926 Schick's method of ascertaining susceptibility to diphtheria, measuring the nature of reaction to an injection of diluted toxin, and the production of active immunity with toxin-antitoxin mixture, had been in general use in Europe and America for several years. However, possibly owing to conflicting reports regarding the keeping properties of both the toxin and the mixture, this prophylactic measure had been neglected in South Africa. Their transportation from Europe proved difficult if the potency was to be maintained.[7]

Immunisation in Cape Town commenced in 1930 with the aim being to immunise every child under 12 years of age. There was a feeling that the African population had a natural immunity to diphtheria, as the incidence of infection in that population was considerably lower than in the European population. A study was done in 1933 to assess the extent and nature of the anti-diphtheria immunity of the African population compared with others. As the immune response was found to be similar to that of Europeans, in that it was acquired general immunity rather than an 'absolute racial immunity', it was concluded that the social factor of conditions of life played an important part in the immunity of Africans against diphtheria. It had been noted in other studies in America that the poorer and more dense the population, the earlier and more regularly diphtheria immunity was developed. It was clear that the so-called natural anti-diphtheritic immunity was acquired as the result of latent but repeated exposure to the diphtheria bacillus, dependent upon the social condition of life and the proportion of the community's daily diphtheritic contacts. It was also observed that the social life of the African infant resulted in far more inter-personal contact than that of the European infant, and certain local customs increased the contact of the infant with different community members. This was thought to be particularly favourable for the establishment of early and rapid antidiphtheritic immunity among Africans, which then accounted for the lower incidence rate of diphtheria amongst that population. The effect of climate on the incidence was not thought to be a significant factor, and if it had any influence at all it was probably because it influenced the social life of the local population promoting more social contact. With Europeans however, it was observed that it was characteristic of Europeans that they:

> Tend to segregate themselves and hold aloof from the rest of the community upon entering new social and climatic conditions, thus maintaining to the greatest possible extent their original mode of life, and thus not exposing themselves to the same epidemiological hazards which confront the indigenous population.[8]

It was postulated that this accounted for the generally observed fact that in tropical and subtropical climates there was a higher rate of susceptibility to diphtheria among the general European population than among the local population, either African or Asiatic. It was concluded that, unlike diseases such as tuberculosis which had been introduced by Europeans and then spread to local peoples, investigations implied that the diphtheria bacillus was already ubiquitous among those populations without any apparent relation to the spread of European civilisation.

The figures for Pretoria illustrated the racial bias in diphtheria with between 22 and 48 European cases occurring annually between 1929 and 1934 and just one or two in Africans. At that time voluntary immunisation was practically non-existent in the city. In special cases contacts were given antitoxin as a prophylactic measure, but the immunity produced lasted not much more than three weeks. It was thought preferable to treat cases early rather than give it routinely to contacts as the antitoxin's effectiveness was less, and it was possibly rendered more toxic, if it had previously been given as a preventive measure. Treatment with antitoxin was given immediately if diphtheria was suspected rather than waiting for a bacteriological report. Active immunisation had by then been proved to be very effective, having been pioneered in New York by Park and Zingher, who instituted wholesale immunisation of school and pre-school children. Deaths in New York from the disease fell from 750 a year to 133 per year following the immunisation drive of 1932-34. Immunisation was recommended for children aged between six months and five years without Schick testing, and for children over five years after Schick testing. However active immunisation had not yet commenced in South Africa and during the 1930s the numbers of cases started to increase with 1,780 cases in 1934.[9] The Department of Health commented: 'That an almost entirely preventable disease like diphtheria should continue to take a heavy toll both by death and crippling of the child population is to be greatly deplored', yet immunisation continued to be inconsistently applied by local authorities across the country.[10] By the mid 1930s the early mixture of toxin-antitoxin used by Park and Zingher had been refined by the use of toxoid preparations which produced fewer side effects. Immunisation continued to be recognised as a need but implementation was still patchy.[11] In 1938 the National Department of Health commenced refunding local authorities for half the cost of immunisation against the disease in order to try and increase the uptake of the vaccine.

There were two outbreaks of milk-borne diphtheria in Cape Town between 1930 and 1945. In both of these virulent diphtheria organisms were recovered from the teats of some of the cows of the milk cows of the herd. Diphtheria outbreaks were linked to ulcerated teats of cows in five outbreaks in Glasgow between 1907 and 1936, and an outbreak in Cardiff in 1928.[12] A study of 276 cases on the Witwatersrand between 1935 and 1939 showed a fatality rate of 8.7%, or 24 deaths, which was a mortality rate of 0.05 per 1,000 population. This was approximately 50% lower than that of England and Wales. The most common strain was the Mitis strain of the disease, which was less virulent than the Gravis type found commonly in Europe. This was considered fortunate as Europe had been experiencing dramatic increases in death-rates from diphtheria.[13] From 1927 a type of diphtheria had arisen which was relatively resistant to antitoxin treatment, appearing first in Berlin and then spreading across Europe. Anderson in England had then shown in 1931 two different types of diphtheria bacteria, the one giving the severe form named Gravis and the milder type named Mitis. In 1933 a third type named Intermediate was identified. The Gravis cases were characterised by greater illness, a high incidence of paralysis and a higher case-fatality rate than the others. They were less responsive to antitoxin treatment and occurred in people who had been actively immunised. The case fatality rate was 13.3% in the Gravis cases compared with 8.6% in Intermedius and 2.3% in Mitis. By 1942 the predominant type in Scotland had changed from Intermedius to Gravis, and the mortality rate increased from 3.4 per 100,000 to 41.8.[14]

In South Africa the events around diphtheria in Europe and changing picture of the disease were giving cause for concern. While the predominant strain in South Africa was still the milder Mitis, the country was at greatly increased contact with at least two areas in which the dangerous Gravis type occurred due to the War. Troops were coming and going between South Africa, Europe and Egypt where the Gravis strain was predominating. The low levels of immunisation and resistance meant that the population were going to be highly at risk should the Gravis strain increase in the country. The disease was one of the three commonest notified diseases and already attacked about 10% of the White child population, of whom around 10% died and many more were permanently disabled.[15]

Murray, in 1942, stated that since 1921 the notified cases of diphtheria had more than trebled, from 1,014 cases in 1921, with 170 deaths, to 3,317 in 1942 with 130 deaths. Following a gradual climb in numbers there had been a steep increase from around 1938 despite the availability of immunisation, with the incidence in Cape Town peaking at 3.36 per 1,000 people for Europeans in 1938-39. The Union Health Department, which subsidized half the cost of the vaccines to local authorities, stated 'Diphtheria forms one of the most serious public health problems of the country…the importance of the subject is not yet fully appreciated; both the public and local authorities are not yet taking sufficiently active steps in connection with the matter'. The highest incidence occurred between birth and five years of age, with the number of deaths highest in the under-four age group, yet immunisation was largely taking place far too late, in the school-age children. After the age of 15 the incidence was low. It therefore pointed to the optimal age of immunisation being less than one year, and around 6-7 months was suggested as ideal. There were also fewer complications from the immunisation at the younger ages, with two doses four weeks apart recommended. It was considered desirable to aim for an immunity of at least 75% of the susceptible population in order to reduce the incidence and mortality of the disease. Murray also recommended the introduction of an immunisation record card, to be given to the parent, and to be 'as jealously guarded as a passport or a birth certificate'. It would include provision for all other vaccines, which at the time included smallpox, typhoid, whooping cough and scarlet fever.[16] He warned that, due to the increasing risk of the Gravis strain, South African should immunize as large a proportion of the European population (that still being the most susceptible) as possible. Schemes were being set up in urban areas for immunisation, but acceptance was voluntary and they touched only a fraction of the children who needed it.

As the War continued and the number of ships arriving increased, bringing with them an increasing risk of infectious diseases, the Department of Health continued to make a plea for immunisation:

> A large number of fatal cases occur each year among children who would otherwise have grown up to be useful citizens, while there is a great deal of invalidity caused by the disease and a considerable amount of chronic ill-health resulting from its after-effects... the immunisation of children against diphtheria should be looked upon by parents as one of their fundamental and essential duties.[17]

Within the railway service diphtheria was the most prevalent of all infectious diseases and they were actively promoting immunisation.

During the period 1941-1946 in Cape Town there were 1,266 cases, of which just 7.4% occurred in children known to be fully immunised. There were 92 deaths in children under 14 years, with the case fatality rate 10 times higher in those who were not immunised.[18] The incidence rate nationally was around 105 per 100,000 population and the death rate around 6.6 per 100,000 in Europeans. This compared with an incidence in Sweden of only 3.5, and in the Netherlands of 15. Even in the relatively badly hit Denmark the incidence was only 28 per 100,000, just a quarter that of South Africa. In 1945 the Union Health Department commented that over the last 10 years there was an average of approximately eight cases notified every day. Pressure mounted for extended immunisation programmes of pre-school children with local authority health visitors and voluntary organisations recommended to assist in 'winning over apathetic or ignorant members of the public'.[19] In the Durban district 515 cases were reported in that year and the Department commented that,

> Until both local authorities and parents awake to their responsibilities to the children of the nation the deplorable toll of death and disease will go on and South African will continue to compare unfavourably with other civilised countries in this respect.[20]

By the 1950s routine immunisation for diphtheria was in place in many countries around the world, and proving so effective that in England the notification and death rates fell by 98.8% between 1941 and 1951 (from 50,797 cases down to 664). France and New Zealand had a 94% drop since 1946 and in Copenhagen, Denmark, the disease had disappeared. However this improvement was not seen in South Africa, where the number of cases had risen from 130 deaths in 1941 to 401 deaths and 3,675 cases in 1952. The rate among Europeans in South Africa was some 30 times higher than in England and Wales. When analysed by race it was found that the hitherto unaffected Non-Europeans, 90% of whom were African, were getting more susceptible to the disease and the incidence had been increasing significantly since the late 1940's. In Johannesburg the incidence had increased from around 30 per 100,000 in 1940 to 86 per 100,000 a decade later, and mortality had increased from 1.8 per 100,000 in 1940 to 16.5 in 1951. 75% of cases were in children less than nine years of age.[21] Similarly in Pietermaritzburg it was noted that from the early 1940's, shortly after the introduction of the immunisation programme, notifications in Africans increased quite dramatically.[22]

Epidemics were reported in 1948 in the Transkei, around Matatiele and Tsolo, deep rural areas set on elevated plateaus to the south east of the country, characterised by hilly, broken ground intersected with deep rugged ravines. Turnbull described the rural area thus:

> The native peoples inhabiting the reserves are mainly Hlubis...who live in circular thatched huts separated from one another. One hut acts as cooking, feeding and sleeping accommodation while in another the mealies are stored. Furniture as such does not exist and the inmates sleep on the floor wrapped in a blanket. Sometimes one blanket covers as many as three children. Three or four huts house a family and a group of families, comprising 20 to 30 huts, comprises a kraal ... the mass of the people still adhere to their animistic beliefs. This is most noticeable in any adversity such as sickness. This is believed to be caused by a spell cast upon the place where the patient falls sick. The 'treatment' is to remove the patient from the bewitched area and call in the witch doctor to exorcize the spell. The ease with which infectious diseases can spread among these people can, therefore, be readily understood.[23]

However he commented that diphtheria had, up until then, been considered rare in African natives. The first cases seen by the District Surgeon at the beginning of March 1948 were then sent back to their homes after receiving one dose of anti-diphtheritic serum, in the belief that it wouldn't spread. Up until this point the biggest outbreak had only affected up to a dozen at a time. But by the 19th March there had been 20 cases and an emergency isolation hospital had to be opened in an old military camp with 40 beds for Africans and two for Europeans. The highest incidence occurred in the 5-10 year age group, although also affecting the 1-5 and 10-15 year age groups, with very few adults. The population had never been immunised and it appeared that the pre-school child was not exposed to the same risk of infection as the older child. There were altogether 142 cases, 57.6% of whom were female, and approximately 25 deaths, although only five of these were in hospitalized patients. Patients struggled to reach hospitals, having to travel by horse, sledge or on their mothers' backs for many miles to reach the nearest road, and it was thought unlikely that all cases were identified, some having died at home without notification.

By the mid-1940s penicillin was being tried as a treatment for diphtheria and the low death rate in hospital was ascribed to the use of penicillin, in addition to anti-diphtheritic serum. Penicillin had also been found effective as a way to eradicate carriers when applied locally to the nose and throat. Throughout the epidemic teams were despatched to immunize as many children as possible but it was hard to reach some of the homes in the deep rural areas, many of them only accessible with horses. It was also difficult to acquire sufficient vaccine due to the lengthy supply route via Durban and the amount required. Many children were immunised at school and ultimately almost 9,000 immunisations were given, with the epidemic finally over after 10 weeks.[24]

The outbreak in Tsolo, on a plateau to the north of Umtata, had 88 confirmed cases with 15 deaths affecting a similar age group. Turnbull again describes the local Africans as he sees them: 'the people are Pondomises and, except in the hilly regions of the south where they are very primitive, they belong to the class known as 'dressed natives'. Their standards of education and intelligence are slightly higher than that of the 'red' or 'blanketed' native. Nevertheless they live in very primitive conditions and witchcraft, with the consequent transference of sick cases, is prevalent'. The outbreak started in February 1948 peaking in May affecting mainly children from 1 year to 15 years, and probably spread partly through school contact. The population had not been immunised and, as in Matatiele, they were treated with a combination of anti-diphtheritic serum and penicillin. Swabs had to be sent to East London, a distance of 150 miles, which took the train – which only ran three days a week - 16 hours, and bacterial confirmation was difficult. However 88 of the 153 suspect cases were confirmed with Mitis strain of diphtheria. In both this outbreak and the Matatiele outbreak it was thought that the infection was predisposed to by an associated streptococcal sore throat.[25]

It was clear that, unlike in European countries, the routine immunisation programme in South Africa was grossly ineffective. It was estimated that an immunisation rate of between 55% and 80% in infants and around 95% in school children would be required in order to eradicate the disease.[26] In South Africa no returns of numbers of vaccinations were submitted by local authorities but it was estimated that the percentage of children immunised was far below 70%, even in urban European areas. In Cape Town the Medical Officer of Health had applied for permission to combine it with whooping cough vaccine and combined immunisation commenced in January 1950, giving a series of three injections at monthly intervals [27] However, the situation still didn't improve with 113 cases in the city in 1955 and 9 deaths.

Johannesburg suffered 510 cases of diphtheria in 1951 and 572 the following year. An analysis of 519 of the cases in Europeans found a case mortality rate of 7.7% and 4% of those who recovered had a residual defect such as abnormal heart function, or paralysis of the palate. The mortality rate was unacceptably high and it was suggested that antibiotics were having little influence in preventing death. The more important treatment was the administration of antitoxin before the fourth day of illness. 75% of the Johannesburg cases were in children under 12 and 32% had been previously immunised against the disease.[28] A further analysis of 1,135 cases in non-Europeans in Johannesburg between 1952 and 1954 was undertaken by Dubb, of which 1,017 were African with 92% under 12 years of age. The case fatality rate was 12.3%, mainly due to acute toxic myocarditis and circulatory failure along with bronchopneumonia and pharyngeal paralysis, and the high death rate was attributed largely to a delay in seeking medical attention. Whether or not they had been previously immunised was not stated, but Dubbs concluded that:

> the tragedy is the large number of cases which made the article possible. In most other countries the scourge of diphtheria has disappeared. In South Africa the battle scarcely seems to have begun. ... the weapon has been in our hands now for many years, but active immunisation is still not practised on a sufficiently large scale.[29]

He recommended compulsory immunisation of infants. Immunisation rates were still lagging behind the necessary levels however. In Johannesburg they estimated their initial immunisation rate at around 66%, with a booster dose rate of only 15%, and it was noted that the diphtheria rate had remained unchanged over a period of 30 years, despite this vaccination programme. The risk of contracting diphtheria in the Witwatersrand area up to 20 years of age was still estimated at between 2.5 and 3%.[30] The incidence stayed static, there being 3,342 cases in 1956. Cape Town, which had a rapidly increasing immunisation programme, had only 49 of these. Immunisation with diphtheria toxoid was recommended from around six months of age given in two doses over a 4-6 week interval. Passive immunisation with antitoxin was used for treatment and also for prophylaxis in contacts. It was also given combined with tetanus and pertussis (whooping cough) vaccine in three doses, with a booster dose two years later and again at school age.

By the end of the 1950's the number of cases however remained stubbornly high at around 3,000 annually which, commented the Department of Health repetitively each year, was appallingly high in comparison with that of other 'civilised countries'. Even Cape Town, with its comprehensive immunisation facilities, was struggling to keep the numbers down. With 87 cases and six deaths in 1960 the Medical Officer of Health, Professor Cooper, stated that it was most disappointing, and due to parents having been lulled into a false sense of security by the progress of the previous twenty years over what was still a dangerous and fatal disease, but warned 'diphtheria will always be a killer in so far as the non-immune is concerned'.[31] Despite vaccinating almost 28,000 children the following year there were still 78 cases in the city, although by 1965 it had reached an all-time low of 12 cases with five deaths, all in unimmunised children, which Professor Cooper attributed to:

> The criminal and callous neglect of indifferent parents ... despite intensive home follow-ups, propaganda and press publicity, a small hard core of parents, through laziness, indifference or for other reasons, are not prepared to have their children protected against the preventable diseases.[32]

In Durban the incidence had been in decline since the peak of 1944, when the notification rate was 209 per 100,000 to 20 in 1957, although it was suspected that only one third of cases in Africans were notified. Over 70% of children in the municipal area were receiving at least the first dose of vaccine. However the overall death rate remained high, with it being observed that the disease seemed to take a more malignant course in Asians and Africans.[33]

The disease continued through the 1960's at only slightly reduced levels with an incidence nationally of around 11 per 100,000 population which was still considered 'alarmingly high, notwithstanding the fact that the very effective vaccine with which children are immunised is supplied free of charge by the Department of Health'. It continued 'the failure of so many parents so ensure the immunisation of their children against this serious disease can only be attributed to ignorance or indifference'.[34] Some of the cities, however, were making significant progress due to their ability to reach out and successfully vaccinate their populations. Port Elizabeth, which in 1964 had had 104 cases and 11 deaths, made progress over the next decade with the Medical Officer of Port Elizabeth commenting in 1975 'Diphtheria has virtually been eliminated from the infectious disease scene in Port Elizabeth. This is an amazing phenomenon if one considers the high incidence in this area not so many years ago'.[35] There was, overall, a gradual reduction in numbers of cases notified across South Africa, with 569 in 1970 falling to 91 in 1979 and 28 in 1983, which was a drop in incidence from a high of 34 in 1944 to just 0.1 in 1983.The number of deaths from the disease followed the downward trend, the case-fatality rate being remarkably constant at around 7%.[36]

While diphtheria globally was on the decline due to the roll out of the Expanded Programme of Immunisation of the World Health Organisation, major epidemics continued to occur when vaccination programmes broke down. Epidemics occurred in Eastern Europe and Central Asia in the late 1980s and early 1990s, with Russia experiencing an epidemic which between 1990 and 1995 had resulted in 125,000 cases and 4,000 deaths. In South Africa however during 1989 only 11 cases were notified, and in 1990 there were 34 cases and one death. The age group most affected were between 5 and 14, although 13 cases were in adults, and they all occurred in the first half of the year. Eight of the 13 adult cases occurred in Europeans in Durban during March, and another cluster of 10 cases in children occurred in Mount Fletcher in the Transkei during the early months of the year.[37] While in the year 2000 there were 30,000 cases of diphtheria in Africa and the developing world with 3,000 deaths, in South Africa the national drive to improve vaccination coverage, driven largely by the goal of eradicating polio as part of the global campaign, lead to the virtual disappearance of the disease. With the national immunisation coverage with three doses of the combined diphtheria/tetanus/pertussis vaccine standing at 98% in 2008, and 107% in 2009, diphtheria had finally vanished from the local scene although, as the Russian experience illustrated, should the vaccination programme falter it may well arise again to repeat the devastation of the past.

ENDNOTES

1. Laidler P.W. and Gelfand M. *South Africa its medical history, 1652-1898: A medical and social study* C Struik, Cape Town, 1971:61
2. Matthews J.W. *Incwadi Yami or Twenty Years Personal Experience in South Africa; 1887*; Africana Book Society 1976:15
3. Mathias J .cited in Gilder S.S.B. 'South African patients and their diseases in the 1880s' *South African Medical Journal* 66(7) August 1984:250-252
4. Murray J.F. 'The significance of C Diphtheriae Gravis on the epidemiology of diphtheria' *South African Medical Journal* 17(21) 1943:337-338
5. Traill David, 'Report of the District Surgeon for Richmond', in *Reports on the Public Health for the year 1902*, Cape of Good Hope, Cape Times Ltd 1903; G66-1903, p130-136
6. Gregory A.J. *Report of the Medical Officer of Health for the Colony on the Public Health for the calendar year 1907*; Cape of Good Hope, Cape Times Ltd 1908; G33-1908; p xxvii
7. Silberbauer S.F. 'The Activity of Schick Reaction Products' *South African Medical Record* 24(9) 1926:207
8. Grasset E. et al, 'Studies on the Nature of Antidiphtheritic Immunity among South African Bantu by means of the Schick Test and Anti-toxin Titrations' *South African Medical Journal*; 7(23) 1933:779-785.
9. Donnolly F.A. and Nelson H. 'Some Observations on the Control of Infectious Disease, *South African Medical Journal* 9(18) 1935:629-641
10. *Annual Report of the Department of Public Health, 1935*, Government Printer Pretoria, UG No 34-'35, p23-24.
11. *Annual Report of the Department of Public Health, 1937*, Government Printer Pretoria, UG No 52-'37, p34
12. Fehrsen F.O. 'Pasteurisation of Milk', Report submitted to the City Council of Cape Town, in *South African Medical Journal* 19(17) 1945:302-305
13. Murray J.F. 'Diphtheria on the Witwatersrand: a bacteriological, clinical and epidemiological survey' *South African Medical Journal* 16(13) 1942:247-250
14. Murray J.F. 'The significance of C Diphtheriae Gravis on the epidemiology of diphtheria', *South African Medical Journal* 17(21) 1943:337-338
15. *Annual Report of the Department of Public Health, 1940*, Government Printer Pretoria, UG No 8-'40, p28.
16. Murray N.L. 'Age for Diphtheria Immunisation in South Africa' *South African Medical Journal* 17(21) 1942:334-337
17. *Annual Report of the Department of Public Health, 1941*, Government Printer Pretoria, UG 46- '41, p21
18. Woodrow A.P. 'Diphtheria Immunisation in Cape Town and its problems' *South African Medical Journal* 20(24) 1946:781-782
19. *Annual Report of the Department of Public Health, 1945*, Government Printer Pretoria, UG No 6-'46, p12
20. *Annual Report of the Department of Public Health, 1946*, Government Printer Pretoria, UG No 18- '47, p14
21. Bokkenheuser V. and Heymann C.S. 'Diphtheria in South Africa' *South African Medical Journal* 28(33) 1954:685-689
22. 'Annual Reports of the Medical Officer of Health', *Pietermaritzburg Corporation Yearbooks*, Pietermaritzburg City Council, 1940-1952

23. Turnbull N.S. 'Diphtheria in African Natives in the Transkei, South Africa' *Transactions of the Royal Society of Tropical Medicine and Hygiene*, 43(2) September 1949:222
24. Turnbull N.S. 'Diphtheria in African Natives in the Transkei', *South African Medical Journal* 23(27) 1949:551-556
25. Turnbull N.S. 'Diphtheria in African Natives in the Transkei, South Africa' *Transactions of the Royal Society of Tropical Medicine and Hygiene*, 43(2), September 1949:215-224
26. Bokkenheuser V. and Heymann C.S. 'Diphtheria in South Africa' *South African Medical Journal*, 28(33) 1954:688
27. *Annual Report of the Medical Officer of Health, City of Cape Town, 1950*, Cape Times Ltd Parow 1950; p25
28. Bokkenheuser V. 'An analysis of 519 cases of Diphtheria in Johannesburg 1951-1952' *South African Medical Journal* 29(20) 1955:461-468
29. Dubb A. 'Clinical Diphtheria in the Non-European' *South African Medical Journal* 29(25) 1955:586-590
30. Bokkenheuser V.' Diphtheria Immunisation in Johannesburg and Boksburg from 1935 to 1955' *South African Medical Journal*, 29(53) 1955:1249-1254
31. Cooper E.D. *Annual Report of the Medical Officer of Health*, City of Cape Town, 1960:4
32. Cooper E.D. *Annual Report of the Medical Officer of Health*, City of Cape Town, 1965:2
33. Bokkenheuser V. and Stephen A. 'Diphtheria in Durban: morbidity, mortality and prevention' *South African Medical Journal* 35(14) April 1961:289-294
34. *Report of the Department of Health for the years 1965, 1966 and 1967,* Published by Authority, 1969, RP 53/1969:17
35. Sher J.N. *Annual Report of the Medical Officer of Health*, Port Elizabeth, 1975, p(ii)
36. Küstner H.G.V. 'Secular trends of selected diseases', *Epidemiological Comments*, 11(3) March 1984:11
37. Department of National Health and Population Development, *Epidemiological Comments*, 18(7) July 1990:168

13   CONCLUSION: A MENACE TO WHOSE HEALTH?

While it appears that infectious diseases at an epidemic level – with the exception of malaria - were virtually unknown in South Africa prior to the arrival of European settlers, subsequent to that event in the 1650s they emerged and took hold on the population to devastating effect. The vast majority were brought on ships, further exacerbated in later centuries by the great increase in shipping and population movements during the various wars. Once they had arrived, these diseases generally moved through the country with great speed as they found their way out of the settler population into the vulnerable local and indigenous peoples, who lacked immunity. Only rarely, as with malaria, do we find the converse situation, where the local population had acquired more resistance and it was the settler population who were the more devastated. One of the few diseases not to spread through the country due to ship-borne arrivals was cholera which, due to quarantine measures eventually introduced at ports to contain other diseases, was successfully held at bay. It was, however, brought in through the mass movements of migrant labour who travelled in from other African countries to the north, and spread it on their way through Mpumulanga and KwaZulu-Natal. Once in the country it showed a predilection for the deep rural areas, without piped water supplies or sanitation, and highlighted the neglect of the development of the rural areas.

In addition, the European population not only brought most of these diseases, which perhaps could be considered an unwitting and unplanned accident of fate, but they then often facilitated their spread throughout the country and to previously unexposed communities. One of the first of these may have been spread inland by the Europeans themselves, as the Voortrekkers carried leprosy into the interior while they migrated across the land. Other diseases spread through the mass movement of African populations across the country, and indeed the sub-continent, brought about by labour policies designed to serve the growing needs of the colonial period. Such diseases as syphilis, influenza, typhoid and typhus were spread in this manner, and people without resistance were brought into malarious areas to work to disastrous effect. These movements were often exacerbated by restrictive legal policies and forced removals, which directly caused the disease to enter new areas of the country as people moved to escape detention - as with leprosy and syphilis - or as people were removed from cities to un-monitored, overcrowded and neglected townships – as with typhoid. The industrialisation of the Witwatersrand and construction of its mining industry was one of the most visible causes of spread of disease, as it created the mass movement of hundreds of thousands of men across the country and region into grossly overcrowded male hostels, which clearly were going to facilitate the spread of infectious disease. The state of medical knowledge at that time was quite sufficient to know that it was an obvious disaster waiting to happen, and their establishment was clearly a direct act of negligence. Its catastrophic impact on other diseases such as influenza, tuberculosis and smallpox were predictable and inevitable. Also predictable was the rise in prostitution and casual sex that happened as a response to the enforced separation of young men from their wives and families, causing the massive increase in syphilis at a time when it was scarcely treatable and had serious, often fatal, health consequences.

Diseases were thus spread not just across the Rand, but from there taken back to rural areas as men migrated backwards and forwards across the country. Hence syphilis and influenza found their way into villages in deep, rural areas. The overall picture created in the rural areas by the reports of the Resident Magistrates of the early twentieth century was one of previously healthy rural communities being increasingly subject to the ravages of illnesses brought back from the mines – tuberculosis, syphilis, pneumonia, the disease later recognised as typhus, influenza, and smallpox. The African rural lifestyle involved sleeping in close quarters in huts and kraals, in poorly ventilated dwellings, which exacerbated the spread of these previously unknown conditions. The overcrowded huts may have been contributed to by the Hut Tax, in which Africans paid tax on each hut, which would have been a disincentive to reduce congestion by building more. This overcrowding was often further exacerbated by the evolving custom of wearing European clothing, without adequate means to wash and dry them – a problem particularly linked with increasing pneumonia, tuberculosis ('sitting around in wet clothes' being frequently mentioned by Magistrates) and typhus - and a gradual change in dietary habits towards less nutritious foodstuffs. Was there ever a country with a more perfect system for the propagation and spread of epidemic disease to the previously innocent and untouched? Yet even at the time of writing, over 120 years later, the hostel and migrant labour system remains in place, albeit at a lower level.

In addition diseases were spread both locally and internationally by mass movements due to war – the movement of typhoid, dysentery, measles, smallpox and diphtheria during the Anglo-Boer War, influenza during the First World War and the spread of polio and new strains of diphtheria in the Second World War are examples. The mass movement of labour to-and-from the mines, and the movement of troops and refugees during the Anglo-Boer War, combined to spread infectious diseases the length and breadth of the country so that by 1902 they were reported regularly by all District Surgeons, Native Commissioners and Medical Officers of Health. Conditions in the insanitary towns and cities were perfect for disease to take hold and spread – report after report details the appalling situation regarding water supplies, sanitation, refuse removal, housing and overcrowding which existed in almost every town and city in the country, with few exceptions. Dire warnings and graphic descriptions – strongly expressed by men who clearly had no fear of town councils or authorities in their desire to speak the truth - were regularly submitted in the Reports, but seemingly ignored (interestingly even after more than 100 years of reporting on the evils of the 'bucket system' it remains in place in some locations of the country).

The implementation of Martial Law during the Anglo-Boer War was of varying effect – in Oudtshoorn the District Surgeon commented 'The Town Council was destitute of any sanitary regulations, due to the negligence of the central authorities, until Martial Law took the matter up, and framed a very complete set of rules and regulations, and it can only be added that the sanitation and general cleanliness of the town was never in such a perfect condition as it was during the period of Martial Law'. He continued in respect of the village of Dysseldorp after Martial Law ended 'The sanitation and general arrangements of the place are fast assuming that primitive order which was the general condition prior to Martial Law and water closets ... are fast becoming dilapidated, whilst pools and ponds etc are being formed in all directions'. However Martial Law also restricted free movement to implement other control measures for infectious disease.[1] In the years after the War there were attempts to improve sanitation, but problems persisted with open, contaminated water courses, inadequate disposal of excrement and no method of refuse or slop water removal, and conditions remained much in the African and Coloured locations.

The insanitary, congested conditions of the towns and cities, exacerbated by the War, also created the conditions for plague shortly after. Once established in the country the response to these epidemic diseases often varied, right from the dawn of foreign settlement, according to the perceived threat to the White population. Responses also were frequently different for each sector of the population, depending on their perceived acceptability at that time – hence if found with syphilis in the early 1800's the Khoikhoi woman would be exiled beyond the Salt River, the slave would be given corporal punishment, and the European woman would be sentenced to bread and water for 10 days. Men appeared to suffer no punishment.

Leprosy was treated in almost all cases by separation and isolation, and the suffering of all races on Robben Island and elsewhere was tragically detailed. Although publicized and argued about, it remained the same for many, many years. With the plague and typhoid the response generally was to eject African people from the towns and cities to inadequate and hastily constructed settlements. For Europeans the policy was to improve housing and sanitary infrastructure, as had been applied in the sanitation revolution in England, and it never seemed to be seriously considered that such an approach may work equally well for Africans. Once ejected to the periphery they remained neglected and in deteriorating slums, such that when the same diseases arose again some years later the Europeans were, rather remarkably, surprised at this natural consequence of their decisions, which then was seen as a serious threat to their health, demanding drastic measures. In addition however, there was the application of tried and tested public health policies – of isolation, quarantine and vaccination where possible, which did have a significant impact in limiting the spread of the diseases in many cases. Still it was largely practised in a 'crisis management' mode, with no coordinated attempt to continue the programmes in rural areas or between epidemics. This was not unobserved by the medical fraternity and District Surgeons however, whose reports often eloquently and vociferously tried to draw attention to the need for concerted efforts on public health interventions.

Notwithstanding that these diseases had been introduced largely by the White community to a previously healthy African population, the attitude of many of the White population was summarised by the Native Commissioner of Carolina in 1910:

> The Natives, through contact with the white inhabitants, are a menace to the health of the white community ... most of the infectious diseases originate in their midst ...[2]

Again and again throughout the twentieth century in South Africa we only see evidence of a response to an epidemic disease when there is a perceived threat to the White population. There was then often a grossly exaggerated, almost hysterical response to the disease – the responses to smallpox, leprosy, the threat of cholera and plague in the major cities, syphilis throughout the first half of the century, and typhus in the 1930s, all displayed levels of over-reaction and gross disregard for the human rights of the African population in order to stop the 'menace to the European population'. The enforced fumigation at the typhus disinfestation stations, public examinations of men for syphilis at the Pass Offices, and forced removals after plague serve as dramatic examples of racially-based interventions which were not, and could not have been, applied to the White population. While it is undeniable that the diseases required determined and well-planned interventions to bring them under control, it was notable that these only became a priority when they approached the European settlements, and were often ignored while smouldering and causing morbidity, mortality and misery in the African locations. Indeed many of the actions taken only served to push the diseases back into the locations by forced removals, where they could remain out of sight and mind until once more becoming visible in White areas. This is clearly exemplified in the example of New Brighton in Port Elizabeth, where the black population was removed to after the outbreak of plague. Some 65 years later it was an outbreak of typhoid that lead to the realisation that the township had languished there, untouched for decades, and deteriorated into a slum.

As a strategy to defeat specific diseases this differentiated treatment of the Black population was also often ineffective, and caused South Africa to fall far behind the countries of Europe in controlling these infections. Only rarely does a glimmer of equitable concern for the welfare of the African population come through, usually contained in the reports of the earlier Medical Officers of Health or District Surgeons, or by an official such as a Magistrate or Native Commissioner stationed deep within the rural communities. It is also, however, highly possible that some of the medical and other officials belaboured the point about the possible threat to the White population in their Reports as a tactical strategy, in order to secure funding for public health interventions from White politicians, knowing that a humanitarian approach on behalf of the black population was less likely to be successful. Funding for improvements to housing, water and sanitation services for the poor was often only forthcoming in many societies, including England, when the interests of the powerful and wealthy were directly at risk, and it would not be the only era in which Medical Officers of Health and public health officials used such a strategy.

Marks and Anderson felt that epidemics highlight the nature of power relations in society. While the officially recognized epidemics may no longer be the former killers of smallpox, cholera and bubonic plague, they comment 'the outbreak of epidemics reveals the concerns of the state and the ruling class in society, both with their own safety and with the reproduction of the labour force'. They continue:

> The presence in South Africa of a conquered and colonized black working class led to the development of policies of racial segregation that also served as a public health strategy to protect white settlers. In the early twentieth century public health officials were in the forefront of the demand for urban residential segregation. For Blacks the experience of public health was by and large authoritarian and repressive. As in the rest of colonial Africa the state intervened when there was danger of disease spreading to the White settlers, and was relatively unconcerned when there was not.[3]

Swanson clearly elucidated these policies in his defining of 'The Sanitation Syndrome' in respect of plague in particular, where the outbreaks were used to motivate the creation of separate residential areas for Africans, and Deacon makes similar points in respect of the unbalanced, racially based treatment meted out sufferers from leprosy and the expansionist agendas of the colonial secretary, Montague.[4,5]

However, when considering the apparently overly-draconian measures which were applied to the control of some of these diseases, an attempt has to be made to put oneself in the context of the times. Before the antibiotic and vaccine era all of them were untreatable and often fatal, or if survived had terrifying sequelae such as gross disfigurement (e.g. smallpox and leprosy) or severe physical handicaps (e.g. polio and diphtheria). Sufferers would often face a chronic and horrific decline over many years (e.g. syphilis) with no hope of recovery. In the present human rights era, when the rights of the infected are often seen to override the rights of the uninfected, it is sometimes hard to recall that drastic public health measures were applied all over the world to prevent the spread of fatal and dreaded epidemic diseases. Still, this was not usually done on such a blatant racially discriminatory basis as in South Africa.

What is perhaps more unforgiveable, as there is not even the mitigating factor of fear, is the uneven treatment meted out to sufferers where effective treatments were known to exist. The deliberate undertreating of syphilis in black patients by the National Department of

Public Health in the 1930s, described at the time by Cluver as 'frankly revolting', was inexcusable.[6] The lack of effort to vaccinate in rural areas until disease once again threatened Europeans in town - applicable to most of the infectious diseases - and the minimal effort to improve living conditions in black areas were indefensible. The dehumanising mass disinfestation for typhus in the Transkei and at the stations, and herd examinations for syphilis as mentioned above, purely to allay White fears, fall into the same category, as do the casual uses of potentially dangerous measures such as dusting with DDT to prevent typhus escaping the Transkei, and the wildly experimental use of drugs and other treatments for leprosy and other diseases. As Bettzieche noted in his study regarding polio, it highlighted early patterns of disease and discrimination in the prevention and treatment which ran along the lines demarcated by Apartheid, and the differences in provision of health services according to race foreshadowed the segregation of health services in the 1960s and 70s.[7] When one looks at the patterns in disease through South African history, their introduction into the country, mode of spread, prevention, treatment and consequences, there is more evidence to suggest that the European population was a menace to the health of the Black population than vice versa, yet the theme of 'White man as Victim' prevails throughout the general discourse.

Whether through racially-biased measures or not, all of the diseases discussed were brought under control at the time of writing. Many factors played a part, malaria for example being brought down significantly by a range of environmental interventions including relocation of dwellings, screening of buildings, planting of trees, draining swamps and canalisation. Similarly it was modification of the environment through water, sanitation and hygiene improvements which reduced the threat and spread of typhoid and cholera in urban areas, and the implementation of rodent control measures which largely defeated plague. These were aided by technological progress such as the discovery of the insecticide DDT and its application to mosquito, flea and lice control and the pasteurisation of milk, which were dramatically effective in their impact on the diseases of malaria, plague, typhus, and typhoid along with other milk-borne diseases.

The use of immunological agents to control epidemics clearly had it first expression in the case of smallpox vaccination, which had its origins in ancient practices in North Africa and India, progressed to 'arm-to-arm' transfer of the vaccine material, and then became refined to a phenomenally effective medical intervention, limited only by the inability of programmes to reach all the population. Vaccines for other infectious diseases followed quite rapidly in the early decades of the twentieth century, of varying efficacy, and not without unfortunate mistakes. However, by the 1960s many of the diseases covered had effective vaccines which, by the late 1990s, had all but eradicated the diseases – polio, diphtheria and measles being examples. Of course this could have happened a lot earlier had they been applied equally across the country from the 1960s. However in the intervening decades South Africa had been applying the principle of separate development for different ethnic or racial groups, which had lead to the existence of some 14 separate Departments of Health by 1994, (for each Province, each 'Homeland', and each 'race') all of which undertook health programmes in different ways or with varying levels of efficiency. In addition South Africa had become increasingly isolated from the rest of Africa and the world, this being illustrated in the comments of Fenner in a World Health Organisation report in respect of the lack of progress in eradicating smallpox, where the country had fallen behind other countries in the region.[8]

Other diseases were controlled largely by antibiotics which came into play from the 1930's, but were dramatically enhanced by the discovery of penicillin during World War 2. It was these antibiotics that made the critical difference in defeating the diseases of leprosy and syphilis and made other diseases such as typhoid, typhus and the plague less fatally threatening.

Another interesting aspect of the occurrence of infectious diseases in South Africa, as indeed in other parts of the world, is the way they arise in a time line of wave after wave of successive diseases. While each is defeated in turn, either by public infrastructure improvements such as water, sanitation, waste management, housing and drainage; or by medical interventions such as vaccines, antibiotics or diagnostic tests; or simply by what appears to be the development of increased resistance in a population, so another disease arises to take their place. This is of particular interest in such epidemics as the emergence of typhus at the beginning of the twentieth century, diphtheria and poliomyelitis in the middle decades, and measles in the latter half of that century. If one were to superimpose incidence graphs of these diseases on top of one another from 1650, one would see the earliest diseases of smallpox and leprosy in the first two hundred years gradually working their way across the country, overlapping with a rising tide of syphilis, typhoid and plague following industrialisation and uncontrolled urbanisation towards the end of the 19th century. In the early years of the twentieth century arise typhus and devastating influenza, seemingly almost from nowhere, and the increasing recognition of malaria as a serious problem which had hitherto been simply avoided. By the middle of that century, when typhus and influenza had faded and progress was being made with syphilis and smallpox, the formidable epidemics of diphtheria and polio had emerged. In fact it had been clearly identified that as progress was made in other areas, such as improved sanitation and lowered infant mortality rate, so the polio attack rate would paradoxically increase. In his address on the State of the Union's Health, on 21 August 1958, Minister M.D.C. de Wet Nel dealt with polio, diphtheria, enteric fever (typhoid), leprosy, malaria and tuberculosis, showing which epidemic diseases were occupying a prominent position in the health of the country.[9] Then as these diseases start to finally come under control in the 1960's emerges measles – hovering in the background for decades but never really identified as a major issue – as a serious cause of morbidity and mortality in African children. This is closely followed by cholera, kept away from the country for hundreds of years, but finally erupting in massive epidemics from 1980 onwards.

By the year 2012 the only problematic epidemic diseases in South Africa out of the twelve presented here were syphilis, mainly due to its relationship with AIDS, and malaria which remains a regional problem due to weaker control programmes north of the border. In addition of course is tuberculosis, which has run a devastating course throughout most of the last 150 years, but which is not considered here as it is an on-going and complex epidemic, rapidly changing in nature. It is a condition which is of major significance to the history of the country and its development, and has been much written about, in respect both of its links with the industrialisation process and migrant labour, and also in its resurgence due to its links with the HIV/AIDS epidemic. All ten of the other diseases in this book have largely disappeared off the radar, although cholera and non-epidemic typhoid may still be waiting in the wings. Yet, despite the absence of these diseases, still mortality rates and life expectancy are getting worse overall due to the impact of what may be called the AIDS/TB co-epidemic. This continues to devastate the population, although it is the subject of a great volume of research and new, more effective treatment regimes for AIDS continue to be developed. Hopefully these will start to bring the disease under control, which will then probably be followed by a decline in tuberculosis. Due to numerous other books on the topic the HIV/AIDS epidemic also is not covered here, but it gives cause to wonder, and perhaps to fear, what may emerge to take its place if it is finally defeated.

ENDNOTES

1. Russell G. 'Report of the District Surgeon for Oudtshoorn 1902' *Cape of Good Hope Reports on the Public Health, 1902*; Cape Times 1903; G66-1903:105.
2. 'Native Commissioner, Carolina', in: 'Public Health Report, Cape of Good Hope', *Blue Book on Native Affairs*, Union of South Africa 1910; U17-1910; p99.
3. Marks S. and Anderson N. 'Typhus and Social Control: South Africa 1917-1950' in MacLeod R. and Lewis M. Disease, *Medicine and Empire, perspectives on Western Medicine and the experience of European Expansion*; Routledge, London, 1988:259.
4. Swanson M.W. 'The Sanitation Syndrome: Bubonic Plague and Urban Native Policy in the Cape Colony 1900-1909' *Journal of African History* 18, 1977: 410.
5. Deacon H. 'Leprosy and Racism at Robben Island' in Heyningen E, *Studies in the History of Cape Town*, UCT Press in association with the Centre for African Studies, Cape Town, 1994:70
6. Cluver E.H. 'Syphilis and the Public *Health*' *South African Medical Journal* 14(23) 14 December 1940:457
7. Bettzieche W.K. *Polio, people and Apartheid: the South African Poliomyelitis Epidemics of the 1940s and 1950s with special reference to the Cape Peninsula* Thesis for a BA Honours Degree, University of Cape Town, 1998:101
8. Fenner F. Henderson D.A. Arita I. Ježek Z, Ladnyi I.D. 'Smallpox and its eradication' World Health Organisation; *History of International Public Health No 6*, Geneva, 1988:984
9. De Wet Nel M.D.C. 'Poliomyelitis: Statement by Minister of Health' *South African Medical Journal* 32(23) 7 June 1958:600.

BIBLIGRAPHY

Publications, Journal Articles and Government Reports

Allen Peter, 'Some general aspects of Poliomyelitis' *South African Medical Journal*, 19(1) 1945:2

Anderson Jasper A. 'Influenza in Cape Town' *South African Medical Record*, 17(3) January 11 1919:36-39

Andrewes C.H. 'Influenza Today and Tomorrow' *South African Medical Journal* 29(1) 1955:3-7

Annecke S. 'Malaria Control in The Transvaal', *South African Medical Journal* 9(1) 1935:3

Anning C.C.P. 'Meteorological factors in the incidence of malaria in Pietermaritzburg' *South African Medical Journal* 8(23) 1934:875-878

Annual Reports of the Department of Public Health, Union of South Africa, Government Printer, Pretoria, years 1927; 1930; 1933; 1935; 1939; 1940; 1941; 1946; 1953; 1959-64.

Annual Reports of the Medical Officer of Health, Cape Town, Cape Times Ltd Parow

Annual Report of the Medical Officer of Health for Port Elizabeth, 1975, Longs, Port Elizabeth 1975

Annual Reports of the Medical Officer of Health, Pietermaritzburg, Pietermaritzburg Corporation Yearbooks, 1940-1952

Anonymous; 'Lepers at the Cape: wanted, a Father Damien' *Blackwood's Edinburgh Magazine*, Vol CXLVI no DCCCLXXXVII September 1889:295

Anonymous; 'More about the Lepers at the Cape, Memorandum for the information of the readers of 'Blackwood's Magazine''; *Blackwood's Edinburgh Magazine*, Vol CXLVI No DCCCLXXXIX November 1889:743-746

Ashe E. Oliver; 'Some Random Recollections of the Kimberley Influenza Epidemic' *South African Medical Record*, 17(1), January 11 1919: 6-9

Bain-Marais C. 'Prevalence of Venereal Diseases', *Debates of the House of Assembly*, 34, 28 April 1939:3714-3754

Baines Gary; 'The Control and Administration of Port Elizabeth's African Population circa 1834-1923' *Contree* 26 1989:16

Baker J. *Submission to the Commission Appointed to enquire into, and report upon, the best means of moving the Asylum at Robben Island to the Mainland*; Saul Solomon and Co 1880

Balfour T. 'TB and Malaria in SADC countries' in: *South African Health Review 2002*, Health Systems Trust Durban 2002:315-320.

Barrett E. *Report of the Department of Native Affairs for the years 1913-1918*, Cape Times Ltd 1919, UG 7-19

Bateman C. 'Cholera: getting the basics right' *South African Medical Journal [online]*; 99(3) Cape Town March 2009:132-136

Baumann E.P. 'Poliomyelitis' *Medical Journal of South Africa*, XIII (6) January 1918:87

Behr S. 'The Treatment of Sulfa-Resistant Gonococci with Penicillin' *South African Medical Journal* 18(21) 1944:369-372

Bekker A.E. *The History of False Bay up to 1795*; Simon's Town Historical Society 1990

Bettzieche W.K. *Polio, people and Apartheid: the South African Poliomyelitis Epidemics of the 1940s and 1950s with special reference to the Cape Peninsula* Thesis for a BA Honours Degree, University of Cape Town, 1998:101

Bickford-Smith, Vivian, *Ethnic Pride and Racial Prejudice in Victorian Cape Town*, Witwatersrand University Press, Johannesburg 1995

Bokkenheuser V. and Heymann C.S. 'Diphtheria in South Africa' *South African Medical Journal* 28(33) 1954:685-689

Bolger James T. 'Report of the District Surgeon for 1902; Cape of Good Hope', *Reports on the Public Health 1902*; Cape Times Ltd 1903, G66-1903;

Blumberg C. *The provision of Medical Literature and Information in the Cape 1827-1973* M Bibl Thesis Unisa, 1974,

Bokkenheuser V. 'An analysis of 519 cases of Diphtheria in Johannesburg 1951-1952' *South African Medical Journal* 29(20) 1955:461-468

Bokkenheuser V. 'Diphtheria Immunisation in Johannesburg and Boksburg from 1935 to 1955' *South African Medical Journal* 29(53) 1955:1249-1254

Bokkenheuser V. and Stephen A. 'Diphtheria in Durban: morbidity, mortality and prevention' *South African Medical Journal*, 35(14) 8 April 1961:289-294

Bonfa A. 'Syphilis and Salvarsan in Country Practice' *South African Medical Record* 15(24) 1917:372-375

Booker C.G. and Annecke S. 'The General Practitioner in the Prevention of Malaria' *South African Medical Journal* 7(3) 1933:80

Botha Graham C, *History of Law, Medicine and Place Names in the Cape of Good Hope*, C Struik Cape Town, 1962

Brain J.B. and Brain P. 'The health of indentured Indian Migrants to Natal, 1860-1911' *South African Medical Journal* 62(20) 1982:739-742

Brincker J.A.H. 'A Historical, epidemiological and aetiological study of measles' *Proceedings of the Royal Society of Medicine.* 31, 1938:807

Brink C.D. 'An Outbreak of Acute Anterior Poliomyelitis' *South African Medical Journal* 8(15) 1934:560-563

Brink C.J.H. 'Malaria Control in the Northern Transvaal', *South African Medical Journal* 32(32) 9 August 1958:805

Brink V. 'Poliomyelitis: Experimental and Therapeutic aspects' *South African Medical Journal*; 11(15) 1937:536-538

Brink Vernon, 'Chemotherapy: Penicillin' *South African Medical Journal* 21(4) 1947:125-131

Brock B.G. 'Syphilis and the Commonweal' *South African Medical Record*, 15(1) 1917:9-25

Brockleby, Dr; 'Surprising instance of the great infectiousness of some diseases, where a free current of air is wanting, even in the most temperate climates'; *The Annual Register*, 8 1765, J Dodsley, 1793:.89

Bryer L. and Hunt K.S. *The 1820 Settlers*; Don Nelson, Cape Town 1984.

Buhrmann M.V. 'Investigation of stillbirths and deaths of children under 5 years of age' *South African Medical Journal* 26(42) 1952:835-839

Bulletin of the World Health Organisation, 10(4) 1954

Burman C.E.L. 'A Review of the Influenza Epidemic in Ladysmith and district with clinical observations' *South African Medical Record*, XVII(1) January 11 1919: 3-6

Burman Jose, *Disaster Struck South Africa*, C Struik, 1971

Cairns P.T. 'Report on an Outbreak of Epidemic Influenza, Philipstown and District, October and November 1918' *South African Medical Record*, 17(2) January 11 1919:219-249

Cape of Good Hope *Reports on the Public Health, 1902*; Cape Times 1903; G66-1903

Cape Town Gazette 25 September 1802 – 30 October 1802.

Cape Town Gazette 25 April 1807

Cape Times January 24th 1919 to March 6th 1919

Cape Times, 19 July 1920

Chais Rev M. translated by Maty M.D.S.R.S. 'A short account of the manner of inoculating the smallpox on the coast of Barbary and at Bengal in the East Indies'

The Annual Register for the year 1769; J Dodsley 1770.
Chronicle of the World Health Organisation, 11(25) 1948
Cliff A. Haggett P. Smallman-Raynor M. *Measles: An historical geography of a major human viral disease; from global expansion to local retreat, 1840-1990,* Blackwell, Oxford
Cluver E.H. 'Syphilis and the Public Health' *South African Medical Journal* 14(23) 14 December 1940:457
Cluver E.H. *Public Health in South Africa* Central News Agency, Fifth Edition (undated)
Cluver F.W.P. 'The Urban and Rural Aspects of Enteric Fever Control' *South African Medical Journal* 11(11) 1937:402-409
Cluver F.W.P. 'Enteric Fever Prevention in Rural Areas' *South African Medical Journal,* 7(9) 1933:290-291
Cluver F.W.P. 'Malaria Control in Natal and Zululand' *South African Medical Journal* 14(6) 1940:113-117
Cluver F.W.P. 'Report on Malaria Control in rural Native Areas by using DDT insecticide' *South African Medical Journal* 20(13) 1946:368-370
Cluver F.W.P. 'Modern Methods of Malaria Control' *South African Medical Journal* 24(18) 1950:327-328
Cluver P.D. *Report of the Influenza Epidemic Commission,* 1919, Cape Times Ltd, UG 15-'19
Cochrane J.C. et al, 'The Influenzal Epidemic of 1950 in Vanderbijl Park' *South African Medical Journal* 25(12) 1951:209-211
Cochrane Robert G. 'Report on Leprosy in the Union of South Africa' in: *Annual Report of the Department of Public Health, Union of South Africa, 1930,* Government Printer Pretoria, UG 40-'30
Coetzee M. et al, 'Malaria in South Africa: 110 years of learning to control the disease' *South African Medical Journal,* 103(10 Suppl 2) 2013:770-778
Coetzee N. Hussey G.D. Visser G. Barron P. Keen A. 'The 1992 Measles Epidemic in Cape Town – a changing epidemiological pattern' *South African Medical Journal,* 84(3) March 1994:145-139
Cole G.D.H. and Postgate R. *The Common People 1746-1946;* Methuen,, London, 1938
Collins V.E. 'Report of the Resident Surgeon Somerset Hospital' in *Reports on the Government and Aided Hospitals and Asylums, 1900,* WA Richards, Cape Town, 1901, G41-'1901
Colonial Secretary's Ministerial Division, *Reports on the Government and State-Aided Hospitals and Asylums,* WA Richards, Cape Town, 1900, G41-'1901
Cooper E.D. and Robertson W.I. 'Problems resulting from the use of live attenuated poliomyelitis virus type 1 in a mass campaign in a large urban area' *South African Medical Journal* 35(11) 18 March 1961:233
Cooper E.D. *Annual Report of the Medical Officer of Health,* City of Cape Town, 1960
Coovadia H.M. *Host Allergic Response variation in children with measles infection* Thesis for Doctor of Medicine, University of KwaZulu-Natal 1977, Durban
Cory G. E. *The Rise of South Africa;* Volume I; Longmans, Green and Co; 1910
Cuthbertson C.C. 'A new town at Uitvlugt: the founding and development of Pinelands 1919-1948' *Contree* 4l 4 July 1978:5-9.
Daneel Jos and Meyer J. 'Major complications of Arsenical Therapy' *South African Medical Journal* 18(14) 1944:247-248
Davison A.R. 'Leprosy in South Africa' *South African Medical Journal* 27(32) 1953:659-661
Day C. and Gray A. 'Health and Related Indicators' in *South African Health Review 2002;* Health Systems Trust 2003, Durban, South Africa
Deacon H 'Leprosy and Racism at Robben Island' in Heyningen E. *Studies in the History*

of Cape Town, UCT Press with the Centre for African Studies, Cape Town, 1994.
Debates of the Legislative Council of Natal, First Session Twelfth Council; December 14 1886; Vol IX
Debates of the House of Assembly, Union of South Africa, Third session 21st January to 23rd June 1955, Vol 87
Debates of the Senate of South Africa, 23 March 1939
De Meillon B. and Gear J. 'Malaria contracted on the Witwatersrand' *South African Medical Journal* 13(9) 1939: 309-312
De Meillon B. 'Distribution of A Gambiae and A Funestus, Report of the Malaria Research Station of the South Afrian Institute for Medical Research' in: *Annual Report of the Department of Public Health, Union of South Africa, 1933*, The Government Printer Pretoria, UG 30-'33, p61-64.
De Villiers C.W. et al, *Report of the Commission on Mixed Marriages in South Africa*, 1939, UG 30-'39
De Villiers J.C. 'The Medical Aspect of the Anglo-Boer War 1899-1902, Part II'; *Military History Journal* 6 (3) June 1984:102-105
De Villiers J.C. 'The Military Significance of Typhoid in the Anglo-Boer War' *Jagger Journal* 2, University of Cape Town Libraries, 1981: 34-41
Devitt Napier, *The Concentration Camps in South Africa during the Anglo-Boer War of 1899 – 1902*; Shuter and Shooter, Pietermaritzburg 1941
De Wet Nel M.D.C. 'State of the Union's Health: Minister's Review', *South African Medical Journal* 32(35) 30 August 1958:876
Dick RJ, 'Report of the Civil Commissioner' *Cape of Good Hope Blue Book on Native Affairs; 1886*, WA Richards, Cape Town
Donnolly F.A. and Nelson H. 'Some Observations on the Control of Infectious Disease' *South African Medical Journal*, 9(18) 1935:629-641
Drewe Frank, 'The Treatment of Leprosy' *South African Medical Journal* 10(19) 1936:655-658
Drewe Frank, 'Some of the Problems of Leprosy' *South African Medical Journal* 19(21) 1945:408-310
Dubb A. 'Clinical Diphtheria in the Non-European' *South African Medical Journal* 29(25) 1955:586-590
Dunley Owen A. 'Notes on Malaria' *South African Medical Record* 16(9) 1918:136-8
Du Preez I.F. *From Mission Station to Municipality*; Municipality of Pacaltsdorp, 1987
Durrheim D.N. et al, 'Cholera–the grim reality of under-development' *South African Family Practice*, 23 (2) February-March 2001:5
Du Toit, G.T. 'The After-care of Convalescent Poliomyelitis cases' *South African Medical Journal* 19(11) 1945:193-195
Dyer J.J. 'Cholera Outbreak Control Programme' *Pietermaritzburg-Msunduzi, Umgeni, Mpofana District Health Services Annual Report 2001*; Msunduzi Municipality, 2002:58-65
Ebden Henry; *Report of the Colonial Medical Committee, 1885*; WA Richards, Cape Town 1886 G2/1886
Editorial: 'Acquired resistance to insecticides' *South African Medical Journal* 28(19) 1954:390
Editorial, 'Penicillin by Prescription', *Natal Mercury* 2nd June 1945
Editorial: 'The Anti-Contagious Diseases Act Agitation' *South African Medical Record*, 15(9) 1917:129-132
Editorial: 'Syphilis in the Union' *South African Medical Journal* 14(23) 1940:452
Editorial, 'Typhoid: The Outlook in South Africa', *South African Medical Journal* 33(31) 1 August 1959:641
Emdin W. 'A clinical and therapeutic survey of an Influenza Epidemic at the

Potchefstroom military camp', *South African Medical Journal* 16(5) 1942:101-107

'Emjanyana Leper Asylum' in: *Reports on the Government and Aided Hospitals and Asylums*, 1900, WA Richards, Cape Town, 1901, G41-'1901 p 154-156

Erasmus Ellis L. 'A Case against the general pasteurization of milk' *South African Medical Journal* 21(12) 1947:432-433

Falconer W. 'Observations on the Leprosy, its Cause and Cure' *The Annual Register for the Year 1791*; J Dodsley, 1795.

Fehrsen FO, Pasteurisation of Milk, Report submitted to the City Council of Cape Town, in *South African Medical Journal* 19(17) 1945:302-305

Fenner F. Henderson D.A. Arita I. Ježek Z. Ladnyi I.D. 'Smallpox and its eradication' World Health Organisation; *History of International Public Health* No 6, Geneva

Finlayson M.H. and Grobler J.M. 'A study of South African Epidemic Typhus strains and the protection afforded by the Zinsser-Castenada vaccine against infection with these strains' *South African Medical Journal* 14(7) 13 April 1940:129.

Finlayson M.H. 'South African Typhus with special reference to the use of an Alum-Precipitated vaccine' *South African Medical Journal* 14,(12) 1940:247-249

Finnemore R.I. 'Report of the Resident Magistrate' *Colony of Natal Blue Book 1883*, Vause Slatter and Co 1884; pGG43

Fisher S. 'Measles and Poverty in Port Elizabeth' *Carnegie Conference Paper No 172*, Second Carnegie Inquiry into Poverty and Development in Southern Africa, Cape Town, 13-19 April 1984

Fitzgerald N.C. 'Report of the Additional District Surgeon, Sub-District of De Aar, 1902' *Cape of Good Hope Reports on the Public Health 1902*, Cape Times,1903, G66-1903

Fitzgerald J.P. *Report on the King William's Town Hospital 1882*, WA Richards, 1883

Fraser, Reith A. 'The Standard of Cure in Syphilis' *South African Medical Record* 20(6) 1922:102-109

Freed L.F. 'Introduction of Syphilis into the Bantu peoples' *South African Medical Journal* 27(6) 1953:112

Freed, Louis F. *The Problem of European Prostitution in Johannesburg: A Sociological Survey*, University of Pretoria 1942.

Gale A.H. *Epidemic Diseases*, Penguin Books London 1959

Gale G.W. 'The Incidence and Control of Venereal Diseases among the Natives of an Urban Area' *South African Medical Journal* 13(8) 1939:265-270

Gear J.H.S. *The Anglo-Boer War of 1899-1902: Enteric Fever and Captain Maxwell Louis Hughes*; Adler Museum Bulletin, 7 (1) March 1981:10-13

Gear James, 'Typhus Fever in the Transkei' *South African Medical Journal* 18(8) 1944:144-148.

Gear J.H.S. 'A note on the use of DDT in Medical and Health Problems' *South African Medical Journal* 19(16) 1945:290-292

Gear James; 'Epidemiological Patterns of Poliomyelitis in Southern Africa' *Medicine in South Africa* Supplement to the South African Medical Journal 1957

Gear J. Measroch V. Bradley J. and Faerber G.I. 'Poliomyelitis in South Africa: studies in an urban native township during a non-epidemic year;' *South African Medical Journal*; 25(18), 5 May 1951:297

Gear J. & Mundel B. 'Studies in Poliomyelitis' *South African Medical Journal* 19(15) 1945:262-264

Gear J.H.S. 'Typhus fever in the Eastern Transvaal, with Special Reference to an Epidemic occurring in 1945' *South African Medical Journal* 21(7) 1947: 214-218

Gilder S.S.B. 'South African patients and their diseases in the 1880s' *South African Medical Journal* 66(7) August 1984:250-252

Gluckman Henry. 'The Treatment of Syphilis' *South African Medical Record* 18 (10) 1920:182-189

Gordon Lennox W. 'Truants of Medicine in South Africa' *South African Medical Journal* 4(1), 13 January 1940:3

Grasset E.et al, 'Immunisation against Typhoid Fever by means of a single injection of Typhoid Endotoxoid Vaccine' *South African Medical Journal* 11(18) 1937:660-662

Grasset E. et al, 'Studies on the Nature of Antidiphtheritic Immunity among South African Bantu by means of the Schick Test and Anti-toxin Titrations' *South African Medical Journal*; 7(23) 1933:779-785

Gregory A.J. *Report of the Medical Officer of Health for the Colony on the Public Health for the calendar year 1907*; Cape of Good Hope, Cape Times Ltd 1908; G33-1908

Gregory Dr, in *Report of the Select Committee on Robben Island Lepers*, 1909, Cape Town, A12-1909

Gumede-Moeletsi N, Suchard M. Schoub B. 'Update on Polio Eradication in Africa' Communicable Diseases Surveillance Bulletin, National Institute for Communicable Diseases, Pretoria, 11(2) 2013:42-47

Hansford C.F. and Muller H. 'Malaria in South Africa 1987-1989' *Epidemiological Comments*, 17(12) October 1990:2-9

Hansford F. Theron D. 'Malaria Update' *Epidemiological Comments* 11(4) April 1984:18

Hanson J. 'An Epidemiological study of the poliomyelitis outbreak in Springs 1944-45', *South African Medical Journal* 19(22) 1945:422-426

Harding Le Riche, 'Smallpox control in the Swartkop Native Location'; *The Medical Officer*, London, No 4; 1945:280

Harrhy W.R. cited in Gilder S.S.B. 'South African patients and their Diseases in the 1880s' *South African Medical Journal*, 66(7) August 1984:250

Hay, George Gray, 'Amaas', *South African Medical Journal* 12(17) 1938:639-641

Hay-Michel A. 'Influenza on the Zaaiplaats mine' *South African Medical Record*, 17(2) January 11 1919:24-26

Haydon F.S. *Debates of the Legislative Council Colony of Natal; First session Twelfth Council, Volume IX;* WM Watson Pietermaritzburg; 1887

Hemson D. et al, 'Still Paying the Price: Revisiting the Cholera Epidemic of 2000-2001 in South Africa; Municipal Services' *Project Occasional Paper No 10; Human Sciences Research Council*, Grocotts, Grahamstown, February 2006

Heymann Seymour, 'Diagnosis and Treatment of Poliomyelitis in the Acute Stage' *South African Medical Journal* 24(20) 1950:373-379

Heyningen E. 'Studies in the History of Cape Town' UCT Press with the Centre for African Studies, Cape Town, 1994

Hill Ernest, *Report on the Plague in Natal, 1902-1903*, Cassell, London 1904

Holland, E.M. 'An Experiment in Slum Clearance Housing in Urban Native Areas', *Race Relations* 7(4) 1940:70.

Hopkins D.R. *Princes and Peasants: Smallpox in History* Chicago, 1983.

Humphries S.V. 'Sulphapyridine as a specific for measles in Adult Natives', *South African Medical Journal* 17(5) 1943:72

Impey S.P. 'Leprosy', Letter in *South African Medical Record*, 22(3) 1924:63-64

Ingram A. & Harvey Pirie J.H. 'Report on Bacteriological Research carried out in connection with Plague during 1925' *South African Medical Record* 24(11) 1926:252-257

Jeal M.E. *The Dell Chronicles 1750-1979*, Parkhurst, 1979

Jeeves Alan, 'The State, the Cinema and Health propaganda for Africans in Pre Apartheid South Africa, 1932-1948' *Southern African Historical Journal*, 48, May 2003:125.

Kaplan L. 'A Discussion on 55 respirator cases in the recent poliomyelitis epidemic of 1956' *South African Medical Journal* 30(45) 1956:1073-1083

Kaplan L. 'Poliomyelitis and Pregnancy: case report of a birth in a respirator during the acute phase of poliomyelitis' *South African Medical Journal* 31(12) 1957:278-279

Kaplan M.W. 'Epidemic Poliomyelitis in Durban' *South African Medical Journal* 19(4) 1945:55-57

Korns R.F. Abstract of Summary Report, Francis T. Korns R.F. et al, 'Evaluation of 1954 Field Trial of Poliomyelitis Vaccine' *South African Medical Journal* 29(19) 1955: 447-452

Kark Sydney, 'The Social Pathology of Syphilis in Africans' *South African Medical Journal*, 23(5) 29 January 1949:77

Kark S.L. 'The management of an enteric fever outbreak in a "Native Territory"', *South African Medical Journal* 17(6) 1943:87-88

Küstner H.G.V. 'Measles Update' *Epidemiological Comments*, Department of Health, 11(6) June 1984:24-31

Küstner H.G.V. 'The six vaccine-preventable diseases' *Epidemiological Comments*, Department of Health, South Africa, 17(10) October 1990:3-18

Küstner H.G.V. 'The measles strategy, South Africa 1991 – an evaluation of its effect' *Epidemiological Comments*, Department of Health 19(7), July 1992:112-127

Küstner H.G.V. 'Downward trend in measles' *Epidemiological Comments*, Department of Health, 22 (4) April 1995:76-81

Küstner H.G.V. 'Poliomyelitis Epidemic in Natal and KwaZulu' *Epidemiological Comments*, Department of National Health and Population Development, 15(3) 1988:2-30

Küstner H.G.V. 'Secular trends of selected diseases' *Epidemiological Comments*, Department of Health, 11(3) March 1984:10

Küstner H.G.V. 'The eradication of Poliomyelitis from South Africa' *Epidemiological Comments*, Department of National Health and Population Development, 17 (8) August 1990:3-9

Küstner H.G.V. 'Analysis of Cholera IV', *Epidemiological Comments*, Department of Health, 11(10) October 1984:5-22

Küstner H.G.V. 'Cholera in South Africa' *Epidemiological Comments*, Department of Health, 18(12) December 1991:268

Küstner H.G.V. 'Cholera in South Africa' *Epidemiological Comments*, Department of Health, 24(1) January 1998:3

Küstner H.G.V. 'Malaria: Problems Old and New' *Epidemiological Comments*, Department of Health, 15(1) January 1988:2-55

Lagden G.Y. *Report by the Commissioner for Native Affairs, Transvaal, for the year ended 30th June 1904*, Pretoria, Government Printing and Stationary office, 1904

Lagden G.Y. et al, *Report of the Contagious Diseases amongst Natives Commission, 1907*, Government Printing and Stationary Office, 1138_25-3-07_750

Lagden G.Y. *Report by the Commissioner for Native Affairs, Transvaal, for the year ended 30th June 1906*, Pretoria, Government Printing and Stationary office, 1906

Lagden G.Y. *Annual Report of the Commissioner for Native Affairs 1905-06*, Government Printing and Stationary office, Pretoria, 1906

Laidler P.W. 'Medical Establishments and Institutions at the Cape', *South African Medical Journal* 11(18) 1937:635-641

Laidler P.W. 'Statistics, Social Disease and Legislation' *South African Medical Journal* 14(4) 1939:71

Laidler P.W. and Gelfand M. 'South Africa its medical history, 1652-1898: A medical and social study' C Struik, Cape Town, 1971

Laing G.D. 'The Public Health Aspect of Typhoid Fever' *South African Medical Journal*, 8(21) 1934:793

Laing G.D. 'The Public Health Aspect of Typhoid Fever in Urban Areas' *South African Medical Journal*, 7(9) 1933:288

Landsberg P. *Report of the Vaccine Surgeon, 1885*, WA Richards, Cape Town G2/1886

Lea J.A. et al; 'A Scheme for the Treatment of Venereal Disease' *South African Medical Record* 16(19) 12 October 1918:296-298.

Leading Article, 'The Influenza Epidemic'; *South African Medical Record*; 16(21) 9 November 1918:317-320

Leipoldt Louis C. *Bushveld Doctor,* Jonathan Cape Ltd London, 1937

Le Sueur D. Sharp B.L. Appleton C. 'Historical Perspective of the Malaria problem in Natal with emphasis on the period 1928-1932', *South African Journal of Science*, 89, May 1993:232-239

Levin S. 'Hospital deaths in non-European children' *South African Medical Journal* 24(48) 1950:993-997

Liebbrandt H.C.V. 'Journal of Zacharias Wagenaer', *Précis of the Archives of the Cape of Good Hope, 1662-1670*, Cape Town 1901

Liebbrandt H.C.V. 'Journal of Governor Willem Adriaan van der Stel 1713'; *Précis of the Archives of the Cape of Good Hope, Journal 1699-1732*; Cape Town 1896

Liebbrandt H.C.V. 'Report of the Commissioners of the Hospital' *Précis of the Archives of the Cape of Good Hope, Journal 1699-1732*; Cape Town 1896

Liebbrandt H.C.V. 'Letters Received 1695-1708' *Précis of the Archives of the Cape of Good Hope*, Cape Town 1896.

Liebbrandt H.C.V. 'Letters Despatched 1696-*1708' Précis of the Archives of the Cape of Good Hope*, Cape Town 1896.

MacLean A. et al, *SARS: a case study in emerging infections*, Oxford University Press, 2005

MacLeod R. and Lewis M. Disease, *Medicine and Empire, perspectives on Western Medicine and the experience of European Expansion*; Routledge, London, 1988

MacNeillie Dr, 'Public Health of the Union', *Cape Times* 30th January 1919:24

Maister M. 'Annual Reports of the Medical Officer of Health' *Pietermaritzburg Corporation Yearbooks* 1944 and 1945

Maister M. 'Epidemiological and Public Health Aspects of the disease: Proceedings of a Symposium on Poliomyelitis, Pietermaritzburg' *South African Medical Journal* 29(18) 1955:416-417

Makubalo L.E. et al, *Annual Report 2007: Prevalence and Distribution of Malaria in South Africa*, Report by the National Department of Health, Pretoria, March 2008

Mansell Prothero R. *Migrants and Malaria*; Longmans Green, London, 1965

Marais Dr, 'Discussion on the Cape Town Influenza Epidemic,' *South African Medical Record*, 16(23) 14 December 1918:353

Marshall, James, 'The Present-day Treatment of Syphilis', *South African Medical Journal*, 23(5) 29 January 1949: 84.

Martens Jeremy C. 'Almost a Public Calamity': Prostitutes, 'Nurseboys' and Attempts to Control Venereal Diseases in Colonial Natal, 1886-1890'; *South African Historical Journal* 45, Nov 2001:27-52.

Martin A.C. *The Concentration Camps 1900-1902: Facts, Figures and Fables*; Howard Timmins Cape Town 1957

Matthews J.W. *Incwadi Yami or Twenty Years Personal Experience in South Africa; 1887*; Africana Book Society 1976; Johannesburg

Maule Clark B. 'Pneumonic Plague: Recovery in a Proved Case', *South African Medical Journal* 17(4) 1943:57-60

Maule Clark B. 'Two interesting South African Typhoid Outbreaks', *South African Medical Journal* 13(24) 1939:806-808

McCall Theal G. *History of South Africa 1486-1691*; Swan Sonnenschein, Lowrey, 1888

McKay Helen M. 'William John Burchell: His Experiences as a Consulting Physician while in the Interior of Southern Africa 1810-1815', *South African Medical Journal*

14(4) 1940:78-80
McLaren T.D. 'Report of the District Surgeon, Herchel for 1902' *Cape of Good Hope Reports on the Public Health 1902*; Cape Times Ltd 1903 G66-1903; p63
Mead, Richard; 'A discourse on the Small Pox and Measles; John Brindley 1748' cited in *South African Medical Journal*, 25(1) 1951:10
Meijer H.B.W. 'Reminiscences of Leprosy and Plague' *South African Medical Record* 21(20) 1923:475-476
Mentzel O.F. *A Geographical and Topographical description of the Cape of Good Hope 1787*; Translated by Marais G.V. and Hoge J. Edited by Mandelbrote H.J. The Van Riebeeck Society, Cape Town, 1944
Merriman Mr, 'Echoes of the Epidemic, Debate in the House of Assembly', *Cape Times* January 28 1919:16
Mitchell J.A. 'Address on Typhus Fever', *South African Medical Record* 15(16) 1917:244-248
Mitchell Dr, 'Address on Venereal Diseases', *South African Medical Record* 15(12) 1917:186-188
Mitchell J.A. 'Typhus Fever ("Black Fever" or "Mtetalala") in the Cape Province', *South African Medical Record* 15(17) 1917:259-262
Mitchell J.A. 'The problem of Venereal Disease; Address given at the Annual Conference of the Transvaal Branch of the National Society for Combating Venereal Disease, Johannesburg 24th February 1921' *South African Medical Record* 19(7) 1921:122-124
Mitchell J.A. 'Venereal Diseases in South Africa', *South African Medical Record* 24(8) 1926:181
Mitchell J.A. 'Plague in South Africa: perpetuation and spread of infection by wild rodents'. *South African Medical Record*, 19(24) 1921:475-477
Moore J.E. and Mahoney J.F. et al, 'Penicillin treatment of early syphilis', *Journal of the American Medical Association,* 126(2) 1944
Mostert H.v.R. 'Leprosy: some aspects of modern research', *South African Medical Journal* 9(13) 1935:459-463
Mugero C. *Cholera Outbreak in South Africa; National Outbreak Committee Situational Report (Sitrep 29);* Pretoria, 11 January 2009.
Muller H. 'Deaths due to Malaria during 1990', *Epidemiological Comments*, Department Of Health 18(4) April 1991:86
Murison, Dr; 'Scheme for Dealing with Venereal Diseases in Durban' *South African Medical Record* 18(19) 1920:371
Murray J.F. 'Diphtheria on the Witwatersrand: a bacteriological, clinical and epidemiological survey', *South African Medical Journal* 16(13) 1942:247-250
Murray J.F. 'The significance of C. Diphtheriae Gravis on the epidemiology of diphtheria', *South African Medical Journal,* 17(21) 1943:337-338
Murray N.L. 'Age for Diphtheria Immunization in South Africa', *South African Medical Journal* 17(21) 1942:334-337
Naidoo S. and Meyers K., 'The Measles Epidemic' *South African Medical Journal*, 84(3) March 1994:125
Nankivell J.H. 'Report of the District Surgeon, Transkei' *Blue Book of Native Affairs 1882*, Cape of Good Hope, Volume 1 part 1, W.A. Richards, Cape Town
Natal Witness, 7 June 1893.
Neame L.E. *City Built on Gold*, Central News Agency Ltd, Cape Town, 1960
Nelson H. 'The Carrier in Enteric Fever' *South African Medical Journal* 21(14) 1947:506-520
O'Malley C.K. 'New methods in the treatment of syphilis', *South African Medical Journal* 15(17) 1941:343-347

O'Malley Kevin C. 'Syphilis in South Africa', *South African Medical Journal* 14(23) 14 December 1940:461

O'Reagan M. *The Hospital Services of Natal*, Natal Regional Survey No 8, University of Natal, Durban, Robinson and Co, 1970

Orenstein A.J. 'Epidemiology', *South African Medical Journal* 11(15) 1937:529-535

Packard R.M. *White Plague, Black Labour: Tuberculosis and the Political Economy of Health and Disease in South Africa* Pietermaritzburg: University of Natal Press 1989

Park Ross G.A. 'Control of malaria in the Union', *South African Medical Record* 20(23) 1922:450

Phillips H, '"Black October': the Impact of the Spanish Influenza Epidemic of 1918 on South Africa', *Archives Year Book for South African History*, Vol 1, Government Printer Pretoria, 1990

Phillips H; 'Cape Town in 1829'; *Contree*, No 8, July 1980:5

Pijper, Adrianus, 'Two and a half years work at an Anti-Venereal Clinic for Natives and Coloured Persons', *South African Medical Record* 22(16) 1924: 369-372

Pijper A. and Russell E.D. 'Malaria treatment of General Paralysis: a Report on 44 cases', *South African Medical Record* 24(13) 1926:292-303

Pijper A. 'Rickettsioses of South Africa' *South African Medical Journal* 12(17) 1938:613-630

'Plague: Control Eradication and Prevention, Extract from a Union Public Health Memorandum' published in *South African Medical Record*, 23(7) 1925:146-150

Pretoria News 10 August 1992

Prinsloo A.J. 'The Eradication of the Namaqua Gerbille and fleas', *Annual Report of the Medical Officer of Health for Port Elizabeth, 1960*, Longs, 1961:50-53

'Public Health Bulletin: Typhus'; *South African Medical Record* 16(19) 12 October 1918:302

'Public Health Report, Cape of Good Hope', *Blue Book on Native Affairs, Union of South Africa 1910*; U17-1910

Pullinger E.J. 'Pasteurisation of Milk in South Africa' *South African Medical Journal* 19(4) 1945:50-55

Purcell F.W.F. 'Syphilis in South Africa', *South African Medical Journal*, 14(23), 14 December 1940:453

Purcell F.W.F. 'Remarks on the treatment of Syphilis' *South African Medical Journal* 8(21) 1934:783

Purcell F.W.F. 'Anti-venereal Prophylaxis', *South African Medical Journal* 14(23) 14 December 1940:462

Purvis Beattie W. 'Influenza and Bacteriological Facts' *South African Medical Record*, 16(23) 14 December 1918:371

Raven-Hart R. *Cape of Good Hope 1652-1702: the first 50 years of Dutch colonisation as seen by callers, Volume 2*; AA Balkema Cape Town; 1971

Report and Proceedings of the Cape Peninsular Plague Advisory Board, WA Richards, Cape Town, 1901, G61-'1901

Report of the Commission on Leprosy; Government Notice No 434 of 1886; The Natal Government Gazette September 28 1886

Report of the Contagious Diseases amongst Natives Commission, (1907) Government Printer, Pretoria

Report on the General Infirmary Robben Island for 1859, Published, 1860, G 11-1860,

'Report of the Influenza Commission', *South African Medical Record* 17(4) 1919:51-55

'Report of the Malaria Commission of the League of Nations', *South African Medical Journal* 7(16) 1933:540

Report of the Native Affairs Department for the Year ended 31st December 1911; Cape Times Ltd, 1911, Cape Town, UG 10-'13

Report of the Tuberculosis Commission, Union of South Africa, 1914, U.G. 34-'14

Reports on the Government and Aided Hospitals and Asylums, 1900, WA Richards, Cape Town, 1901, G41-'1901

Rhodes W.F. 'Typhus-like fevers in the Union of South Africa' *South African Medical Journal* 8(21) 1934:797-799

Ross W.H. 'Report of the Acting Medical Inspector 1902'; Reports of the Medical Inspectors on the working of Part 1 of the "Contagious Diseases Prevention Act, 1885"; in Reports *on the Public Health ; Cape of Good Hope, 1902,* Cape Times Ltd 1903; G66-1903:275.

Ross W.M.H. *Robben Island Infirmary Annual Report for 1885,* Cape Of Good Hope, WA Richard, Cape Town, 1886 G2/1886

Russell P. 'An account of Inoculation in Arabia, in a letter from Dr Patrick Russell at Aleppo to Dr Alexander Russell' *The Annual Register for the year 1776*; J Dodsley 1770:82

Sapieka N. 'Modern insecticides: their toxicity and control', *South African Medical Journal* 33(50) 12 December 1959:163

Saville Lewis J. *Annual Report of the Medical Officer of Health for Port Elizabeth, 1964,* Waltons, Port Elizabeth

Saville Lewis J, *Annual Report of the Medical Officer of Health for Port Elizabeth, 1965,* Longs, Port Elizabeth

Sax Sidney, 'The Introduction of Syphilis into the Bantu peoples of South Africa', *South African Medical Journal* 26(27) December 1952:1037-1039

Schaffer R. and Shapiro B.G. 'Studies in Influenza', *South African Medical Journal* 15(5) 1941:83-91

Scott Millar J.W. *Report of the Medical Officer of Health on the Public Health and Sanitary Circumstances and Housing in Johannesburg during the period 1st July 1953 to 31st December 1957,* City of Johannesburg 1957,

Scott Millar J.W. *Report of the Medical Officer of Health on the Public Health and Sanitary Circumstances and Housing in Johannesburg during the period 1st January to 31st December 1959*; City of Johannesburg. 1959

Scott Millar J.W. *Report on the Health of Johannesburg in 1961,* City of Johannesburg, 1961,

Scott Millar J.W. 'Poliomyelitis in Johannesburg' *Public Health* 13 May 1949.

Scully W.C. *A History of South Africa* Green and Co; 1922

Searle C. *The history of the development of nursing in South Africa 1652-1960* The South African Nursing Association; 1980

Seedat M.A. 'Cholera in South Africa', *Modern Medicine of South Africa,* 7(9) September 1982:81

Seeff Harry, 'The Dietetic Treatment of Typhoid Fever' *South African Medical Journal* 7(9) 1933:291

Sheldon H.F. 'Leprosy', *South African Medical Record* 23(20) 1925:447-453

Shepherd A.J. et al 'Studies on Plague in the eastern Cape Province of South Africa', *Transactions of the Royal Society of Tropical Medicine and Hygiene,* 77(6) 1983:800

Shorten J.R. *The Johannesburg Saga,* JR Shorten for Johannesburg City Council, 1970

Silberbauer S.F. 'The Activity of Schick Reaction Products', *South African Medical Record* 24(9) 1926:207

Simpson W.J. *Memorandum dated 10 February 1901 to the Cape Peninsular Plague Advisory Board,* WA Richards and Sons, Cape Town, 1901,G61- '1901

Sinclair G.S.et al, 'Determination of the mode of transmission of cholera in Lebowa', *South African Medical Journal* 62(21) 1982:753-755

Sitas F. *An investigation of a Cholera outbreak at the Umvoti Mission Reserve, Natal. A Non-Water Borne epidemic?* Second Carnegie Inquiry into Poverty and Development

in Southern Africa, Carnegie Conference Paper No 151, 1984
Slome R. 'Immunization', *South African Medical Journal* 31(18) 1957:422
Smith Andrew B. 'The Origins and Demise of the Khoikhoi: The Debate'; *South African Historical Journal*; 23, December 1990:13.
Smuts F. *Stellenbosch: Three Centuries* The Town Council of Stellenbosch; 1979
Spencer H.A. 'Malaria as it Occurs upon the Middelveld of the Transvaal' *South African Medical Record* 20(18) 1922:342-249.
Spencer H.A. 'Malaria on the Lowveld', *South African Medical Record* 21(1) 1923:3-7
Spencer H.A. 'The Treatment and Prevention of Malaria', *South African Medical Record* 21(4) 1923:84
Spencer I.W.F. *Various Studies in the Prevention of Disease,* Thesis for Doctor of Medicine, University of Witwatersrand, 1969, Johannesburg
Stockenstrom A. *Parliamentary Debates, Cape of Good Hope, 1854* published by The State Library, Pretoria, Reprint 33, Volume 1 1968, debates dated 11th September, 14th September, 22nd September and 16th August 1854,
Stokes J.H.et al, 'Action of Penicillin in late syphilis', *Journal of the American Medical Association*, 126(2) 1944:
Sunday Times 3rd October 1937
Swanson, Maynard W. '"The Asiatic Menace": creating segregation in Durban, 1870-1900' *International Journal of African Historical Studies*, 16(3) 1983:416
Swanson M.W. 'The Sanitation Syndrome: Bubonic Plague and Urban Native Policy in the Cape Colony 1900-1909' *Journal of African History* 18, 1977
Swift E.W.D. 'General Paralysis of the Insane and its treatment', *South African Medical Journal*, 24(6) 1950:122
Tait K.R. 'Report of the District Surgeon of Colesberg 1902' *Cape of Good Hope Reports on the Public Health 1902;* Cape Times Ltd 1903; G66-1903
Taylor J. 'Meaningful Learning and Social Change: the case of the Eshowe cholera crisis in South Africa' *African Wildlife* 59 (2) 2005:12-14.
'The 12th National HIV/Syphilis sero-prevalence survey of women attending public antenatal clinics in South Africa 2001' *Epidemiological Comments*, 5(1) Jan-March 2002:1-15.
Theal George McCall; *History of South Africa from 1873 to 1884: twelve eventful years*; George Allen and Unwin Ltd, London; 1919
Tobias J.M. 'The problem of Venereal Disease in the Transkei,' *South African Medical Journal* 18(8) 1944:142
Traill David, 'Report of the District Surgeon for Richmond', in *Reports on the Public Health for the year 1902, Cape of Good Hope*, Cape Times 1903; G66-1903:130-136
Tren R. Bate R. *Malaria and the DDT story*, Institute for Economic Affairs London, 2001
Turnbull N.S. 'Diphtheria in African Natives in the Transkei, South Africa' *Transactions of the Royal Society of Tropical Medicine and Hygiene* 43(2) 1949:215-224
Turnbull N.S. 'Diphtheria in African Natives in the Transkei', *South African Medical Journal* 23(27) 1949:551
Turner R. 'Active Immunization against Poliomyelitis: A review' *South African Medical Journal* 29(36) 1955:833
Turner R. 'Some Epidemiological and Public Health Aspects of Poliomyelitis' *South African Medical Journal* 19(1) 1945:2
Turner R. 'The Role of the Laboratory in the diagnosis and control of typhoid fever', *South African Medical Journal*, 33(31) 1 August 1959:647
Turner R. 'Vaccination against Typhoid Fever' *South African Medical Journal* 33(31) 1 August 1959:639
Van Heerden J.R. *Annual Report of the Medical Officer of Health for East London 1968*, Griff-Stan East London, December 1976.

Van den Ende M. et al; 'The 1950 influenza epidemic in Cape Town' *South African Medical Journal*; 25(26) 30 June 1951:445

Van Heyningen E. 'The Social Evil in the Cape Colony 1868-1902: Prostitution and the Contagious Diseases Acts' *Journal of Southern African Studies*, 10 (2) 1984:170-197

Van Heyningen, E. 'Epidemics and Disease: Historical writing on Health in South Africa' *South African Historical Journal* 23; 1990:122

Viljoen, Russel; 'Disease and Society: VOC Cape Town, its people and the smallpox epidemics of 1713, 1755 and 1767' *Kleio* 27; 1995:22

Wade M.M. Straws in the Wind: early epidemics of poliomyelitis in Johannesburg, 1918-1945'; Thesis submitted for M.A. degree, UNISA, December 2006

Wannenburg H.R.J. 'Administrative Aspects of poliomyelitis in isolation hospitals' *South African Medical Journal*, 33(4) 24 January 1959:76

Watt T, *First and Second Reports of the Select Committee on Treatment of Lepers*, Cape Times Ltd Government Printers 1918, S.C.10-'18

Watt, Thomas, 'Public Health of the Union', *Cape Times* 30th January 1919 p24.

Webb E.M. 'Leprosy today: World Situation and South Africa' *Epidemiological Comments*, Department of Health, 20 (4) April 1993: 55

Weekly Epidemiological Record 67(21) 1992:153-160

Welsh Alex R. 'Report of the Civil Commissioner', *Cape of Good Hope Blue Book on Native Affairs*; 1886, WA Richards, Cape Town

Westwood M.A. and Gear J. 'A laboratory study of the Influenza Epidemic which occurred in South Africa in the winter of 1950', *South African Medical Journal* 25(47) 1951:862-864

Westwood M. Smit P. and Oberholzer D. 'Asian Influenza in South Africa, A laboratory and clinical study of an outbreak on the Simmer and Jack mine' *South African Medical Journal*, 32(8) 1958:216

Willcox R.R. 'Early Syphilis: some modern advances in its treatment with antibiotics', *South African Medical Journal* 23(52) 1949:1040

Woodrow A.P. 'Diphtheria Immunisation in Cape Town and its problems', *South African Medical Journal* 20(24) 1946:781

Worden N.and Groenewald G. *Trials of Slavery: selected documents concerning slaves from the criminal records of the Council of Justice at the Cape of Good Hope, 1705-1794*; Van Riebeeck Society for the publication of South African historical documents; Cape Town 2005

*World Health Organisation Technical Report Series No 64:*1953

INDEX

Acriflavine 23
Acute Flaccid Paralysis 239
Albert 109
Alepol 19
Alexander L.L. 234
Alexandra County 10
Alexandra Township 43, 75
Aliwal North 8, 80
Alma Ata Declaration 218
amaas 71, 73
Amapepeta 9, 10
Amatikulu Leper Institution 19, 20
American Typhus Commission 138
Anglo-Boer War 13, 22, 35, 71, 82, 85, 105, 108, 110, 143, 180, 210, 212, 242, 257
Annecke S. 188
Anti-malarial measures 185, 187, 188, 190, 192-196
antimony 37
anti-toxin: diphtheria 243, 244, 250, 251
anti-diphtheritic serum 248
apartheid 62, 175
Arab traders 5
arsenic 37, 42, 46, 49, 52, 53, 55, 89
arsenical poisoning 211
artificial respiration 225, 231
Ashe Dr 147
Asian Flu 160, 161
aspirin 50
aureomycin 53, 98, 140

Bain-Marais Mr. 43
Ballinger Mrs 43
Barkley East 110
Barkley West 30, 139 182
Barry, Dr James 4
Basotholand *see* Lesotho
Baumann E. P. 223, 224
BaVenda 34, 71
Behr Dr 49
Beredska pill 113
Bethlehem 156, 228
Birtwhistle Dr 5
bismuth 42, 46, 52, 53
black fever 129, 130
Blackwood's magazine 10, 12

blindness
    in leprosy 16
    and measles 215, 218
    in syphilis 33
Bloemfontein 72, 95, 96 105, 150, 151, 154, 224, 225
Bochem Leper Institution 15,19,21,34
Boer laagers 210
Boer Commandoes 106-108
Boksburg 234
Bothaville 93, 96, 97
Bradfort Mr, 85
Brakpan 120
Brandfort 48, 21
Brickfields 91
British Empire Leprosy Relief Association 19
Brock B.G. 35
brothels 28, 32, 36,
bucket system 109, 111, 113, 115, 116, 119, 123, 125, 170
Bulwer Sir Henry 9
Burchell 143, 208
Burdett Coutts W. 106
Burgersdorp 92
Bushmen 15

Cadman Rev. Miles 43
Caledon 4, 8, 115
Calvinia 8
Camps:
    Concentration 107, 108, 180, 210, 211, 242
    Congella 145
    military 212
    plague 13
    quarantine 83, 84
    refugee 22
    segregation 34
    squatter 219, 217
    typhoid fever 120, 121
Cape Peninsular Plague Advisory Board 82
Cape Flats 84-86, 98
Carnegie Enquiry into Poverty 217
carriers: typhoid 111-113, 118, 120, 122
cemeteries 86, *and see* Maitland cemetery
chancroid 57
Chamber of Mines 39, 153, 154
chaulmoogra oil 13, 15, 21, 22

chicken pox 69
Children's Act 156
Chlamydia trachomatis 57
chloramphenicol 53, 121, 167
chlorine gas 68
chloroquine 196, 199, 200
cholecystectomy 121
Ciskei 139, 140, 217
Clanwilliam 8
Cluver E.H. 46, 47, 112, 261
Cochrane Robert 19, 20
Coega 99
Coetzee N. 220
cold chain 238
Colenso 109
Colesberg 71
Coloured Labourers Health Regulations 144
Commissions of Enquiry:
    Anglo-Boer War 106
    Influenza 154
    Leprosy 6, 7, 9, 10, 16
    Public Health 75
    Robben Island 5
    Venereal diseases 43
compulsory vaccination:
    smallpox 73
    measles 220
    polio 234, 237
    diphtheria 250
Congella 166
congenital syphilis 42, 56
conscientious objectors (vaccination) 73
Contagious Diseases:
    Acts (Cape) 28-30, 32, 34-36, 38
    Amongst Natives Commission 32-34, 37
    Bills 10, 30-32
Contagious Diseases Commission 27
convalescent serum 212, 213, 225, 231
copper sulphate 226
Cooper Prof 214, 215, 251
Coovadia H. 216
cowpox 67
Cradock 72, 211, 226
cremations 89
Cronjés
    Fever 107
    Laager 107
Cutter incident 233
cyanide 131

Cyclone Demoina 199
cyfluthrin 202

Daneel J. 49
Danielson 20
DDT 97, 99, 137-141, 194-203, 233, 261
De Aar 72, 242
De Beers Diamond Company 147
Delagoa Bay 82, 179
    railway line 185
Delmas 125
deltamethrin 202
De Meillon 190
desquamation 152
De Wet C. 233, 235, 263
De Wit Nel Mr, 23
District Six 147
Docks location 148
Doornfontein 105
Drewe Frank 21, 22
drought 63
Dubb A. 250
Duncan Patrick 36
Dunstan John, 17
Durban 20, 41, 43, 44, 56, 68, 72, 73, 88-90, 93, 94, 118, 132, 145, 149, 151, 154, 158, 159, 166, 167, 172, 180, 181, 192, 211, 227, 228, 230, 232
Dutch Reformed Church 65
dysentery 27, 118

East Griqualand 9
East London 22, 87, 88, 92, 124, 146, 149, 154, 211, 232, 234,
Edendale 74, 116, 117
Elim 34
Emanjanyana Leper Institution 14, 15, 19, 21
Empangeni 172, 173
encephalitis 49, 214, 232
erythromycin 57
Eshowe 171-175
exfoliative dermatitis 49
Expanded Programme on Immunisation 218, 220, 252
Expert Committee on Influenza 160

Falconer, Dr W. 3
Fehrsen F. O. 118, 119
Felstead's disease 69

Fenner F 77, 78, 262
Fingoland 8
Fingoes 33, 68
Fitzgerald J.P. 68
flaccid paralysis 224
flag system 150, 166
fleas 82, 89, 93-97, 133, 135, 137, 138, 195
flies 17, 75, 112, 113, 115, 117, 123, 138, 194, 195, 223, 224, 228, 232, 233
forced removals 84-87, 90, 91, 110, 116, 132, 256, 258
Fordsburg 92
Fort Beaufort 8
Franco-Prussian War 104
Franschoek 3
Fraserburg 242
Frontier Medical Association 30
fumigation 68, 69, 71, 94, 131, 132, 145, 187, 192, 259
funerals 136

Gale G.W. 45
gall bladder 112
Gazankulu 215, 237
Gear J. 137
General Paralysis of the Insane 39, 40
George 105
gerbils 93-95, 97, 99
German measles *see* rubella
Germiston 42, 145
Girdwood Dr 129
Glen Grey 72, 93, 96, 130, 133
Global Malaria Eradication Campaign 197
Global Polio Eradication Initiative 238
Gluckman Sir Henry, 37
gonorrhoea 28, 29, 33, 49, 51, 52, 54
Gordon Mrs E. 230
Graaff Reinet 92, 228
Grahamstown 5, 9, 28
Gray Colonel 36
Gregory Dr 14
Grey's Hospital 74
Greytown 188
Griquas 5
Groblersdal 197
Gubbs location 87
Guild Keith 8

Haarhy W.R. 30

Haffkine's Prophylactic 85, 90
Hansen 8
Hanson Mr 85
Hanson Dr, 228
Harding 186
hares 94, 95
Harries 182
Harrismith 228
Hay G. 71
Haydon 180
Heidelberg 22
Hemel-in-Aarde 4, 5
Hemson D. 175
Henderson 78
hepatitis 50
Hermanus 4
herpes simplex 57
Herschel 8, 14
Hertzog A. 236
Heymann S. 230
Hill, Ernest 88-90
Himeville 22
HIV/AIDS 56, 57, 263
Hlabisa 57, 171, 199, 237
Hobhouse Emily 108, 211
Hopetown 8
hostels 51, 144, 145
Hottentots *see* Khoikhoi
Hughes Captain 109
Huguenots
Hulett J.L. 31
Humphries S.V.
hydnocarpus oil 13, 19, 21

Icelandic disease 232
Immigration Restriction Act 167
Immorality Laws 35
immunisation *see* vaccination
Impendle 18
INAH *see* isoniazid
indentured Indian labourers 9, 68, 166, 167
Indian
    barracks 72, 167
    Immigration Board 10
    Relief Committees 154
Industrial and Commercial Workers Union 133
infant mortality 43, 213, 215
infantile paralysis 223
influx control 54
Ingwavuma 199, 200

inoculation *see* vaccination
insanity 30
iron lung 225, 231, 234
Isipingo 188
isolation centre 76, 77
isoniazid 23

jackals 93
jaundice 49
Jenner Edward 67
Johannesburg 34, 43, 44, 46, 55, 56, 75, 91, 105, 145, 159, 172, 223, 225, 236, 250
Johannesburg Chamber of Mines 39

Kalahari desert 97
Kalk Bay 84, 85
KaNgwane 168, 200
Kaplan L. 227
Kark Sydney 41, 54, 117
Karoo 22, 98
Kentani 129
Khoikhoi 7, 28, 62-65, 128, 129, 179, 258
Kimberley 29, 33, 34, 48, 69, 105, 114, 117, 143, 145-149, 151, 152, 154-156, 242
King Williams Town 28, 55, 68, 70, 88, 92, 93, 107
Klerksdorp 22, 33, 69, 76
Klipspruit 92
Kliptown 92, 116
Knutsford Lord 32
Knysna 92
Kokstad 73
Korsten 88
kraals 17, 68, 75, 90, 99, 115, 134, 248
Kroonstad 93, 107
Küstner H.G.V. 219
KwaNdebele 56

Labour Importation Ordinance 144
Ladies Commission 108, 181
Lady Frere 140
Ladysmith 106, 109, 145, 152, 186, 188
Laing G.D. 111, 112
Landsberg P. 70
Langa 157, 161
League of Nations 46
Lebowa 168, 169, 218, 237
Leipoldt Louis 153, 189, 190

Leitner 4
Leonard Wood Memorial Conference 20
Leprosy Acts 14
Leprosy Advisory Committee 18, 21, 22
leprosy belt 24
Leprosy Commission 4
Leprosy Repression Act (Cape) 8, 9, 18
Lesotho 5, 8, 18, 33, 99, 131, 134, 145
lice 128, 129, 131, 135, 136
Lichtenburg 134
Liesching Dr. 4
lithium carmine 23
Little Soweto 217
Local Health Commission 117
Lock hospitals 29, 30
Loeffler 242
Louch F.W.B. 30
lunatics 6, 10, 16
Lusikisiki 137
Lydenburg 179
lynxes 93

Maclear 133
Magersfontein 105
Maister Dr 74, 75, 232
Maitland 86, 87
    Cemetery 151
Malan D. 189
Malan F.S. 157
Malarial Control Programme:
    Southern African 203, 204
    LSDI 203
Malaria committees 193, 194
malarial treatment for syphilis 40, 55
malathion 99
Malawi 27, 76, 144, 177
Malmesbury 8, 129
malnutrition 22, 43, 133-135, 137, 139, 143, 191, 213, 215-217, 227
Mansell Prothero 198
marboran 76
Marshall 53
martial law 257
Matatiele 130, 248, 249
Mathias J. 242
mass immunisation (polio) 232, 237
Matthews Dr J.W. 6, 8, 12, 166, 180, 242
McNeillie Dr 37
Mead R. 63

Measles strategy 218
Mehliss Dr 33
Meijer H.B.W. 15
Mentzel O.F. 27, 65, 179
mercury 29, 39, 42, 46, 47, 94, 151
mercurochrome 21, 226
methylene blue 21, 226
miasmatic influences 143
Mice 92, 93, 99, 226
    leprosy and 9, 11, 15
Middelburg 22, 93, 138, 180, 182, 194
migrant labour system 41, 51, 54, 56, 137, 140, 143, 144, 167, 171, 198, 256, 263
military isolation hospital 145
milk 21, 111-113, 117-119, 121, 122, 137, 139, 147, 226, 245, 161
mine compounds 29, 245, 147, 161
mining 29, 33, 35, 39, 41, 42, 48, 51, 56, 69-71, 113, 114, 130, 143-147, 153, 155, 159, 161, 168, 171, 180, 198, 242
mines:
    Durban Deep 114
    Zaaiplats 147
Mitchell Dr J. A. 36, 38-40, 130, 131
Mkambati Leper Institution 15, 19-21
Mkomati river 199
Mkomazi 124
Modder river 69, 105, 107
Molaba Chief 33
Moll Marius J 40
mongoose 94, 95
Montague Mr, 5, 260
Moore pads 168, 171
Moravian Missions 3, 4
Mossel Bay 92
Mostert H.v.R. 20
Msinga 187
Murison P. 90
Murray J.F. 246
Musina 176

Namaqualand 8, 65
naphthalene oil 135
Natal Assembly 30
Natal Mercury 50
Natal Witness 70
National Council for the Prevention of Venereal Diseases 36
National Malaria Organising Committee 198

National Outbreak Committee 176
Natives Urban Areas Act 39, 43
Naudé Minister 233, 234
Ndabeni 82, 132, 148, 157
neoarsphenamine 47
neosalvarsan 39, 188
neurosyphilis 52
New Brighton 55, 88, 98, 211, 259
Newlands 148
Newtown 91
notifiable disease 18, 43, 215, 216
notification 69, 214, 218, 220, 225, 236, 248
nursemaids 31, 34, 35, 41, 44

O'Malley C.K. 49
opium 150
Oudtshoorn 257
overcrowding 21, 22, 43, 54, 89, 107, 123, 128, 149, 155, 157, 209, 217, 235, 256, 257

Paardeberg 107
Paarl 131, 156,
Pacaltsdorp 105
pail system *see* bucket system
paludrine 195
para amino salicylic acid 23
paralysis 224, 225, 227, 229-233
Parden Island 67
Park Ross 180, 181, 184, 185
Passes 121
pass office 44, 45, 72, 92, 112, 259
pasteurisation 111, 118, 119, 121
Paulpietersburg 193, 194
penicillin 47, 49-55, 57, 120, 167, 249, 262
Peri Urban Areas: 115, 116
    Health Board 75
Pfeiffer 143, 159
Philips Howard 151
Philipstown 152
phosphorus 37
Pietermaritzburg 10, 30, 44, 45, 54, 72, 74, 88-90, 110, 116, 118, 145, 154, 172, 175, 187, 193, 209, 210, 212-214, 228, 232, 248
Pietersburg 15, 33, 181
Piet Retief 71, 191
Pigeons 9
Pilgrim's Rest 155, 180
Pimville 92

Pinelands 77, 157
Plague Administration Committee, (Durban) 88
Plague and Health Committee (Eastern Province) 99
Plague Board, (Port Elizabeth) 87
Plague Committee (Rand) 91
plague hospital, Durban, 88
plasmoquine 188
pneumonia 71, 107, 134, 137, 149, 150-152, 162, 181, 182, 211, 213, 215, 216, 218, 256
Polela 22, 117
polio eradication 237, 252, 262
Polio Expert Committee 238
Polio Research Foundation 230, 232, 234
Pondoland 15, 40
Pongola 191, 197
Potchefstroom 93
Port Elizabeth 3, 5,7, 22, 28, 44, 55, 56, 76, 87, 91, 96, 98, 99, 105, 107, 110, 118, 121, 123, 137, 140, 146, 180, 210, 215-217, 237, 252
Port Shepstone 171, 188, 237
potassium iodide 29, 39, 151
potassium permanganate 39, 226
Potgietersrus 33, 185
Pretoria 15-18, 20, 38, 40, 44, 56, 112, 118, 120, 146, 147, 158, 212, 213,
Pringle Dr, 64
prisoners 107
prostitutes *see* sex workers
Protein Shock Treatment 21
Prowazek 130
Public Health Act 38, 47, 69, 73, 85, 94, 156, 209, 224, 243
Public Health Act (Natal) 90
Purcell F.W.F. 46, 47
pyrethroids 202
pyrethrum 195
pyrimethamine 197, 200, 202, 203
pyrexial treatment (syphilis) 40, 49, 52

quarantine 62, 68-71, 75, 76, 83, 87, 90, 97, 146, 158, 166, 167, 208, 214, 255
   station 69
   camp 83, 84
Queenstown 72, 88, 93, 130, 133, 140
quinine
   influenza and 152

malaria and 180-196
syphilis and 40
typhus and 137
Qumbu 133

Red Cross Society 39, 44, 226
Red Location 88, 123, 140
Report:
   On the Natal Plague (Hill) 89, 90
resistance:
   bacterial 49, 51
   insecticides 196
Richmond 243
Rietfontein hospital 55
Rietfontein Lazaretto 33, 34
Robben Island 5, 7, 9-14, 16-19, 21, 208, 258
Robinson J 31
Rondebosch 8, 76, 83, 84
Rosebank Depot 146
Ross Dr R. 7, 8
Ross W.M. 36
Royal Army Medical Corps 109
Royal Commission:
   on Venereal Disease 34, 35
   on Vaccination 70
rubella 136
Russell P. 66
Russian Influenza 143
Rusternburg 191

SADC 203
Saldanha Bay 8, 68
Salisbury Island 20, 88
salmonella 118, 119
Salt River 28
salvarsan 37, 40, 42, 45, 46
sanitation 9, 14, 16, 91, 104, 108, 110, 111, 114, 116, 150, 155, 170, 175, 177, 179, 229, 255, 257, 262
SARS 162
Saville Lewis J. 55
Sax Sidney 29, 54
scarlet fever 118
Schick test 243, 255
schools
   measles in 213
   polio and 225, 226, 232
Scottsville 75
Second World War *see* World War 2
Seedat 168
segregation 17, 22, 34

Senekal 34
sex workers 28-34, 36, 39, 46, 47, 51, 54-56, 256
Shand Alex 84
Shangaan 34
Sheldon H.F. 18
Shepstone Sir T. 9
Sher J. N. 55, 215
Shongwe hospital 168
Sierra Leone 145, 156
silver bromide 37
Simonstown 28, 65, 84, 104, 107, 148, 208
Sitas F. 170, 172
Smuts General J. 42, 43
Somerset Hospital 107
Somerset Lord Charles 4
South African Institute for Medical Research 190
South African Malaria Advisory Group 202
Spanish Flu 145, 147, 150
Spencer 182, 183, 185, 214
Springs 41, 228
Stainbank H.E. 31
Standerton 180, 194
Stellenbosch 68
Sterkstroom 131-133
St Helena 208, 223
Stijn 28
streptomycin 51, 53
Stuttaford Clr Richard 157
slave lodge 27, 28, 62, 209
slaves 27, 28, 62, 64, 65, 67, 68, 104, 258
Society for Combating Venereal Disease 39
Solomon Saul 29
Somerset, Lord Charles 4
South African War *see* Anglo-Boer War
squirrels 94
Standerton 22
Stanger (town) 169
Stockenstrom Sir A, 6
streptomycin 23, 98, 120
sulphonamides 23, 49, 98, 159, 167, 213, 214
suricats 94
Swanson M.W. 91, 260
Swellendam 5
Swellengrebel 189, 190

Sydenham T. 208
syndromic approach to STDs 57
syphilis 19, 20, chapter 2

taxation 10, 181, 182,
    hut 256
Taylor J. 174
Theal McCall 128
The Times 106
Thornton Commission 43
throat lozenges 50, 52
Tongaat 72
tonsillectomy 233
traditional healers 23,186
tracheostomy 13, 215
Transkei 9, 15-17, 22, 24, 48, 55, 56, 70, 72, 75, 124, 129, 130, 139, 14, 149, 183, 186, 210, 218, 220, 227, 229, 252
Trichardt Louis 179
trypan blue 21
Tsolo 133, 248, 249
Tuberculosis Commission of 1914 35
Tudhope Mr, 12
Tulbagh Governor, 65
Turner Dr 33
Turner R 226
Tyler Dr 67
Tzaneen 185, 190, 191, 193, 199

Uitenhage 5, 76, 93, 96, 98, 99, 146
Uitvlugt 13, 83, 84, 157
Ulundi 172
Umvoti Mission Reserve 170
Umzinto 37, 75, 186
undulant fever 118
uranium 42
Urbanised Areas Administration Committee 117
Utrecht 75

vaccination
    campaign, polio 232, 236, 239
    cholera 167
    committee 67
    diphtheria 242-246, 249, 250
    measles 216, 219, 220
    poliomyelitis 225, 227, 231, 233-235, 238
    smallpox 19, 29 33 62-81, 85
    typhoid 113, 114, 119, 120, 122
    typhus 135

Vaccine
    anti-pneumonic 149, 151
    Edmonston Zagreb 219
    influenza 159, 161, 162
    Institute 75, 77
    measles 214, 217
    MMR 220
    Sabin 236, 237
    Salk 232, 233, 236
    Schwarz 216
    smallpox: chapter 3
    Zinsser Castenada 135, 136
vaccine coverage rate 238, 239
vanadium 42
Van Beitenbach 129
Van der Stel, W.A. 62
Van der Waal 210
Van Heerden J.R. 124
Van Rieebeck J. 103
variola minor 71, 74, 76-78
Veale Dr 33
Venda 56, 218 (*see also BaVenda*)
Venereal Disease Advisory Committee 44
Ventersdorp 134
Vi agglutination test 122
Volksrust 145, 180
Voortrekkers 5, 179, 180, 209, 211, 255

Wade M. 229, 230
Wagenaar Mr 129
Walmer location 77
Wannenburg 236
Warm Baths 17
war *see* Anglo Boer, World War 2, World War 1
warfarin 98
War Production Board 50
Wasserman test 32, 34, 39, 42, 48, 53
Waterberg 22, 33, 37, 72, 185
water disconnections 173
water vendors 169
Weigl 136
Weil Felix test 131, 137
Welsh A.R. 70
Wessels J.H.B. 156
West Fort 18-23
Wheelwright 181
Widal test 111, 131
Witbank 139
Withenshawe Mr. 85

Witwatersrand 29, 32, 35, 104, 168, 193, 194, 245
Witwatersrand Native Labour Association 33, 39
Woodstock 84, 145
World Health Assembly 62, 197
World Health Organisation 53, 77, 78, 160, 173, 176, 196, 202, 203, 218, 232, 238, 239, 252, 262
World Influenza Centre 161
World War 1, 109, 145, 146, 156, 157, 212, 223, 257
World War 2 46, 49-51, 74, 97, 122, 137, 159, 194, 196, 213, 227, 246, 247, 257, 262
Wortley Montague, Lady Mary 66
Wright Sir Almroth 109
Wynberg 87, 148
Wynne Dr. 9

Xhosas 33, 134, 135

yaws 30
Yonge Sir George 67
Yzerplaat 84

Zimbabwe 175-177, 197, 203, 204
Zionist faith 75
Zoutpansberg 33, 185
Zwartkop 10

ABOUT THE AUTHOR

Julie Dyer (née Hanwell) grew up in England, studying Medicine at Leeds University, and Tropical Medicine and Hygiene at Liverpool University. After working in Sierra Leone she came to South Africa, studying Public Health at the University of Natal. She was Medical Officer of Health for the Development and Services Board, and then for the City of Pietermaritzburg (Msunduzi Municipality) from 1994 until 2005. Her first book, 'Health in Pietermaritzburg 1838-2008: a history of urbanisation and disease in an African city', was published by the Natal Society Foundation in 2012. She has two children, Jack and Carmen.

www.ingramcontent.com/pod-product-compliance
Lightning Source LLC
Chambersburg PA
CBHW051800170526
45167CB00005B/1815